Dave,

Please think carefully about how you use your tools.

Cordially,

Bill Havens

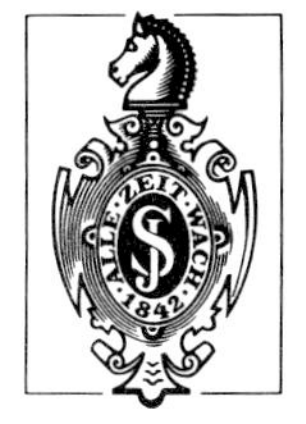

Georg Eisner

EYE SURGERY

An Introduction to Operative Technique

With an Introduction by Peter Niesel
Translated by Terry C. Telger

With 357 Figures, Most in Color
Drawings by Peter Schneider

Springer-Verlag
Berlin Heidelberg New York 1980

GEORG EISNER, MD, Professor of Ophthamology
Universitäts-Augenklinik Bern

PETER NIESEL, MD, Professor of Ophthamology
Universitäts-Augenklinik Bern

PETER SCHNEIDER, Medical Artist
Abteilung für Unterrichtsmedien der Universität Bern

Translator:
TERRY C. TELGER, 3054 Vaughan Ave., Marina, California 93933/USA

Title of the German Edition:
Georg Eisner, Augenchirurgie

ISBN 3-540-08371-5 Springer-Verlag Berlin Heidelberg New York
ISBN 0-387-08371-5 Springer-Verlag New York Heidelberg Berlin

ISBN 3-540-09922-0 Springer-Verlag Berlin Heidelberg New York
ISBN 0-387-09922-0 Springer-Verlag New York Heidelberg Berlin

Library of Congress Cataloging in Publication Data. Eisner, Georg, 1930– Eye surgery. Translation of Augenchirurgie. Bibliography: p. Includes index. 1. Eye-Surgery. I. Title. [DNLM: 1. Eye-Surgery. WW168 E36a] RE80.E3813 617.7′1 80-10856

Printed in Germany.

Typesetting, printing, and bookbinding by Universitätsdruckerei H. Stürtz AG. Würzburg
2123/3130-543210

Hans Goldmann:

"...I am not manually skilled by nature,
so when it came to surgery
I had to carefully ponder,
and try to understand
rationally, each step of
the procedure..."

(From a casual conversation)

Preface to the English Edition

The reactions to the German edition of this book have been most contradictory. While some readers found the book absolutely unnecessary ("Surgery is learned from practice, not from theory"), others were enthusiastic ("Just the sort of book I have always needed"). In my opinion the divergent reception of the book is best explained by the comment of my friend, BALDER GLOOR*, who called the book a "grammar of eye surgery".

Indeed there are people who can learn a language by practice alone, and there are others who do better by knowing its grammar. In learning by mere practice to be sure, proficiency will be long in coming, because it will be more difficult to recognize, and thus to correct, whatever errors are made, whereas a knowledge of grammar will reveal the basic structures and shorten the learning process.

Similarly, surgery can be learned purely from practical experience. Yet the trial-and-error quest for experience is not compatible with the interests of the patient. A knowledge of "surgical grammar", on the other hand, not only shortens the time for learning but also helps us to compare different surgical techniques and to weigh their advantages and disadvantages. It is also helpful in developing new surgical methods, for the general rules can always be applied to novel situations where experience, of course, is lacking.

This book, therefore, does not comment on individual procedures and methods, just as the grammar of a language is little concerned with what should be expressed in it. It does not show *what* should be done, but only *how* it should be done.

These basic ideas determine the structure of this book. The emphasis placed on certain chapters does not necessarily correspond to their importance in everyday surgical practice. The chapter on iris surgery, for example, deals extensively with the size and shape of excisions even though present surgical practice allows considerable tolerance in this regard. But interpreted in a broader sense, the chapter illustrates the general behavior of highly extensible and resilient tissues and thus touches on problems involved in new surgical fields such as surgery of the vitreous. On the other hand, retinal surgery is not dealt with specifically, because surgical manipulations affect only the ocular wall and can thus be derived from the principles discussed in the chapter on that subject.

Likewise, vitreous surgery and phacoemulsification are not described in special chapters. These techniques can be derived from the principles discussed in extenso elsewhere, that is, in the chapters on the cutting of tissues, on space-tactical problems, and on modern ways of combining tissue- and space-tactical procedures with microinstruments.

---

* Professor of Ophthalmology at the University of Basel, Switzerland

The English edition of this book contains some major changes from the German version. The continuous surgical progress with the development of new instruments (e.g., a point-blade trephine), the development of visco-surgical methods, and the increasing experience with the combined tissue- and space-tactical microinstruments are reflected in the extensive revisions of the chapters concerned. In addition many other illustrations were added or replaced.

Translating the book into English was a difficult matter due to the specific technical language involved. The rendering of novel terms and concepts requires a keen sense of language and idiom. Fortunately, a translator was found who possessed the necessary expertise. His interest in didactic aspects also contributed much to a clear presentation. The reader will see for himself the care with which Mr. C.T. TELGER undertook his task. The credit is his if the book has become readable for the English reader. I must confess that I am actually more pleased with this English version than with my own original German text, and for this he has earned my sincere thanks.

Bern, Summer 1980 G. EISNER

Preface to the German Edition

This book is the culmination of many years of collaboration which began as a teacher-student relationship between PETER NIESEL and the author and has evolved into an amiable partnership.

The first reason for writing down the results of numerous conversations and discussions, in which Prof. HANS GOLDMANN often played a guiding role, was actually a coincidence in that the impending transfer of PETER NIESEL awoke the author to the need to put into writing the many principles that had been derived in conversation. In 1967 this material was assembled into a manuscript for the operative training of residents and was distributed as a mimeographed pamphlet for internal use.

We received many requests thereafter to put the material into book form, thereby making it accessible to a wider audience. That this has finally been done is due largely to yet another coincidence: An accident gave the author the leisure time necessary to revise and update the material in the light of experience. Preparation of the manuscript and illustrations, however, proved much more difficult than anticipated and took several years to complete.

During this time I could always count on the generous help and advice of PETER NIESEL, who not only worked out the basic concept for Chapter I.2, but also aided the development of the book with his stern criticisms. I am much indebted to him for these efforts, and for consenting to write the Introduction, thereby documenting his contribution to this book.

I am also grateful to my illustrator, Mr. PETER SCHNEIDER, who not only rendered excellent drawings based on our sketches but contributed his own ideas for portraying the problems in the clearest manner possible. The reader will appreciate the success with which Mr. SCHNEIDER has accomplished this task.

Much of the material in this book is usually presented orally to the medical student by his instructor. Much is found scattered throughout the ophthalmologic literature of many decades. Many valuable ideas were obtained from works by ELSCHNIG, CERMAK, BARRAQUER and LEONARDI. In the early phase of writing the manuscript I was greatly assisted by Mr. ERNST GRIESHABER and his successor, Mr. HANS GRIESHABER of Schaffhausen, who, as manufacturers of surgical instruments, offered valuable technical insights.

But a book which is primarily didactic in nature also requires the criticism of its intended readership. For this I am indebted to three colleagues who reviewed the manuscript and made corrections where needed: Dr. MARLISE ALBRECHT, a resident at our hospital, did this from the standpoint of an ophthalmologist in the early stages of her operative training; Dr. PAULUS DE JONG, chief surgeon at the Oogheelkundige Klinik of Amsterdam, from the standpoint of a colleague who must himself train young surgeons; and Dr. HEINZ BAUMANN of Lucern, who suggested revisions from the standpoint of a practicing eye surgeon and also made valuable contributions in many casual conversations.

But how could this book have been completed without the patient assistance of Miss CHRISTINE LEHMANN, who typed the manuscript. The unflagging good will with which she undertook the many textual revisions helped greatly to create an atmosphere in which corrections could be freely suggested.

My special thanks go to the staff of Springer-Verlag, who made every conceivable effort in the publication of this book. This fact will, I believe, be evident to the reader.

Finally, I wish to thank my wife SUSANNE and my children DANIEL, MIRIAM and SIMONE for their patience and understanding in coping with the many encroachments upon family life which were unavoidable during the publication of this book.

Bern, Fall 1977 GEORG EISNER

Contents

Introduction

Ophthalmic surgery is, as its name implies, a handicraft. I learned how greatly the sensible application of handcrafting principles can contribute to the solution of surgical problems while a young resident under Prof. E. LEONARDI in Rome. This became even clearer to me when I myself was given the task of training young residents in this field of ophthalmology. I found considerable individual differences in the skills of the residents training under me, but in the case of *one* colleague my task was greatly simplified. After working together for some months, we hit upon a key to rapid mutual understanding: Having both had prior experience in woodworking, we developed a "code" based on handcrafting concepts. Later on, we attempted to make this code a basis for the training of other residents. We were pleased to find that they not only mastered surgical techniques more rapidly by this method, but also gained the ability to adapt these techniques to novel situations – a skill essential for their later independent work and further training.

We thus see what this book is intended to do, and what it is not: It is intended to represent the basic problems of ophthalmic surgery and their solutions as handcrafting activities. In other words, it will focus on methodology rather than methods.

Much of the material will already be familiar to the experienced surgeon, having been learned through careful observation of instructors, intuitive skill, and the interpretation of successes and failures. He will know intuitively when to use a special-purpose scalpel for opening the eyeball, or a general-purpose razor blade; when to use this forceps or that for grasping tissue; and when optimal wound closure requires a continuous or interrupted suture, and whether plastic monofilament or twisted silk should be used.

However, purely intuitive skills are difficult to analyze. The underlying causes of success or failure remain obscure. This may be why the operative methods described by one author are often less successful in other hands: While the method has been learned, the craftsmanship has not. Experience, dexterity and intuition are not conscious processes and are thus difficult to transfer to others.

The present book is concerned with finding a rational basis for specific surgical manipulations. The operator will be shown how to plan and successfully carry out surgical measures, such as determining the number and position of corneal sutures, deciding the form and size of an iridectomy, and applying the proper force during lens deliveries; and he will not have to rely upon intuition to acquire these skills, but will learn them on the basis of specific geometric and physical principles. Success should depend as little as possible on such factors as experience, dexterity and intuition.

One thing remains to be said about the use of this book: The beginner will not be able immediately to translate pure theoretical knowledge into practice in a complex surgical situation; the sheer number and diversity of the problems would confuse him. Whenever possible, he should use models to try his hand at the problems discussed, for only by experimentation can theory and practice be reconciled. In time, he will improve his ability by subjecting every failure – stemming from an error in a *single manipulation* – to retrospective analysis. He will then be able to solve the problem the next time and avoid repetition of his error. It is hoped that in this way surgery will become for him a part of ophthalmology, and that his planning and actions will be governed by logic and reason, as in any clinical endeavor. If this book also enables the experienced surgeon to view his actions in a new light, it will have exceeded our expectations.

PETER NIESEL

I Instruments and Their Use

1 General

Instruments are *energy transmitters* through which mechanical, thermal and electromagnetic energy is applied to tissues.

Every instrument has, by virtue of its construction, specific *functional characteristics* which determine its optimal range of use. By knowing these characteristics, the surgeon can make the best use of the instrument to achieve the desired result with a minimum of traumatizing side-effects. If optimal use of the instrument is not possible, knowledge of its functional behavior will enable the surgeon to estimate the side-effects in advance, to allow for them in the operating plan, and thus to find at least the best compromise.

A knowledge of the functional characteristics is also important for revealing defects in the construction of an instrument which might impair its function. It is the basis for quality control, which begins when a device is procured and must continue for the duration of its use.

In the chapters that follow, we shall discuss the basic types of instruments and operative manipulations. Special-purpose instruments will be described later in connection with the special problems they are designed to solve.

2 The Application of Mechanical Energy

Mechanical forces are vector quantities which have magnitude and direction. The amount, or magnitude, of the force that can be transmitted is limited by the "stability" of the instrument used. If increasing force is applied to an instrument which is not sufficiently resistant to deformation (i.e., less resistant than the tissue), this force will act to deform the instrument rather than work at the tissue, and the instrument will deviate from the direction intended. To "transmit his will to the tissue," therefore, the operator will always select the *most stable* instrument which anatomical conditions will allow.[1]

As a general rule, *forces which are not to influence each other must be applied at right angles to each other*. This **"rule of vector separation"** must be taken into account in the design of instruments in order to separate the actual working motion from subsidiary motions, and these in turn from the guiding motion through the tissue (Fig. 1).[2]

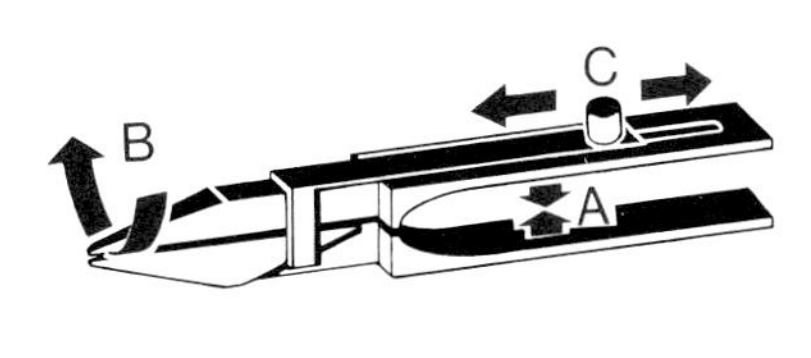

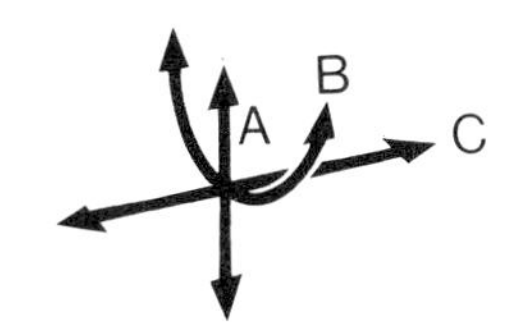

Fig. 1. **Rule of vector separation,** shown here for a needle holder. The working vector of the needle holder (*A* grasping the needle) is perpendicular to the direction of needle guidance *(B)*. Perpendicular to both is the subsidiary vector (*C* motion of slide catch), so arranged that it will not interfere with instrument operation

2.1 Instrument Handles

2.1.1 Manually-Operated Handles

The handle transmits forces from the fingers to the tissue, and is an important element in the feedback system between the working end of the instrument and the surgeon: It relays information on tissue resistance back to the fingertips, so that the forces to be transmitted to the tissue can be precisely regulated.

The sense of touch is most sensitive when the fingertips are largely freed of their weight-bearing function.[3] **Long-handled** instruments satisfy this requirement in that the weight is borne by the metacarpus, and the fingers play only a guiding role.[4] Moreover, there is support at three points which gives a better feel for the spatial position of the instrument. In the case of **short handles** which can be held with only two fingers, some load can be taken off the fingers by the use of a broad holding device. However, such handles are poorly suited for transmitting large forces.

In the case of a **one-piece** handle,[5] the working and guiding motions are identical. Instruments with **two piece** handles[6] consist of two parts connected by a joint. The working motion consists of rotation about this joint and so is separate from the guiding motion.

---

[1] This contradicts the widely held belief that fine instruments are automatically superior to coarser instruments due to their smaller dimensions. In suturing, for example, too small a forceps for holding the wound edge cannot offer sufficient resistance to the advancing needle and will bend. The tissue will be deformed, and consequently the needle will deviate from the intended path.

[2] There is also the possibility of temporal separation, whereby motions that are not to interfere with each other are performed at different times. Examples:
- separation of working and guiding motions during cutting with scissors; closing motion not simultaneous with swiveling motion.
- separation of guiding and checking motions as an instrument is advanced within the tissue: raising the needle point to check its intramural position (e.g., in the sclera) before or after, but not during, movements to advance the needle.

[3] $\Delta J/J$ according to the Weber-Fechner Law.

[4] Example: a pencil.

[5] Example: knives, spatulas, hooks.

[6] Example: forceps, scissors.

The **magnitude of the force** that can be transmitted from the handle to the working part of the instrument (jaws) varies with the length ratio of the lever arms. If the lever arm of the handle is much longer than that of the jaws, very large forces can be produced. But this places correspondingly higher structural demands on the joint, which must stabilize the transmission of force and ensure precise closure of the instrument. The shorter the lever arm of the jaws in relation to the handle, the longer the joint must be (Fig. 2).

If larger forces are applied to the instrument than its construction provides for, its blades will bend and its jaws will not appose correctly.[7] In precision instruments, therefore, stops must be provided to limit the force that can be applied (Fig. 3).

Angulation of the handle and working end is necessary when anatomical obstacles are present (Fig. 4) or for special viewing requirements (microscopy). It complicates the guiding motions, inasmuch as simple rotation of the working end now requires a swiveling motion of the handle (Fig. 5). This larger amplitude makes fine corrective movements difficult; on the other hand, it helps to maintain a given direction of guidance, since tiny inadvertant lateral movements of the handle produce only minimal effects at the working end.

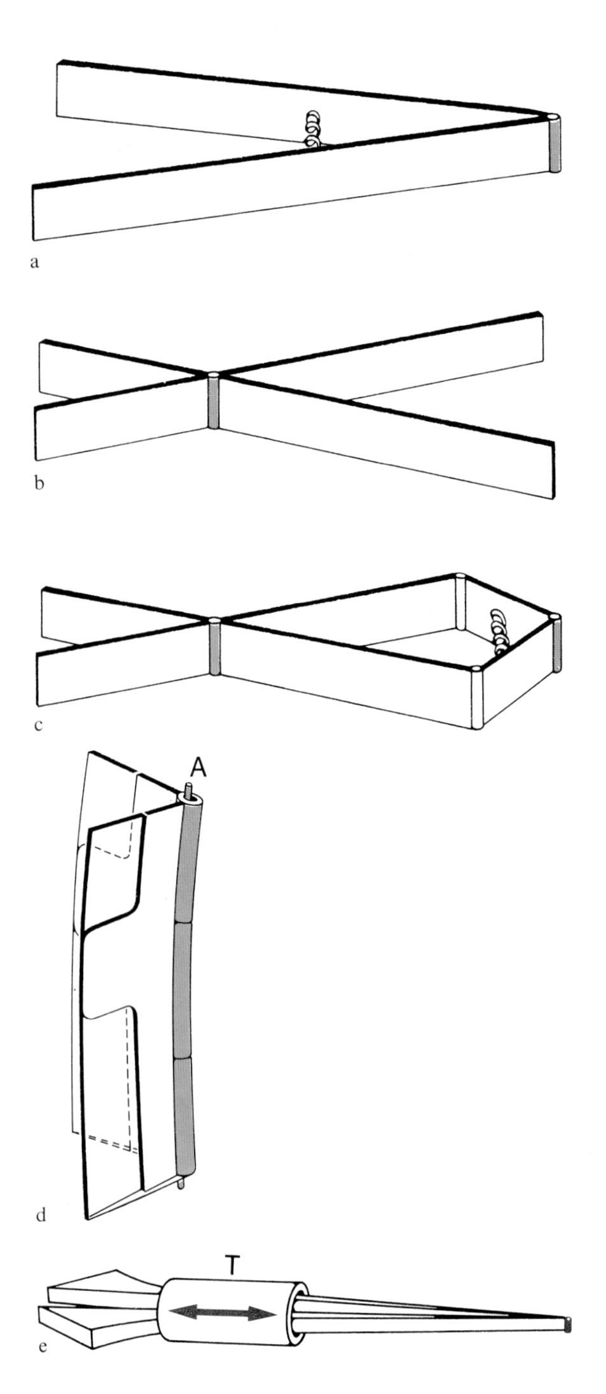

2.1.2 Motorized Handles

Cutting instruments with motorized motion are advantageous when finger control alone cannot guarantee sufficient precision, i.e., when the excursion of the cutting edge is either extremely long or extremely short.

[7] The jaws and handle may require different material properties. The instrument then is made from two parts soldered together, e.g., brittle steel for the jaws and flexible steel for the handle. Of course, the melting point of the solder limits the sterilization temperature.

Fig. 2. **Instrument handles**

a *Simple forceps handle.* The working part and handle are identical. Force is transmitted from the fingers to the jaws without benefit of a stabilizing joint. The precision of closure thus depends entirely on the stable and precise construction of the blades.

b *Scissors handle.* The joint is short in relation to the blades, and so precision depends largely on precise finger movements.

c *Spring handle.* Closure of the blades is made more precise by an extra joint.

d *Hinge handle.* The joint length is maximal, i.e. equal to that of the entire handle. The lever of the handle is about as long as that of the jaws. The "spring tension" necessary for opening is produced by slight flexure of the joint *(A)*.

e *Tube handle.* Very fine forceps blades are enclosed in a stabilizing guide tube *(T)*, which is slid forward to close the blades

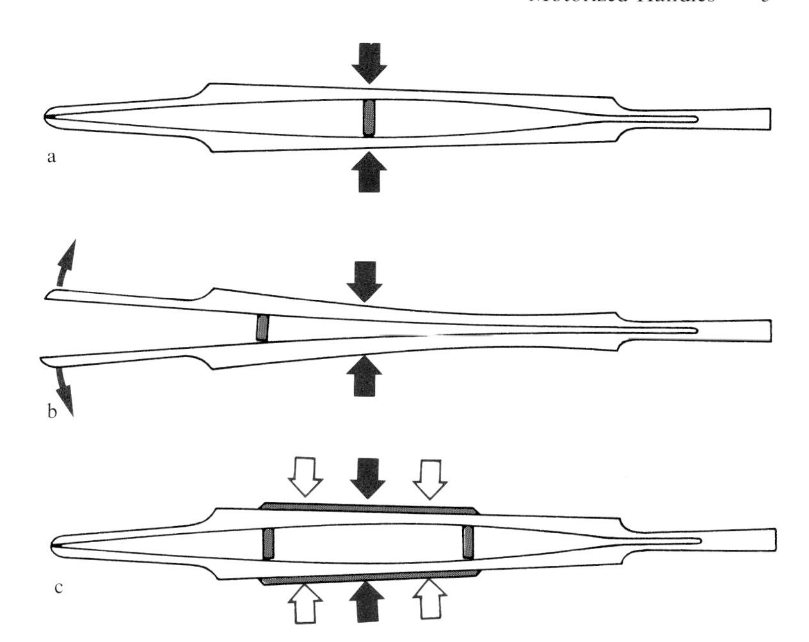

Fig. 3. **Regulation of force by stops.** The stops limit the pressure applied to the instrument handle.

a To work properly, the stops must be located directly below the point of finger contact.

b If the fingers grip the handle behind the stop, the jaws will gape as pressure is increased.

c The permissible area of finger contact can be increased by providing two stops connected by a rigid "bridge"

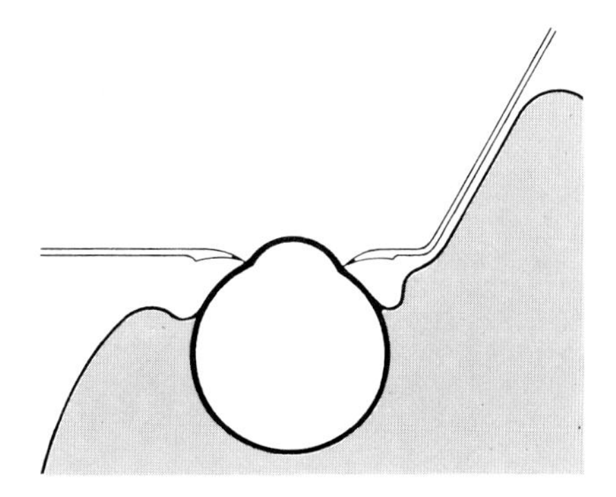

Fig. 4. **Angled handles.** The handle and working end must be angled where the orbital margin or bridge of the nose obstruct access

In **rotatory knives** (trephines, circular knives), the tissue fibers are subjected to an "infinitely" long blade movement. Inertial effects of the instrument are useful, as they contribute to a more stable blade motion. In rotatory motion, however, fibers which have not been sectioned are entrained by the blade along with adherent tissue from adjacent areas.

Oscillatory knives have short single excursions and so must be operated at a high speed in order to produce a cutting action. Inertial effects of the instrument limit its frequency. Frequencies above 18 Hz impair the visibility of individual blade movements (Fig. 6). Hence the cutting process cannot be monitored in the usual way by observing the motion of the blade itself, but only by watching its effect on the tissue.

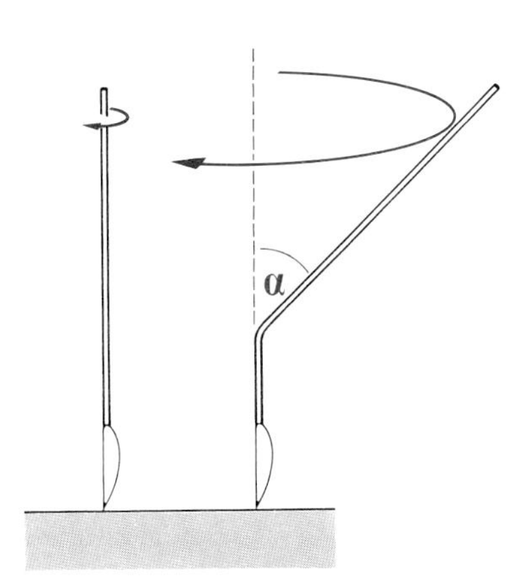

Fig. 5. **Movement of angled handles.** In the straight handle, rotation of the working end requires an identical rotation of the handle *(left)*. In the angled handle, this must be done with a swiveling motion whose extend depends on the value of the angle α *(right)*

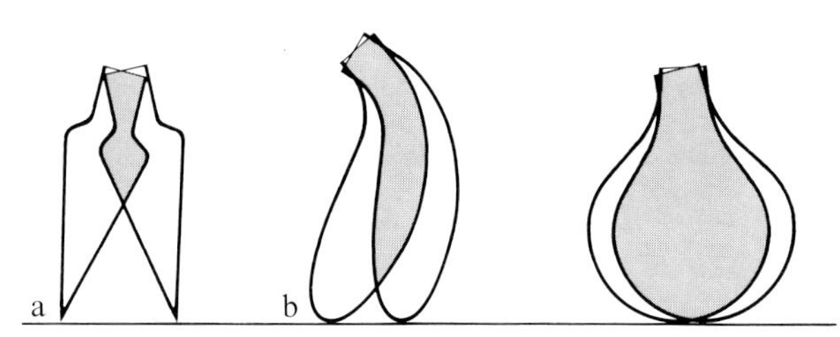

Fig. 6. **Oscillatory knives.** At high frequencies the single movements of the blade are invisible, and only those portions of the knife are seen which overlap (gray). Therefore in **a** and **b** the blade tip in contact with the tissue is invisible during working motions

2.2 The Grasping of Tissues

In the grasping and pulling of tissues, the working motion must produce a resistance between tissue and instrument high enough to withstand the forces of the guiding motion (Fig. 7). This "frictional resistance" is determined by:

- the *force* exerted on the substrate;
- the *area of blade contact*;
- the *angle* between the vector of the grasping force and that of the guiding motion.

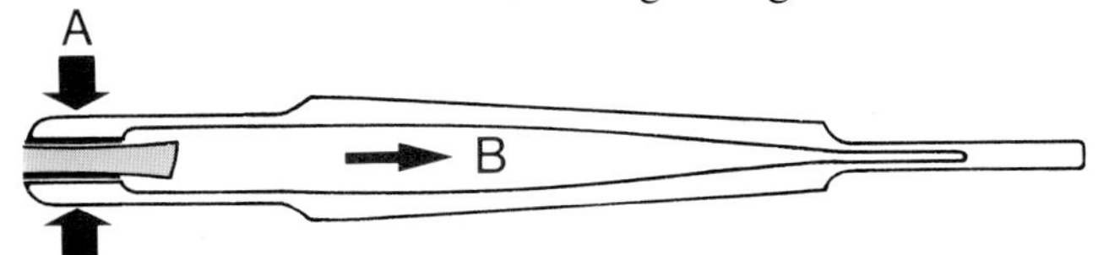

Fig. 7. **The principle of grasping.** To grasp and manipulate tissue, a "frictional resistance" must be created by the working motion *(A)* between instrument and substrate which is higher than the force of the guiding motion *(B)*

To spare delicate structures during the grasping of **tissues,** a high pressure will be avoided wherever possible, and the necessary resistance will be created by the other two factors, i.e., by increasing the area of contact (non-toothed forceps) and by deforming the tissue surface to produce optimal vectors of attack (forceps with teeth or grooving). A high pressure is employed only when gripping **needles and suture material,** since here the other two factors cannot be varied.

2.2.1 Non-Toothed Forceps

In forceps with a **variable grasping surface** (Fig. 8), the flexibility of the blades determines whether increased digital pressure will result in an enlargement of the contact surface or a higher grasping pressure. If the blades are very rigid, the pressure increases considerably before the grasping surface becomes large

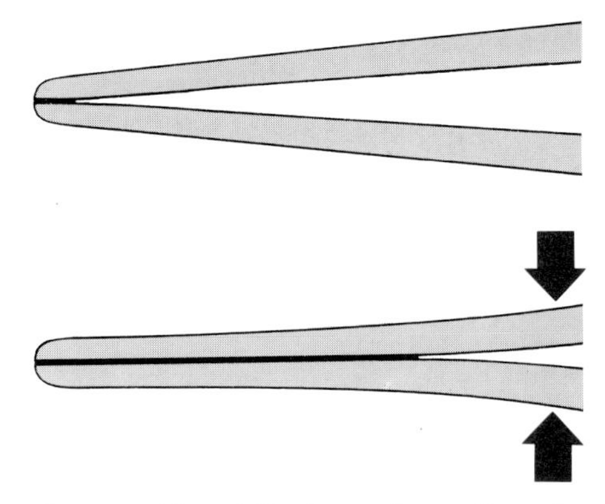

Fig. 8. **Plane forceps with undefined grasping surface.** As increasing force is applied to the blades, the grasping area increases. The pressure between the blades (=force per unit area) does not increase accordingly, but the effectiveness of the instrument is improved by increasing the area of contact (and with it, the friction)

enough, and the tissue is crushed. If the blades are relatively flexible, on the other hand, the pressure remains low, and little friction develops despite the large grasping surface.[8]

In the case of forceps with a **predetermined grasping surface** (Fig. 9), the blade pressure also must be defined by the construction. If the pressure on the blades is too low, only the tips will touch; if it is too high, the jaws will gape. Pressure-regulating devices are necessary, therefore (Fig. 3).[9]

The "friction" of non-toothed forceps can be increased considerably by **grooving** the opposed surfaces (Fig. 10). But grooving is effective only for soft tissues into which the grooves can penetrate (Fig. 11). If the substrate is rigid,[10] grooving will actually impair the grasping ability of the forceps.

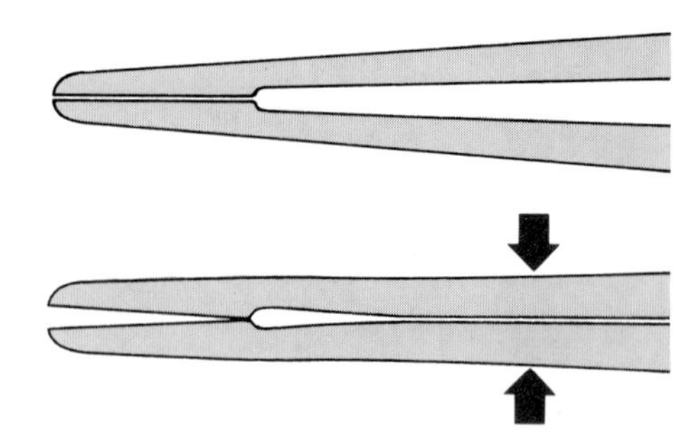

Fig. 9. **Plane forceps with predefined grasping surface**

a Grasping surfaces come into contact only at a defined blade pressure.

b If this pressure is increased beyond the design point, the grasping surfaces begin to gape

[8] Function is tested by a load test with material of known weight and surface roughness.

[9] Function is tested by visual inspection of the jaws as digital pressure is increased.

[10] Example: sclera, needles, suture material.

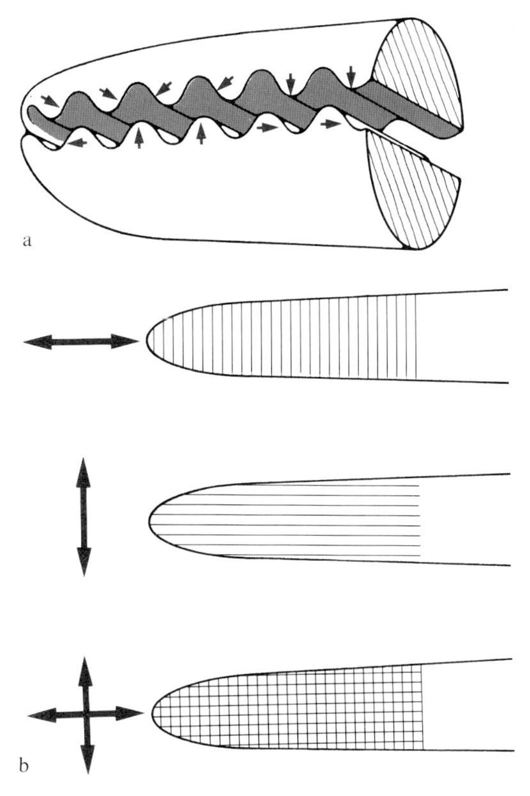

Fig. 10. **The principle of grooving**

a Grooving both increases the contact area and alters the angle of attack at the substrate.

b The ability to exert traction depends on the direction of the grooving. Cross-grooving provides resistance to traction in the direction of the handle *(top)*, while longitudinal grooving resists transverse traction *(middle)*. Forceps with criss-cross grooving offer resistance in all directions *(bottom)*

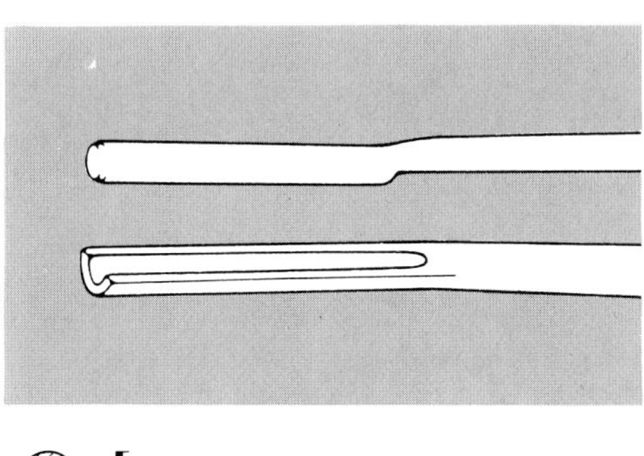

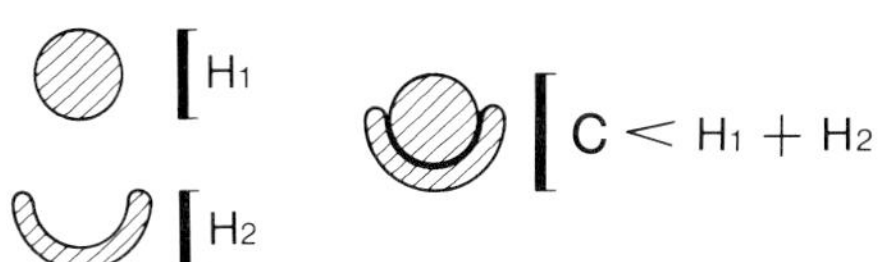

Fig. 12. **Forceps with a hollowed blade.** One blade is trough-shaped, the other cylindrical. The stability of each blade depends on its height *(H)*. Since the two blades interlock, the total cross-section *(C)* is smaller than the sum of the blade heights *(H)*. Owing to the curvature of the grasping surfaces, the advantages of grooving are present

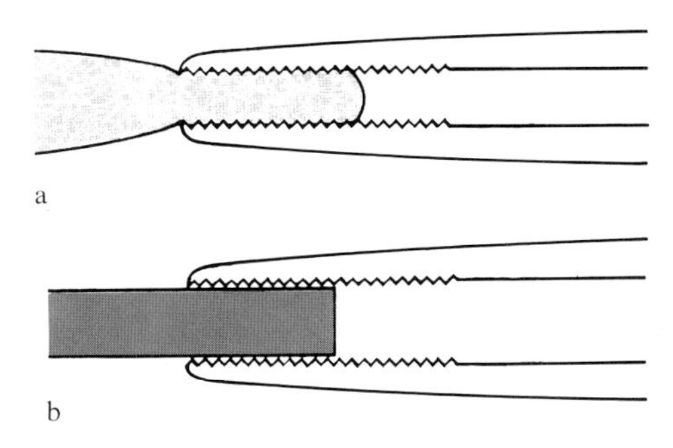

Fig. 11. **Conditions necessary for grooving to be effective**

a The grooves can penetrate into nonrigid material.

b Only the elevations come into contact with a rigid substrate, thereby reducing the area of contact. The varying angles of attack have no effect

The very finest untoothed forceps can be fitted with a *hollowed blade* as shown in Fig. 12. Despite their small cross-section, the blades are stable, have a relatively large grasping area, and have the advantage of varying angles of attack.

Another special type of forceps is the *ring forceps*, which actually is equivalent to circular grooving. Its large contact surface makes it suitable for grasping delicate structures; its circular shape permits traction in all directions (Fig. 13).

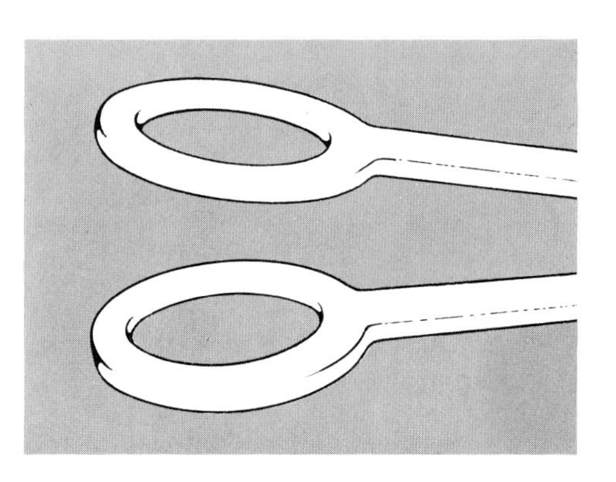

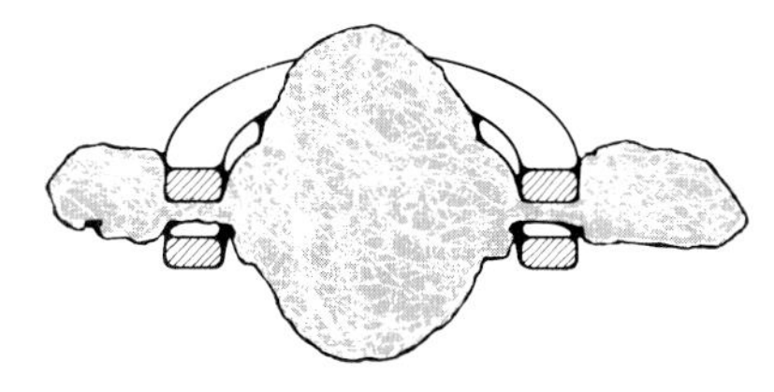

Fig. 13. **Ring forceps.** The enclosed material has a larger cross-section than that compressed between the blades. This prevents the tissue from shifting in any direction

2.2.2 Toothed Forceps

Toothed forceps produce their grasping resistance mainly by *surface deformation*. Despite their small grasping area, they provide good traction and are thus suited for precise "point" grasping and fixation. Their applications are determined by the force vectors of the teeth.

Forceps with **teeth set at right angles ("surgical forceps")** (Fig. 14) are, owing to the direction of the main vector, suited for grasping material that can be brought directly *between* the branches (Fig. 15). Since no vectors are outward-directed, the outer surface of the forceps can be ground smooth.[11] When closed, it forms a blunt instrument which slips harmlessly past delicate tissues (e.g., in the interior of the eye) (Fig. 16).

The *size and sharpness of the teeth* must be suited to the thickness and quality of the tissue (Fig. 17). Once the teeth have seized the tissue, the working motion is completed, and further action is limited simply to maintaining this position while the instrument is guided. Thus, complete closure of the jaws is not a criterion for grasping and can be prevented if necessary by the presence of stops (Fig. 17).

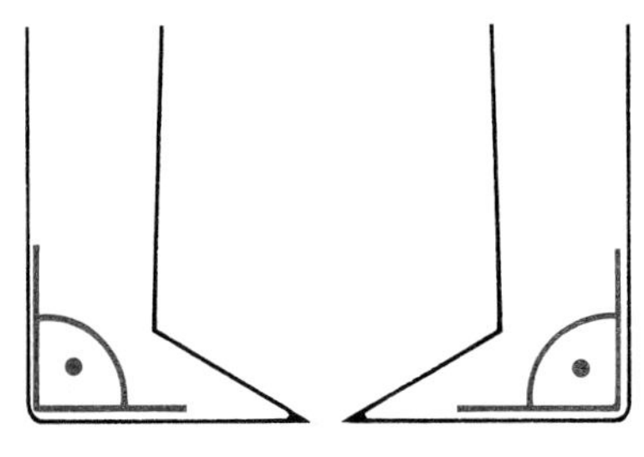

Fig. 14. **"Right-angle" teeth**

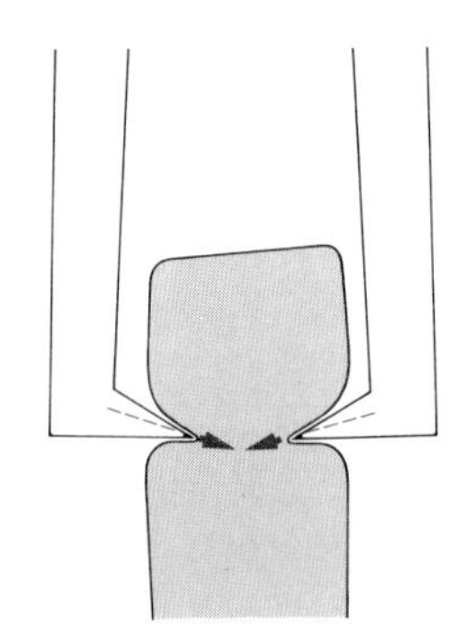

Fig. 15. **Vectors created by right-angle teeth.** The thrust vectors are directed inward to seize material lying between the blades

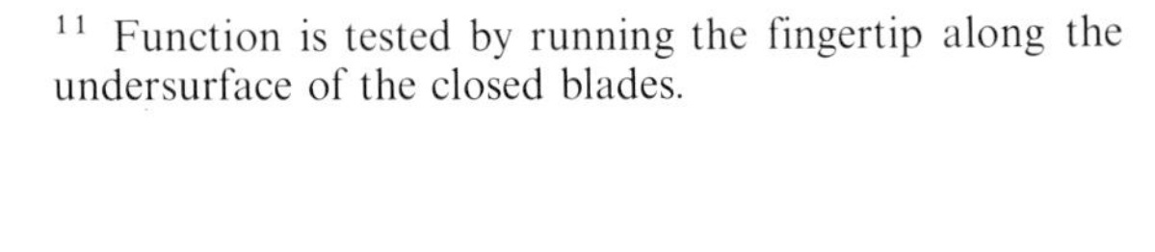

[11] Function is tested by running the fingertip along the undersurface of the closed blades.

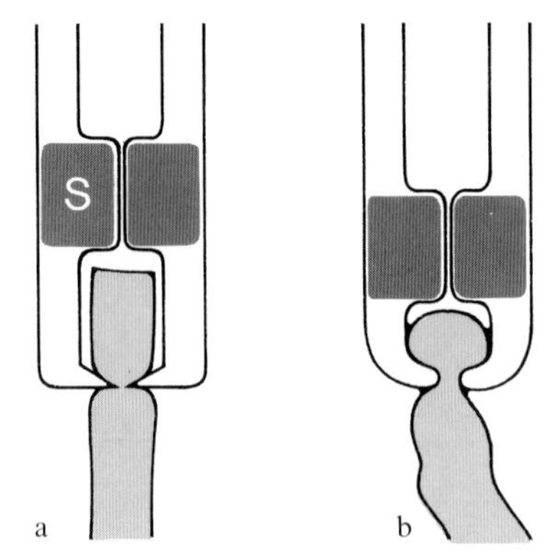

Fig. 17. **Tooth shape and tissue quality**

a For tough material, such as the cornea and sclera, the teeth must be sharp enough to penetrate.

b For soft material, such as the iris and conjunctiva, blunt, nonlacerating teeth can be used. Stops (*S*) prevent tissue trauma

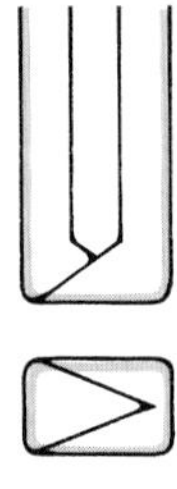

Fig. 16. **Closed forceps as a blunt instrument.** Forceps with right-angle teeth can be ground such that their outer surface is completely smooth when the blades are closed

Forceps with **angled teeth ("mouse-tooth forceps")** have a forward-directed vector component (Fig. 18). The teeth therefore can seize tissue lying *in front of* the ends of the branches

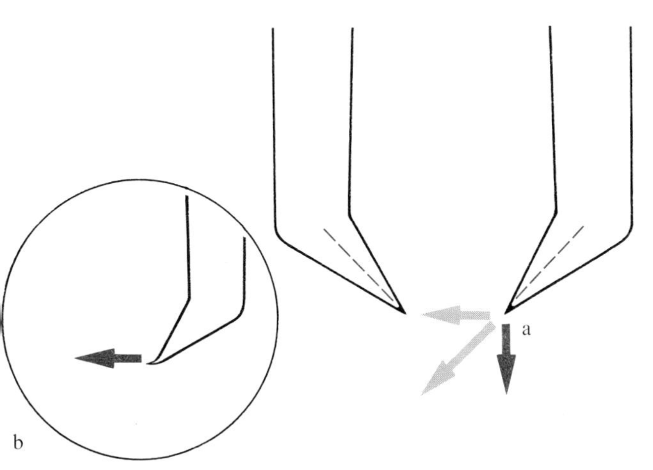

Fig. 18. **Angled teeth**

a One component of the thrust-vector is forward-directed (*dark red*).

b If the tooth is bent, the thrust vectors deviate from the normal working direction

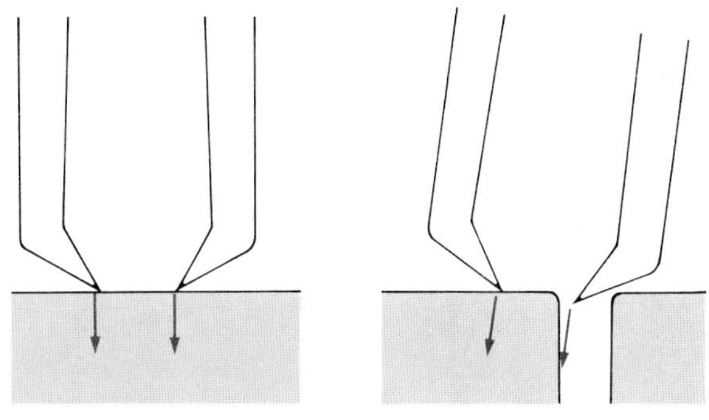

Fig. 19. **Possible points of attack of the thrust vector.** Owing to the forward-directed vector, mouse-tooth forceps can grab into flat surfaces *(left)* or penetrate into the space between wound edges *(right)*

(Fig. 19). However, the forward vector component requires that a force of equal direction be applied during closure of the forceps, so that the working motion is always coupled with a "thrusting" motion *forward.* This thrusting motion may meet with a sizable resistance if the teeth of the mouse-tooth forceps are not absolutely sharp. If the teeth are dull or bent, the forceps can at best be used as a surgical forceps (Fig. 18b). Thus, mouse-tooth forceps require as much care in their manufacture and maintenance as *cutting instruments.*[12]

With regard to its function, the mouse-tooth forceps can be likened to a claw, anchor or trident (Fig. 20), its various *applications* depending on the blade spacing when the instrument is applied:

As a *claw*, it is particularly suited for grasping wound edges at an angle, with the advantage that the teeth bite more easily into the tissue than with ordinary surgical forceps. When used to grasp smooth surfaces, it produces a fold.[13]

As an *anchor,* it includes a minimal tissue volume in its grip and can thus grasp surfaces with a minimum of deformation.[14]

As a *trident* it can, without penetrating the tissue, produce a friction that can withstand weaker forces.[15]

The properties of mouse-tooth forceps can be combined with those of blunt grasping plates to create a special forceps with a variety of applications (Fig. 21).

[12] Function is tested by visual inspection of the tooth shape or by the presence of reflections at the tooth tip (a sign of dulling, see also footnote 20).

[13] A typical example of its "claw" function is the grasping of a muscular insertion transconjunctivally (see Fig. 157). In contrast, when the sclera is grasped the resulting tissue fold decreases the volume of the eye and thus raises the intraocular pressure.

[14] Unlike the claw, the anchor is suited for grasping the sclera. It can fixate this tissue "at a point".

[15] This resistance, which is quite low in itself, may be sufficient for passing sutures with an extremely sharp needle. Here the trident has the advantage that the teeth need not penetrate into the wound edge.

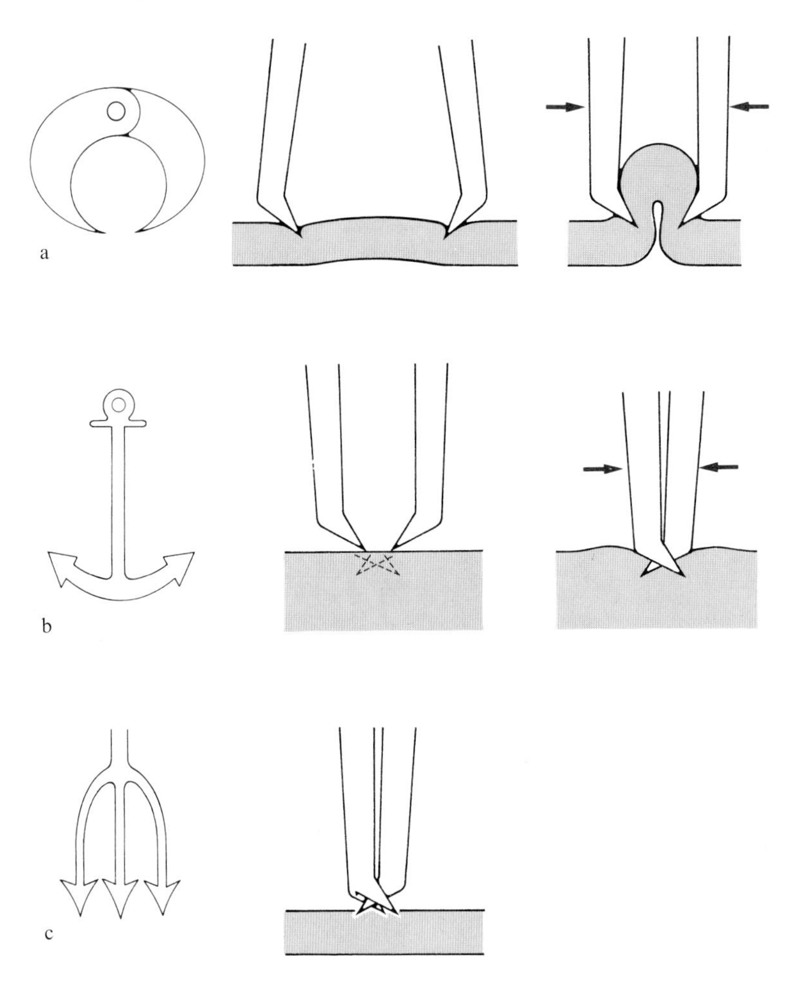

Fig. 20. **Possible applications of mouse-tooth forceps**

a Large blade spacing: *Claw*. Closure of the blades produces a fold.

b Small blade spacing (about one tooth width): *Anchor*. Note: The forceps must be held perpendicular to the tissue surface for all the teeth to penetrate uniformly.

c Closed: *Trident*. The trident is formed by the teeth as they project beyond the surface of the closed forceps tip

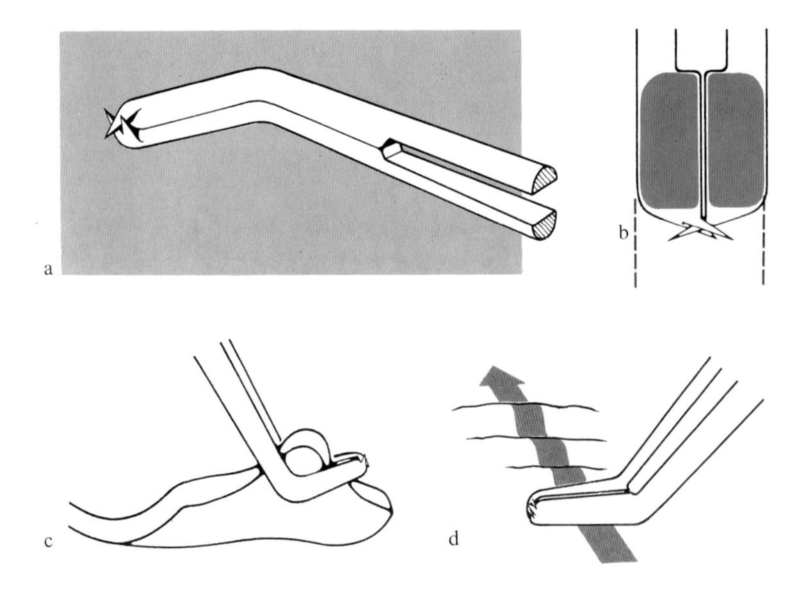

Fig. 21. **Possible applications of a combination forceps ("colibri" forceps after Barraquer)**

a Blades with mouse teeth, grasping plates and handle angled at plates. The teeth have the claw, anchor and trident functions described above.

b The grasping plates at the end of the forceps can be used for suture tying, provided they extend far enough laterally beyond the teeth to prevent fouling.

c The angulation of the grasping plates creates "half-ring" blades which can be used to apply traction at the edges of delicate tissues.

d When closed, the instrument forms a spatula whose roughness can be varied by adjusting the position of the teeth

2.2.3 Needle Holders

If a needle is to pass through tissue, its resistance in the holder must be greater than in the tissue. The only practical means of creating this resistance is to increase the grasping pressure on the needle[16] (see 1.2.). This requires a needle holder of rigid and stable construction.[17]

If a high pressure is exerted on the needle, there is a danger that it will slip or bend in the holder. This places certain constraints on the **shape of the jaws**. The danger of needle bending or breakage can best be avoided through congruity between the curvature of the needle and the cross-section of the jaws. This would require a special holder for each needle type; for practical reasons, of course, compromises are sought (Fig. 23).

Slippage of the needle is a danger if the pressure is not applied precisely at right angles to the needle axis, as in a V-shaped jaw opening (Fig. 22). Oblique force vectors can also cause tilting if the needle is not gripped such that the distance between the points of contact is minimal (Fig. 24a). Thus, the shape of the jaw determines the angle at which a needle can be grasped relative to the handle (Fig. 24b, c, d).

The demands on jaw construction are less stringent if only a slight grasping pressure is required, as in the suturing of soft tissues or when an extremely sharp needle is used.[18]

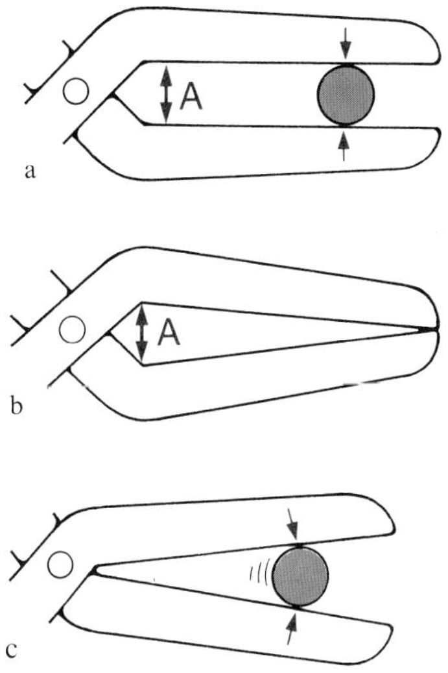

Fig. 22. **Direction of force vectors in a needle holder**

a When the blades are parallel, the forces are applied at right angles, and the needle is held securely.

b When such a holder is closed empty, a gap is left near the joint (A) whose dimensions determine the diameter of the needle which can be held.

c If this gap is absent, the blade aperture becomes V-shaped when the needle is grasped; the force vectors are oblique, and the needle is pushed out

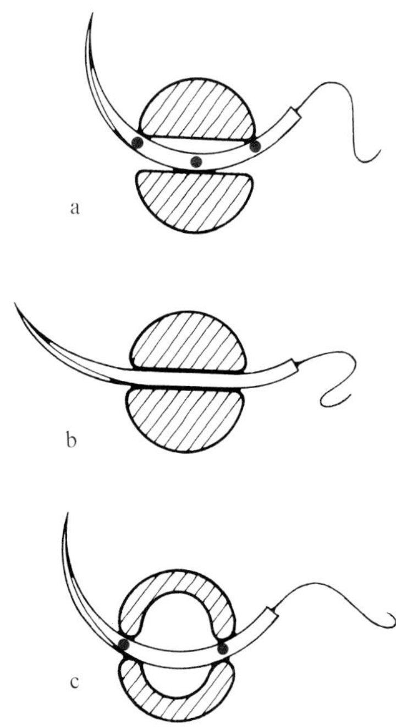

Fig. 23. **Cross-section of jaws**

a If the inner jaw surfaces are flat, they will contact a curved needle at three points.

b When the jaws are closed, the needle may be bent or broken, the danger varying with the ratio of the blade width to the needle curvature.

c Hollowed jaws make contact at only two points, and the danger of needle damage is reduced

---

[16] There is no room for large contact surfaces, and roughening or grooving can be effective only at the cost of needle damage.

[17] The fingers can be freed from maintaining a high pressure by the use of lock mechanisms. But in fine work such mechanisms are a hindrance and are unnecessary, since then the tissue resistance and thus the necessary grasping pressure are low.

[18] When the conjunctiva is sutured with sharp needles, for example, a simple forceps makes a satisfactory needle holder.

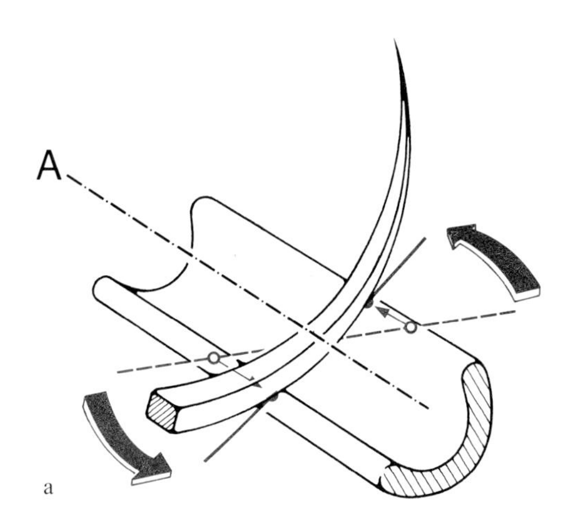

Fig. 24. **Longitudinal section of jaws**

a When grasped, curved needles have a tendency to shift until the distance between contact points is minimal, i.e., until they are perpendicular to the jaw axis *(A)*.

b With straight jaws (i.e., a straight jaw axis), the angle *(α)* at which the needle can be grasped is determined by the angle between the jaw axis *(A)* and handle axis *(B)*.

c With curved jaws (i.e., a curved jaw axis), the needle can be grasped at various angles (α, β, γ) to the handle axis. However, a different contact area must be used for each angle (that at which the needle is held perpendicular to the jaw axis).

d With hemispherical jaws (spoons with a "point" axis), the distances between contact points are equal in all directions. The needle can therefore be held in the same spot at various angles to the handle axis

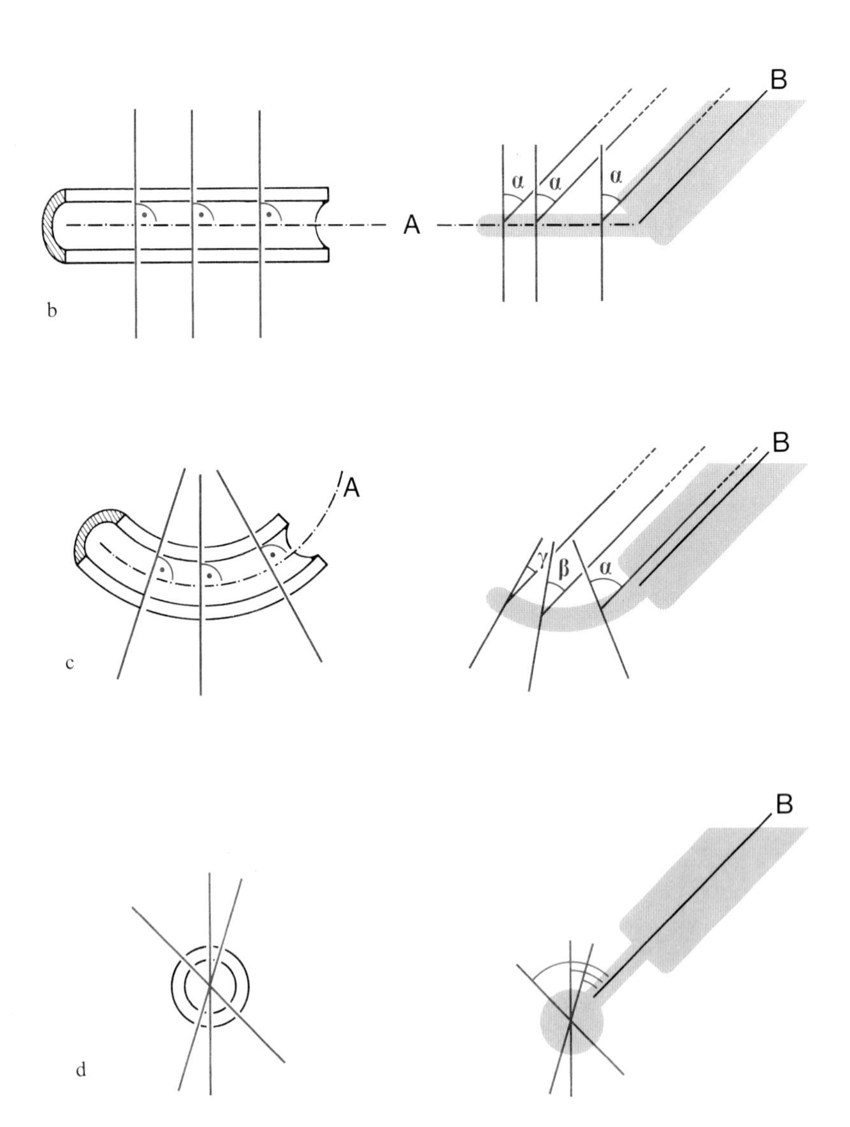

2.2.4 Tying Forceps

To avoid damage to delicate suture material, tying forceps must have carefully rounded edges. At the same time, the tip should have sharp edges (Fig. 25) so that threads lying on the tissue surface can be grasped.

It is essential, therefore, that the forceps be *properly held* if suture damage is to be avoided. The tip area is used only for picking up the thread. For further handling, the threads are passed over the rounded side edges. Of course these can also act as "cutting edges" if strong (especially sudden) tension is exerted on the threads. So if a high tensile stress is required, the threads should not be stretched over spots with a small radius of curvature (Fig. 26).

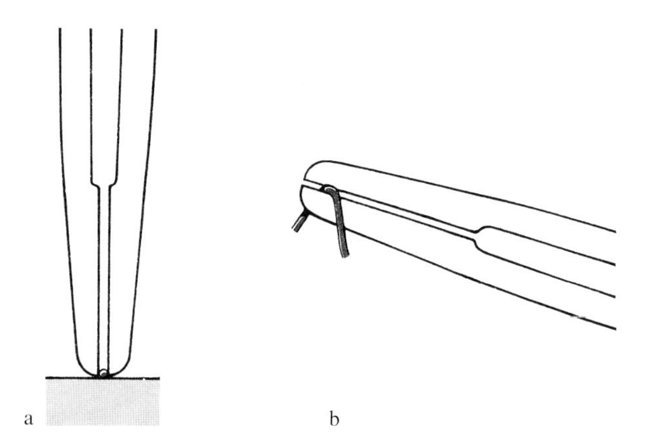

Fig. 25. **Tying forceps**

a Threads lying on smooth surfaces can be grasped only if the jaws come into contact up to the very tip (sharp edges).

b For handling, the thread is passed over the rounded side edges

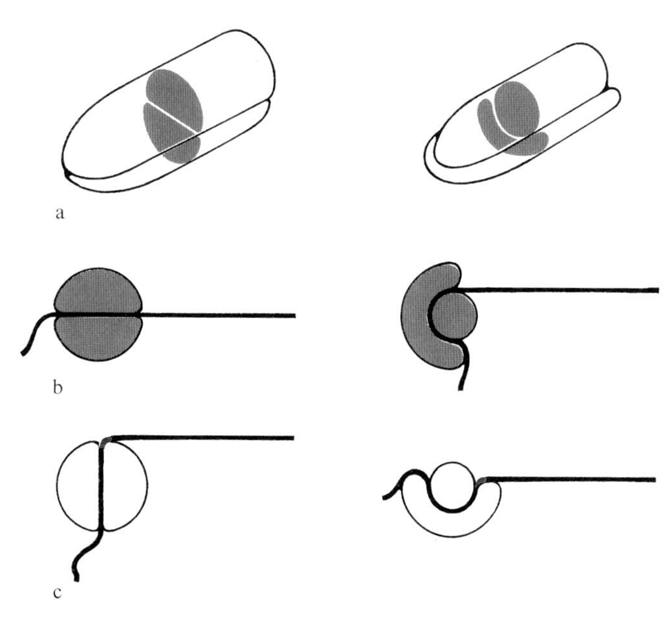

Fig. 26. **The proper holding of tying forceps under a high suture tension.** *Left:* plane forceps; *right:* hollowed-blade forceps.

a Jaw configurations; (cross-section: *gray*)

b Thread is preserved by passing over the largest radius of curvature.

c Thread passed over spots with a small radius of curvature *(red)* is more prone to breakage

2.3 The Division of Tissues

2.3.1 Division Techniques

Processes such as sawing, drilling and burning involve the **removal of material** lying between the parts to be divided (Fig. 27). When the divided parts are reunited, the tissue cannot be fully restored to its original state due to this loss of material. Therefore, such processes generally are used in ophthalmic surgery only if the goal of the operation is *dehiscence*.[19]

In the **splitting procedure**, tissue fibers are overstretched in a longitudinal direction. Where preformed tissue spaces are present, characterized by varying strength in different directions, the split can be made by means of a wedge (Fig. 28). The wedge pushes the more resistant layers apart, while causing the loose intervening fibers to rupture without coming in direct contact with them. Thus, the properties of the cutting edge play a role only in the search for a suitable level at which to initiate the split, but not in the splitting process itself. The latter, incidentally, can be controlled by neither the shape nor the movement of the wedge, but depends primarily on the *anatomical path of the tissue space*. Splitting, or "*blunt dissection*" is therefore used when the surgeon wishes to be guided by the properties of the tissue itself, without "imposing his will upon it."

In **cutting**, the tissue fibers are divided by a concentrated application of pressure. Only those fibers touched by the cutting edge are divided ("*sharp dissection*") (Fig. 29). Thus, the surgeon can directly control the cutting process by guidance of the cutting edge.

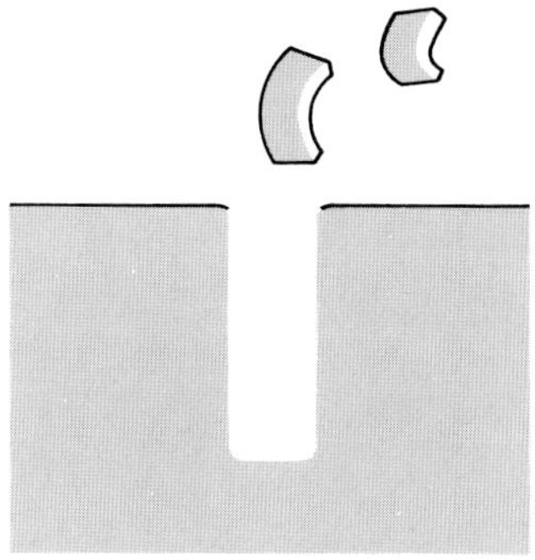

Fig. 27. **Processes which divide tissue by removal of material.** Division is achieved by creating a "channel" in the tissue

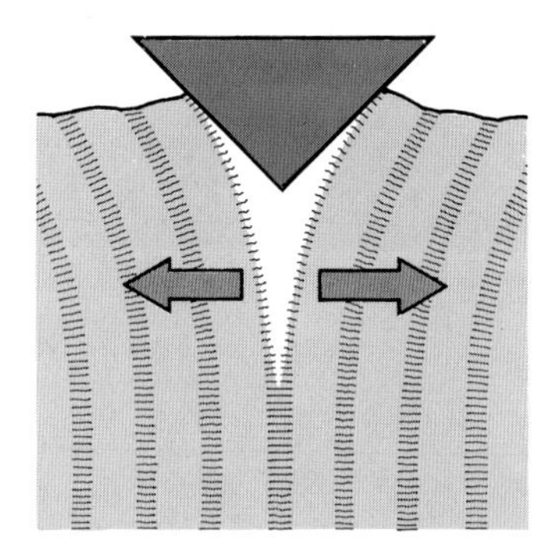

Fig. 28. **Splitting (tearing).** Splitting is done by driving a wedge into a preformed tissue space. The effect depends on the width of the wedge and the properties of the tissue; the tip of the wedge does not touch the fibers to be divided and plays no role in the splitting process

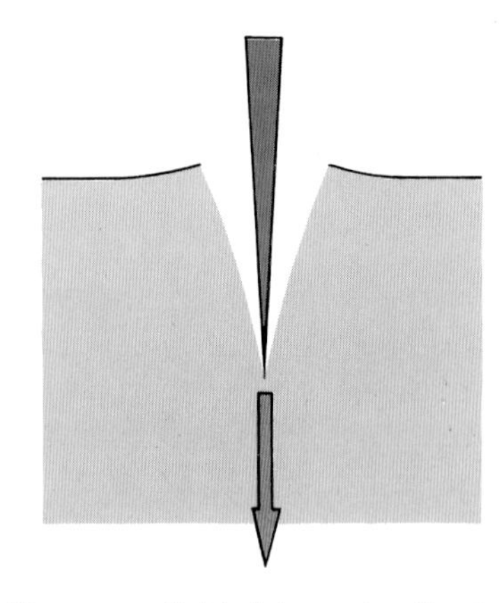

Fig. 29. **Cutting.** The fibers are divided by a localized pressure (pressure of the cutting edge and counterpressure of the tissue), the effect achieved depending on the degree to which the pressure can be localized. The direction in which the division proceeds is determined by the movement of the cutting edge

[19] For example, burning with a cautery, diathermy knife or laser to create fistulae in glaucoma operations.

2.3.2 Cutting

Three factors are involved in the cutting process: The *shape of the instrument*, its *guidance* by the surgeon, and the *properties of the tissue*. All these factors play a role both in regulating the effective "sharpness" of the cutting edge and in determining the shape of the resulting cut.

Sharpness, or the ability to divide tissue, is a product of the *cutting ability* of the instrument and the *sectility* ("cuttability") of the tissue. These are not determined strictly by the properties of the instrument and tissue; they can be varied as needed by the guidance actions of the surgeon.

The **cutting ability of instruments** (Fig. 30) is determined chiefly by the properties of the cutting edge. If the edge has the property of a geometric point or line (i.e., zero surface area), the pressure becomes infinitely high when any force is applied, and the *resistance* of the edge (i.e. the cutting resistance proper) becomes infinitely low.[20]

Cutting ability is also influenced by the tissue displacement of the structure that bears the cutting edge (the "carrier"). The amount of resistance that occurs here, or the *lateral resistance*, depends on the angle formed by the carrier surfaces (Fig. 30 b).

Guidance motions can further improve cutting ability: When the blade is "pulled through", i.e. guided parallel to the cutting edge, each tissue fiber is submitted to numerous cutting points.

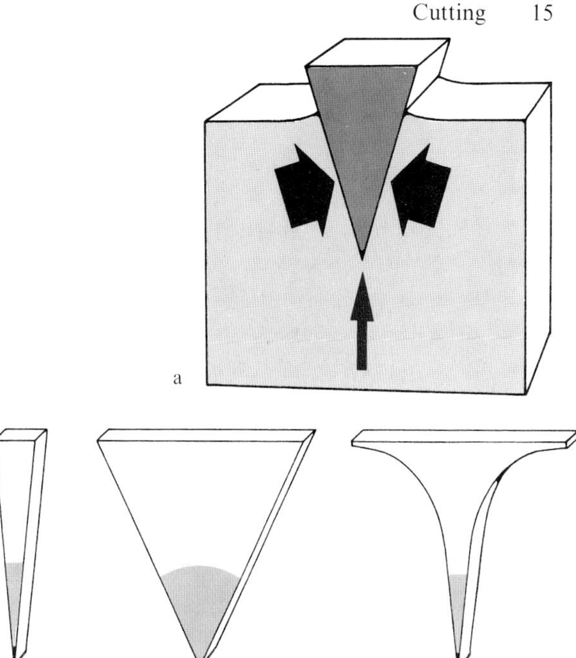

Fig. 30. **The concept of cutting ability**

a A cutting instrument consists of a cutting edge and its carrier. The resistance to the cutting edge *(red arrow)* determines the actual cutting ability of the instrument, while the resistance to the carrier (lateral resistance: *black arrows*) determines the ability of the instrument to penetrate into tissue.

b The narrower the wedge, the lower the lateral resistance, but the lower the blade stability as well. The concave blade *(right)* combines high sharpness (low lateral resistance) with high stability (broad back)

The **sectility of the tissue** depends on the degree to which the fibers are shifted, rather than cut, by the blade (Fig. 31 a). If a blade is passed through tissue layers of *varying sectility*, only the layers with high sectility are cut, while those of low sectility will remain intact (Fig. 31 b).[21]

This principle is exploited to control sharpness through *selective tension*, which allows sectility to be confined to the zone lying directly in front of the cutting edge (Fig. 32) while adjacent fibers are spared.

In general, sectility can be enhanced by the use of *mechanical supports* or increased *tissue tension* to prevent the tissue from shifting under the action of the cutting edge (Fig. 33). The *speed* of the guidance motion can also be utilized to hinder tissue shifting through inertial effects.[22]

[20] Function test: The absence of surface area on a properly ground cutting edge is manifested visually by the absence of reflections from it, regardless of the angle of light incidence. If a ground edge reflects light, this is an indication that it has a definite surface area and thus is dull.

[21] This principle can be utilized to prevent damage to displaceable tissue layers while layers with a high sectility are cut. Example: Incising the cornea without damaging the more mobile iris by employing small-amplitude cutting movements (e.g., with a vibratory knife). The iris is protected from lesion as long as its mobility is not restricted by incarceration between the cornea and lens or by synechiae.

[22] Note that a rapid blade motion is safe only if the thrust vector terminates in empty space after the target is reached (example: needle, Graefe knife), or if its magnitude is limited by the construction of the instrument (example: vibratory knives, including those that operate at ultrasonic frequencies).

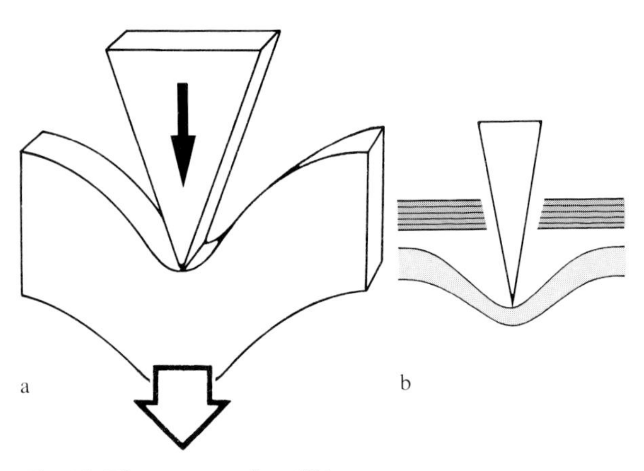

Fig. 31. **The concept of sectility**

a Tissue which is displaceable can shift ahead of the blade and is not sectioned. If sectility is low, even "sharp" blades become dull.

b The significance of sectility: If superposed layers of different sectility are cut, only that of high sectility is sectioned, while that of low sectility is merely shifted and remains intact

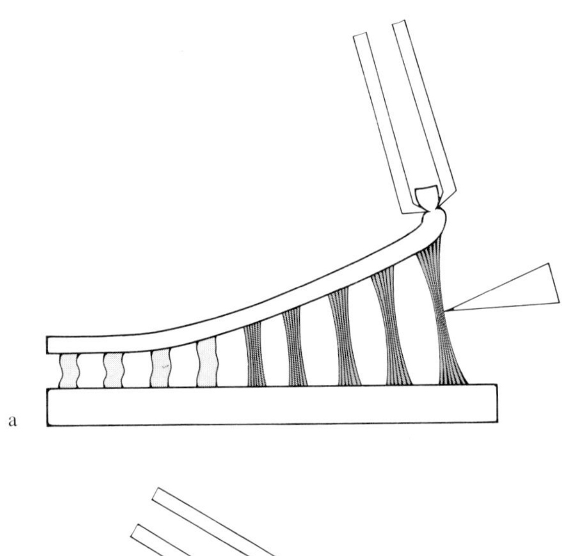

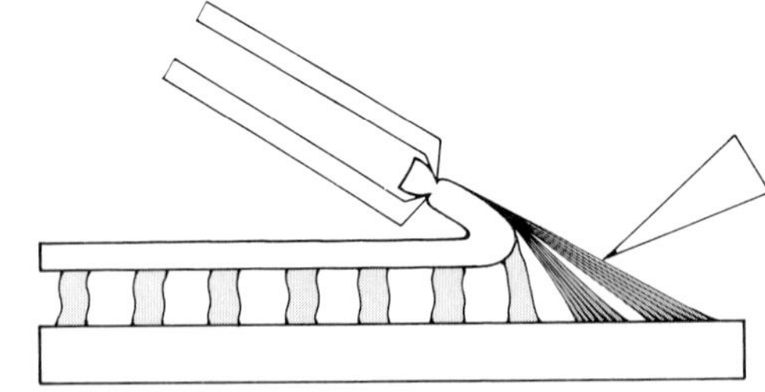

Fig. 32. **Regulation of tissue sectility**

a Diffuse tissue tension: The tissue layer which transmits forceps traction to the target fibers is lifted vertically away from the underlying layer, so that tension is exerted on a great number of fibers. This produces good sectility over a large area.

b Selective tissue tension: The layer which transmits the traction is drawn back so that tension is exerted only on the most peripheral fibers. The remaining fibers and the overlying layer have poor sectility and are thus protected from inadvertant lesions

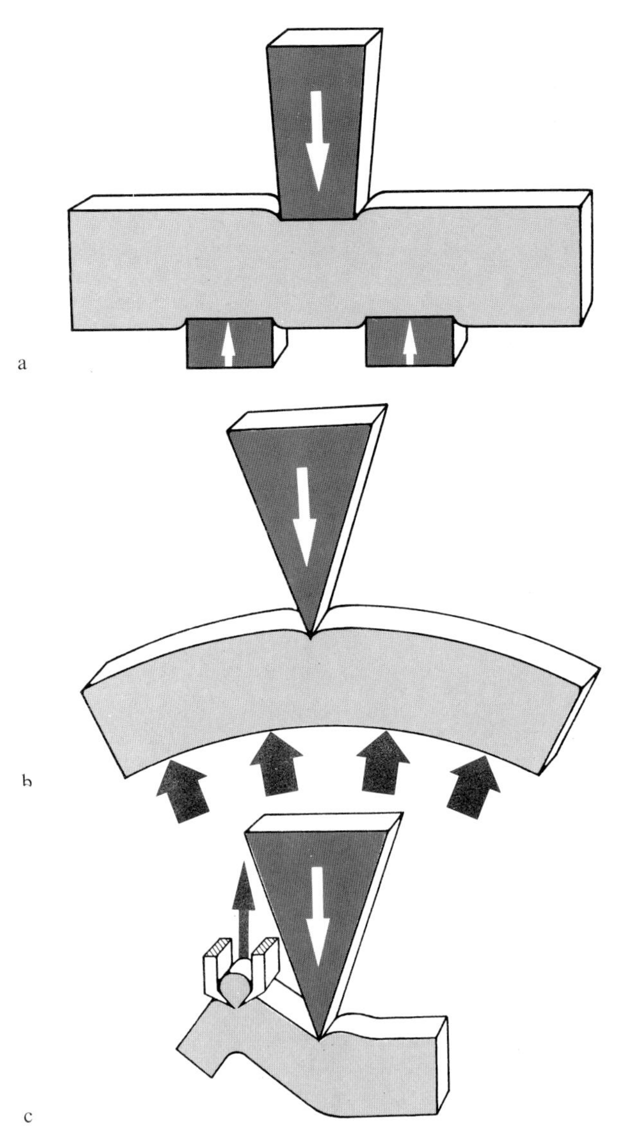

Fig. 33. **Means of improving sectility**

a The instrument can be constructed so as to support the tissue from below (here: the punch principle). See also Fig. 56.

b Tissue tension is increased by a high intraocular pressure.

c By applying countertraction with forceps, the tissue tension can be varied. However, this technique may involve tissue deformation which requires corrective blade movements in order to obtain the intended cut (see Figs. 256, 258c)

The **shape of the resulting cut** is defined by the path followed by the cutting edge through the tissue. This path also is influenced by the three factors mentioned earlier: the construction of the *instrument* (the path the cutting edge tends to follow by virtue of instrument construction), its guidance by the *surgeon*, and

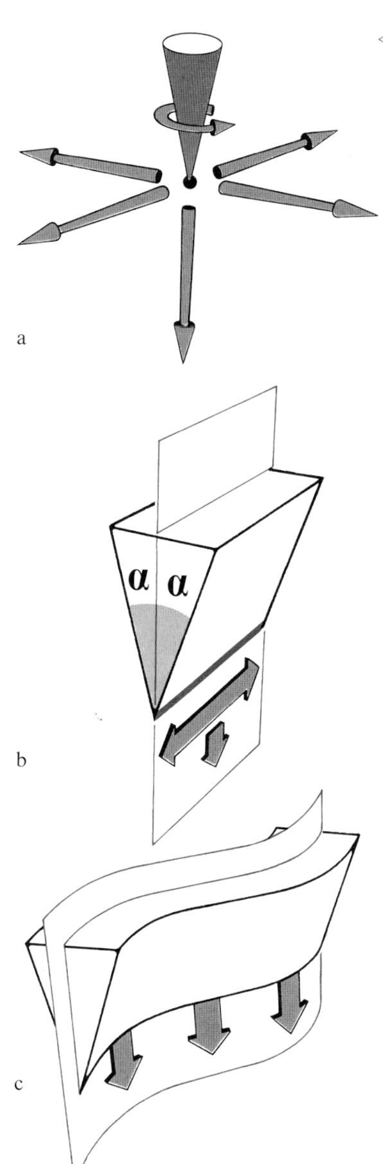

◁ Fig. 34. **Motions with symmetrical lateral resistance**

a The mobiluty of a single cutting point is theoretically unlimited. In practice, it is limited by the lateral resistance of its carrier.

b A linear cutting edge describes an imaginary surface as it moves. If the lateral resistance is symmetrical, its motion follows the bisector of the carrier surfaces, which we shall call the "preferential path." If this path is a plane (knife) or the surface of a body of revolution (trephine), there are two motions with a symmetrical lateral resistance:

- motion perpendicular to the cutting edge (thrusting motion)
- motion parallel to the cutting edge ("pull-through" motion).

c If the preferential path is a surface with an irregular curvature, the only motion with a symmetrical lateral resistance is the thrusting motion, since a pull-through motion creates vectors perpendicular to the preferential path. Blades of this shape can only be used in punch-like mechanisms

Fig. 35. **Motions with asymmetrical lateral resistance**

a Vectors pependicular to the preferential path ▷ give rise to an asymmetrical lateral resistance.

b, c Asymmetrical lateral resistances arise if the cutting edge is not guided along the preferential path. These motions have rotatory components about either the cutting-edge axis (**b**, also see Fig. 52) or the axis perpendicular to the cutting edge (**c**, also see Fig. 51)

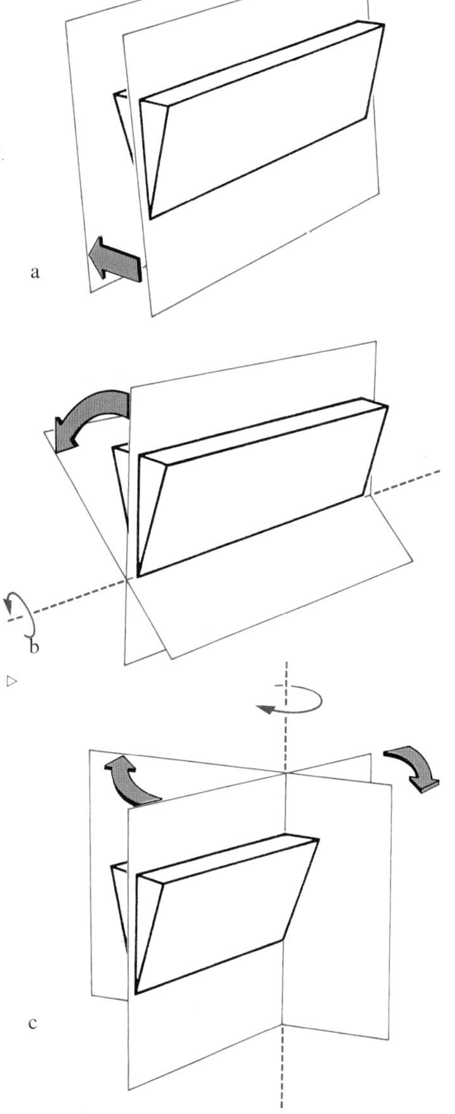

the behavior of the *tissue* (its tendency to shift ahead of the advancing cutting edge).

The **path of the cutting edge** is influenced by the lateral resistance acting at the carrier surfaces (Fig. 34). The *preferential path* of the cutting edge is that in which the lateral resistance is symmetrical, i.e., along the bisector of the carrier surfaces. This bisector is an imaginary plane which coincides with no real carrier surface and characterizes the path which a cutting edge tends to follow by virtue of the instrument's construction.[23] Cutting motions along the preferential path of the instrument can be resolved into components perpendicular to the cutting edge (*thrust vectors*) and components parallel to the cutting edge (*pull-through vectors*, Fig. 34b). The *thrusting motion* constantly brings each cutting point of the edge in contact with new substrate, so that the cut proceeds in the direction of thrust. The *pull-through motion* brings several cutting points past the same point on the substrate and thus improves cutting ability without deepening the incision.

All *other motions* give rise to vector components perpendicular to the preferential path (Fig. 35). This causes increased lateral resis-

[23] If the cutting edge is a point, the preferential path of the instrument is a geometric line.

tance on one side, and the instrument is pushed back to its original position by the tissue. To overcome the increasing lateral resistance, a greater application of force is required for motions incongruent with the preferential path.[24]

During **guidance motions made by the surgeon**, each cutting point follows a line, and each linear cutting edge a plane, which we shall call the *guidance path*. This path characterizes the intentions of the operator. Precision is greatest when the guidance path (of the surgeon) is congruent with the preferential path (of the instrument).[25] If this condition can be met, it is useful to maximize the lateral resistance (either by the selection of blade shape or the manner of holding the blade), because this makes it easier to continue the cut in a given direction and lessens the danger of inadvertant deviations (Fig. 51).

[24] They may lead also to a deformation of the edges of the incision which causes the wound to gape (e.g., in the case of the anterior chamber: drainage).

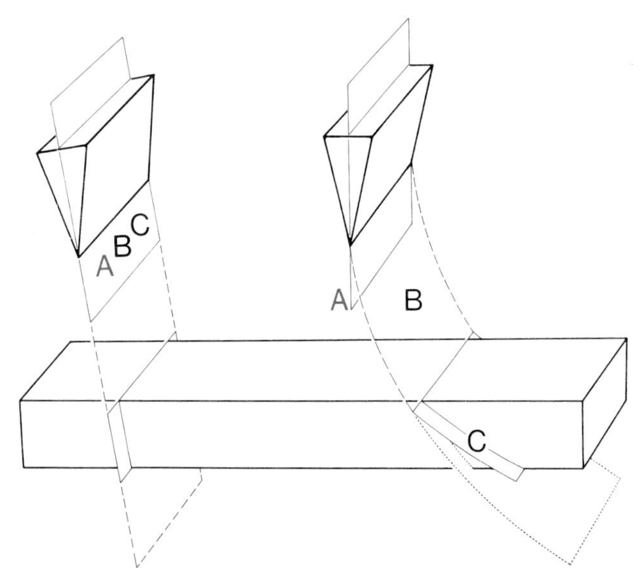

Fig. 36. **The cutting process described in terms of preferential path, guidance path and cut surface.** The three factors – instrument, surgeon and tissue – can be characterized geometrically by three surfaces.

Preferential path A: Path the instrument tends to follow owing to its construction.

Guidance path B: The actual path of the cutting edge as directed by the surgeon.

Cut surface C: The result of the cutting process in the tissue.

Ideally *(left)*, all three surfaces coincide; the cut surfaces then correspond exactly to the surgeon's intentions. In reality *(right)*, the surfaces are usually incongruent since

- guidance path ≠ preferential path if the surgeon does not guide the cutting edge precisely along the bisector of the carrier surfaces
- cut surface ≠ guidance path if the tissue shifts ahead of the cutting edge

If the cutting edge cannot be guided along its preferential path, as when curved incisions must be made for which there is no congruent blade, the lateral resistance becomes asymmetrical. The attendant disadvantages can then be minimized by making the lateral resistance as *low* as possible. This is done by selecting a blade with a small carrier surface and guiding it such that only a small portion of the blade enters the tissue.

The shape of the cut – the result of the cutting process – should in theory coincide with the guidance path of the surgeon (Fig. 36). But this congruence can exist only if the tissue does not shift ahead of the cutting edge. Otherwise deviations will occur, and the shape of the cut surface will not correspond to the surgeon's intentions. However, if the **shifting tendency of the tissue** is known in advance, it can be allowed for in the operating plan and can even be exploited to achieve specific results.

If the lateral resistance is *symmetrical*, the tissue will be shifted by the cutting edge in the direction of blade motion; the cut will proceed in the direction intended. If the lateral resistance is *asymmetrical*, the tissue will be shifted toward the higher resistance. The cutting edge thus encounters more and more tissue from the region of lower resistance, with the result that the cut deviates in the direction of the lower resistance.

Asymmetrical lateral resistances may on the one hand result from *guidance motions* which are inconsistent with the construction of the instrument (i.e., *guidance path ≠ preferential path*, Fig. 37).

Asymmetrical lateral resistances may also arise from the sectile characteristics of the *tissue structure*, which causes incisions to devi-

[25] Examples: A plane guidance path for Graefe knives or keratomes; a cylindrical guidance path for trephines.

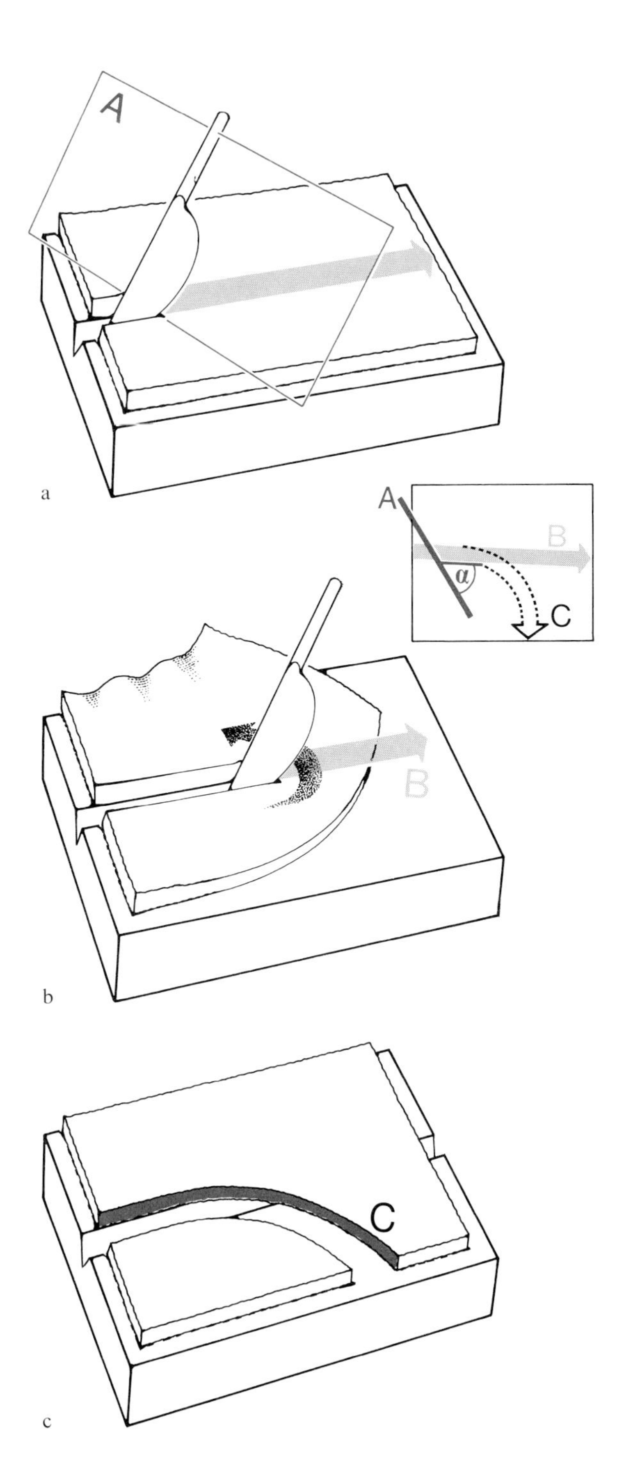

Fig. 37. **Deviation of cut during guidance motions with asymmetrical lateral resistance.** If the blade is guided such that the guidance path *(B)* forms an angle with the preferential path *(A)*, the resulting incision *(C)* deviates from the direction intended *(inset)* and increasingly follows the direction of the preferential path (where the lateral resistance again becomes symmetrical)

a Blade guided at an angle to the preferential path (outlined in red).

b The tissue in front of the edge is shifted toward the side with the higher resistance.

c Deviation of the cut results

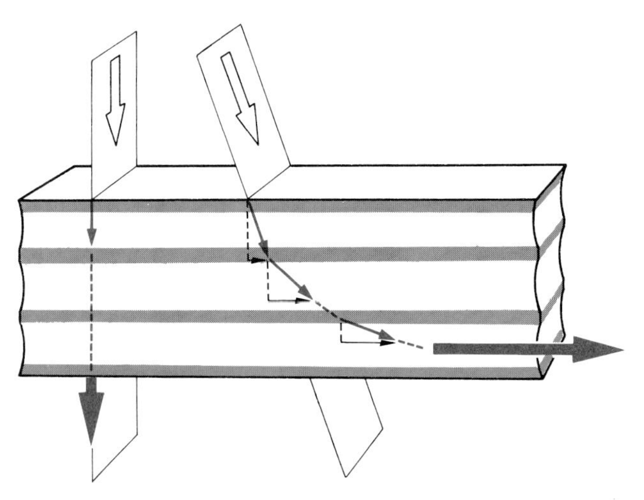

Fig. 38. **Lamellar deflection.** Lamellar tissues consist of a regular arrangement of layers with varying resistances. If a blade is applied to the lamellae at right angles *(left)*, it encounters a symmetrical lateral resistance and can advance in the direction intended. If the blade is applied obliquely *(right)*, the lateral resistance becomes asymmetrical. The incision deviates until it terminates in loose interlamellar tissue, where the lateral resistance is again symmetrical

ate in typical ways. In **lamellar tissues**, for example, the incision is gradually deflected into an intermediate layer with lower resistance, or in the *lamellar direction* (Fig. 38). This tendency depends on tissue resistance. It can be controlled by the surgeon by regulating the effective "sharpness" of the cutting process. The *lamellar deflection* is most pronounced when the cutting edge is dull or the sectility low.[26] It is exploited if the operative goal is the dissection of lamellae, but should be avoided if the lamellae themselves are to be divided.[27]

Other typical sectile characteristics are found in **compliant, resilient tissues**. When under uniform tension, these tissues tend to *shift forward* ahead of the blade (Fig. 39), and the resulting incision is shorter than the distance traveled by the cutting edge.[28] To achieve a

[26] Example: Lowering the intraocular pressure by medication or by puncture of the anterior chamber in lamellar keratoplasty.

[27] Example: If the anterior chamber must be opened when the intraocular pressure is low, lamellar deflection may prevent the blade from reaching the anterior chamber at all. Intraocular pressure must be restored, therefore.

[28] Penetrating foreign bodies "cut" openings that are smaller than their own diameter. To remove the foreign body through the entry wound, this wound usually must be extended.

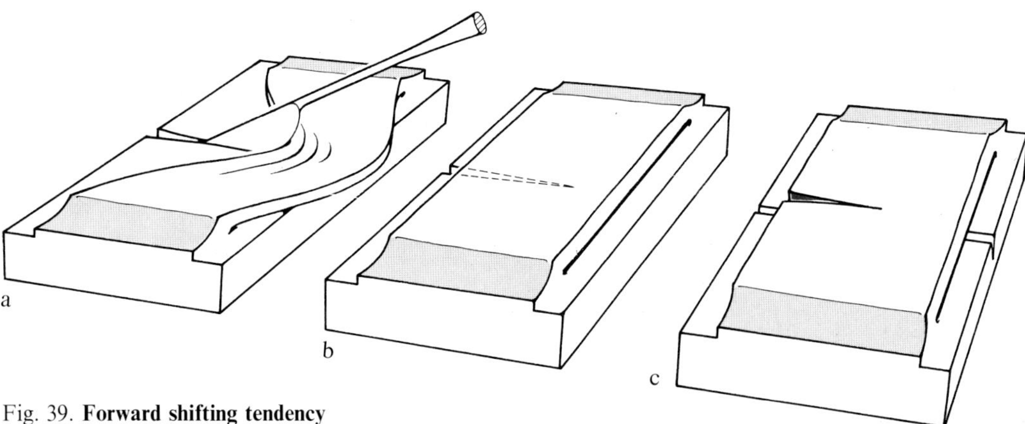

Fig. 39. **Forward shifting tendency**

a Compliant tissue is shifted ahead of the blade.

b Short cutting movement: In firm tissue (the sublayer in the figure), the length of the resulting incision equals the distance traveled by the cutting edge. The displaceable layer, however, is not divided by a short cutting movement (see also Fig. 31b).

c A longer cutting movement incises the displaceable layer as well, but this incision is shorter than the distance traveled by the cutting edge.
Note: Under symmetrical tissue tension, the cut follows the guidance path
(*gray*: zones of fixation)

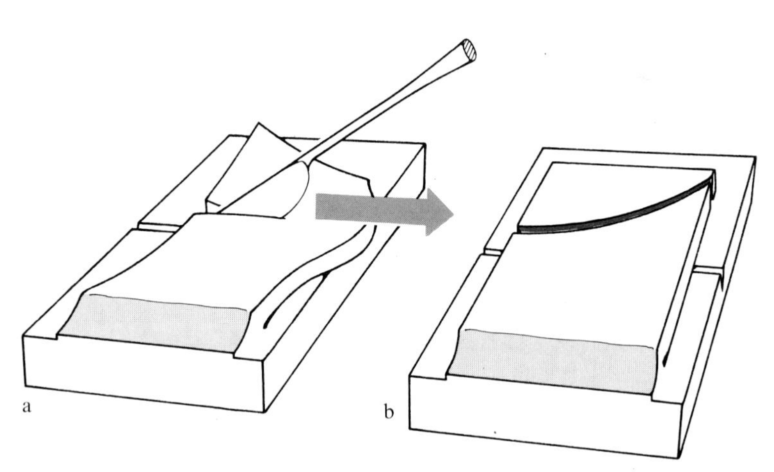

Fig. 40. **Lateral shifting tendency.**
a If tensions on the tissue are asymmetrical, the tissue will shift ahead of the cutting edge toward the side of higher tension, i.e., toward the fixation *(gray)*.

b The resulting incision in the displaceable layer deviates toward the opposite side and away from the fixation. In the firm layer, on the other hand, it coincides with the guidance path

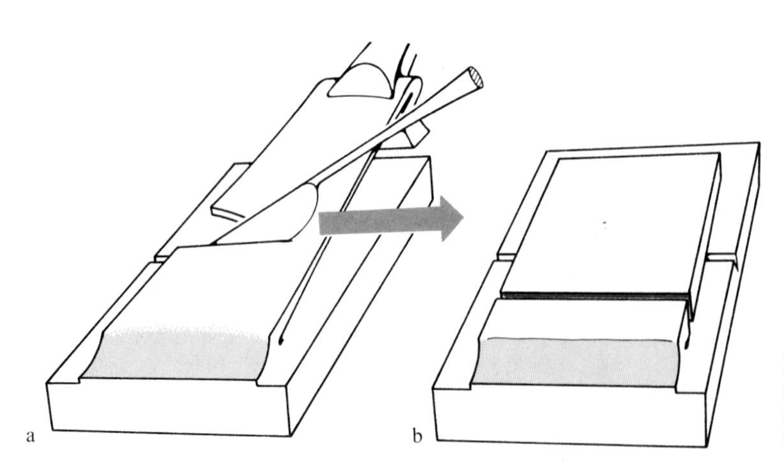

Fig. 41. **Tendency of retraction.** If tissue is divided while stretched (**a**), the resulting incision will be shifted toward the zone of fixation after tension is released (**b**)

certain length of incision, therefore, it is necessary to guide the blade beyond the target.

If compliant, resilient tissue is under asymmetrical tension, it tends also to *shift laterally*, with a resulting deviation of the incision toward the side of lower tension (Fig. 40). Such asymmetrical tensions are encountered wherever loose tissue is fixed unilaterally, whether by its anatomical structure[29] or by scars, or by the surgeon himself with fixation instruments.

These shifting tendencies can be reduced by making the tissue tense before cutting, thereby increasing its sectility. This, however, causes the cut to deviate from the guidance path by yet another mechanism: the *tendency of retraction*: If traction is applied to compliant, resilient tissue, the tissue will be stretched. When released, it will return to its former shape, and all distances will again be shortened in proportion to the degree of stretch (Fig. 41). Incisions made in stretched tissue are thus shifted from their original position toward the zone of fixation,[30] and excised areas are diminished in size. This *tendency of retraction* may become the source of unanticipated changes in the shape and position of incisions, but can also be exploited as an important aid in achieving specific operative goals.[31]

2.3.3 Blades with a Point Cutting Edge

Owing to their great freedom of movement, "point" cutting edges (Fig. 42) can produce incisions of any shape desired. The preferential paths of the instrument and the guidance paths are identical in all directions, and an incision line is made wherever the blade is directed (Fig. 43). An areal effect is achieved by making several incision lines in close proximity (Fig. 44).

But as soon as the blade penetrates more deeply into the tissue, the *lateral resistance*,

[29] Example: Fixation of the conjunctiva at the limbus, fixation of the iris at the iris root.
[30] Example: Shifting of incisions toward the limbus or iris root.
[31] Example: Iridectomies.

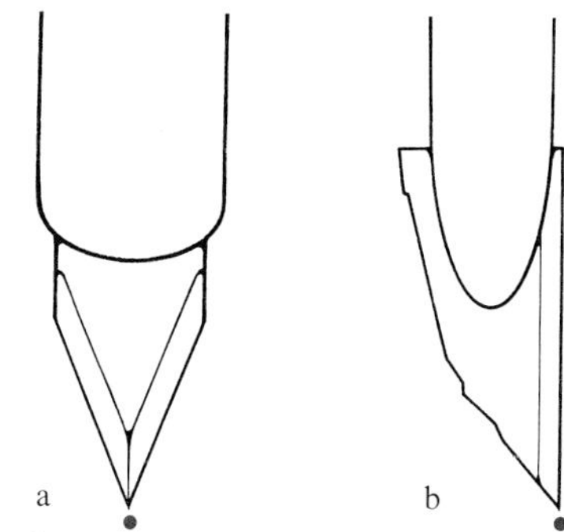

Fig. 42. **Blades with point cutting edges**
a Diamond knife.
b Razor-blade fragment in holder

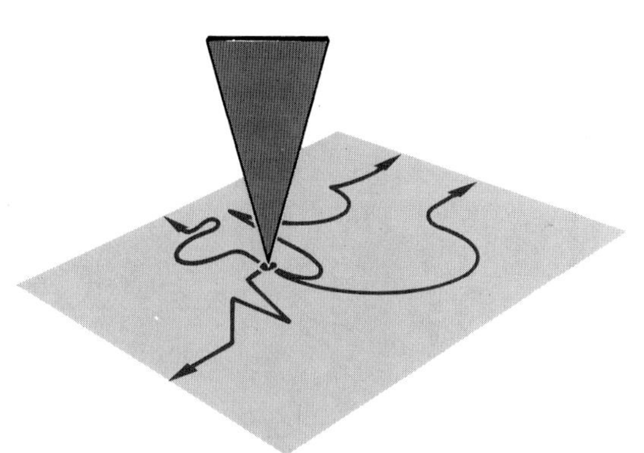

Fig. 43. **Cutting characteristics of a point cutting edge.** As long as a blade is used purely as a point cutting edge (i.e., as long as it does not penetrate so deeply into the tissue that the shape of the carrier becomes a factor), it will encounter a symmetrical lateral resistance in any direction, and the number of preferential paths is infinitely large. Cutting conditions are ideal in almost all guidance directions, i.e., the preferential path and guidance path are congruent. The surgeon can thus use the point cutting edge like a pencil to "draw" linear incisions of any shape desired

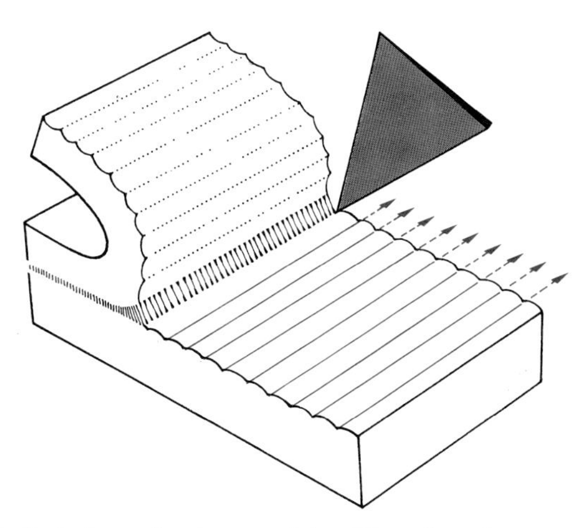

Fig. 44. **Technique of using a point cutting edge.** A cut surface is produced by making a closely-spaced series of linear incisions. The resulting surface has a "hatched" appearance

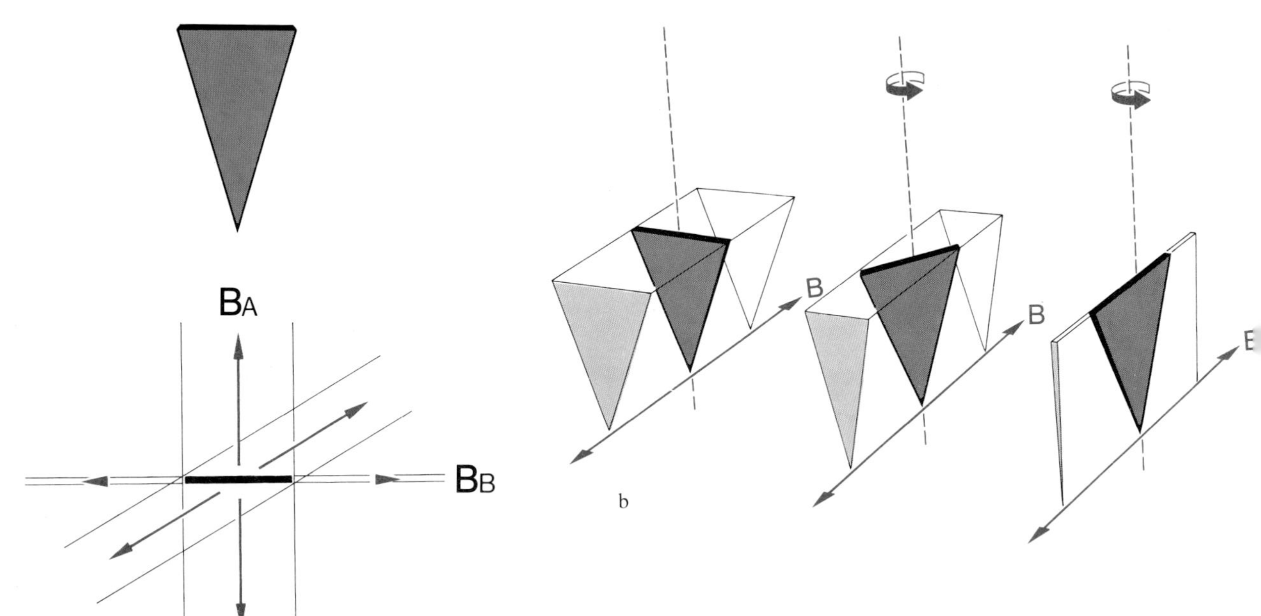

Fig. 45. **Lateral resistance of blades with a point cutting edge**

a With a prismatic carrier, the lateral resistance increases with the width of the blade surface as projected in the guidance direction *(B)*. Thus, the lateral resistance is maximal when the widest blade surface is perpendicular to the guidance direction *(BA)*, and minimal when the widest blade surface is parallel to the guidance direction *(BB)*.

b Simple rotation of the blade is sufficient to change the lateral resistance from maximal *(left)* to minimal *(right)*. *B* guidance direction

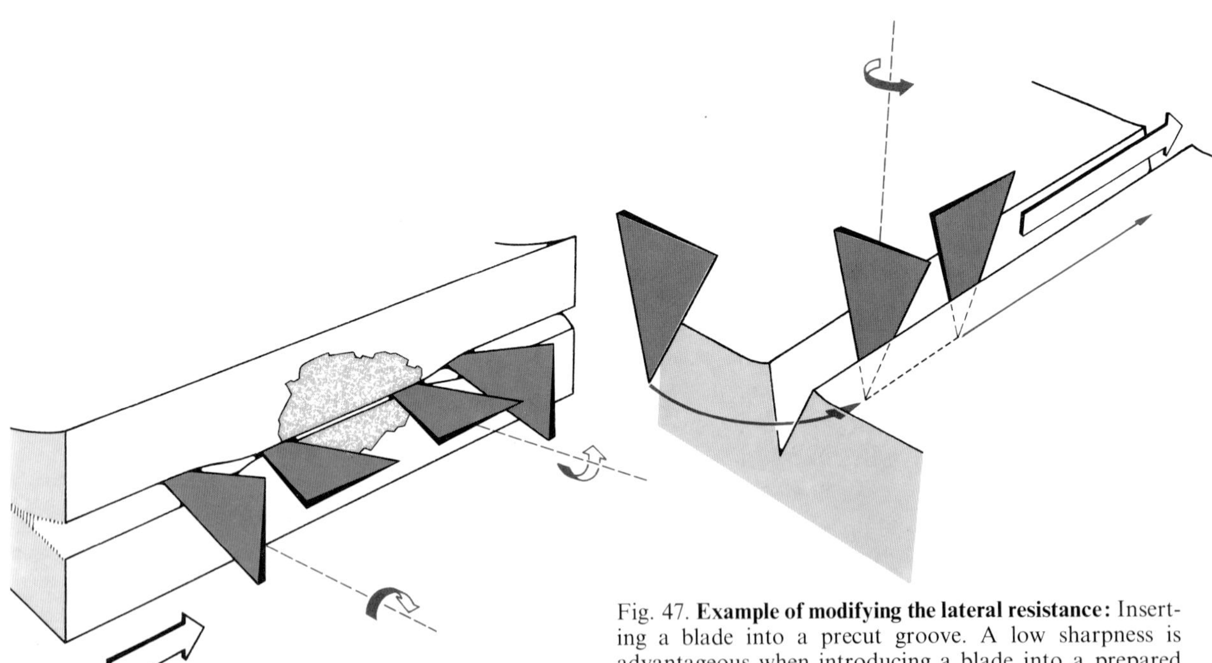

Fig. 46. **Example of modifying the lateral resistance: dissection of lamellae.** To keep the blade within a particular layer in the loose interlamellar tissue, the sharpness should be minimal, so the blade is directed "bluntly." If structures with a higher and irregular resistance are encountered (scars, for example), sharpness can be increased by rotating the blade *(red arrows)*

Fig. 47. **Example of modifying the lateral resistance:** Inserting a blade into a precut groove. A low sharpness is advantageous when introducing a blade into a prepared incision so that the cutting edge can pass to the base of the groove without injuring the walls. The blade behaves as a blunt instrument if its broadest surface is held perpendicular to the guidance direction. When the base of the groove is reached, maximal sharpness is required to continue the incision: This is achieved by rotating the blade until its broadest surface is parallel to the guidance direction *(red arrows)*

and thus the shape of the carrier, becomes a factor. If the carrier is conical, this resistance is equal in all directions. If the carrier is prismatic, the resistance depends on the *position of the largest carrier cross-section relative to the guidance direction* (Fig. 45). By rotating the blade, therefore, the surgeon can vary the resistance and thus modify the "sharpness" of the blade as needed (Figs. 46, 47).

Thus, blades with a point cutting edge are extremely versatile cutting instruments and are so adaptable in terms of sharpness and mobility that the surgeon can achieve an optimal result even in unusual and unexpected situations. But they are also quite delicate and prone to rapid wear. The blades are therefore constructed of material which is highly resistant (diamond blades) or easily replaced (razor-blade fragments).[32]

[32] If the point cutting edges are used exclusively in the "thrusting" mode, such as the points of keratomes, Graefe knives or needles, the problem of wear is lessened.

2.3.4 Knives with Linear Cutting Edges

Knives are characterized by linear cutting edges and a preferential path in the form of a *plane* (Fig. 50). The cut surface they produce under a symmetrical lateral resistance is also a plane, therefore ("straight incision").

Different blades (Fig. 48) differ on the one hand in the longitudinal profile of the cutting edge, which determines the angle at which each cutting point attacks the tissue (Fig. 49), and on the other in the form of the carrier surfaces, which determines the lateral resistance.

To obtain *plane cut surfaces*, it is necessary to position the blade such that a maximum amount of blade surface comes between the edges of the incision. In *curved incisions*, on the other hand, it is desirable that only a small amount of blade surface enter the tissue (Fig. 51). Changing the direction of the cut is facilitated by turning the blade so that the cutting edge itself forms the axis of rotation (Fig. 52); otherwise the cut surfaces would be facetted.

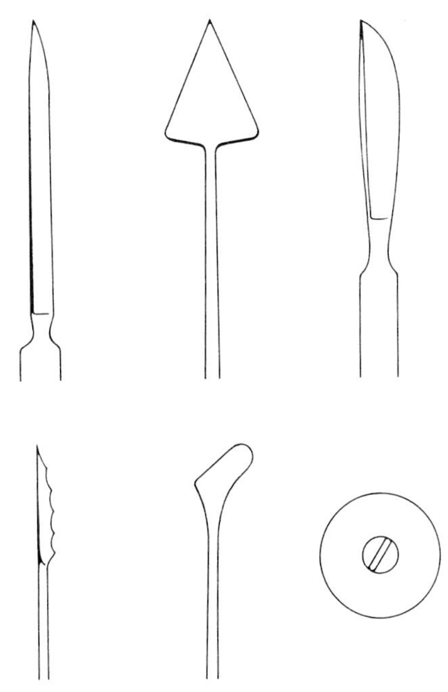

Fig. 48. **Knives with linear cutting edges**
Top row: Cataract ("Graefe") knife, keratome, scalpel.
Bottom row: Serrated knife, hockey knife, circular knife

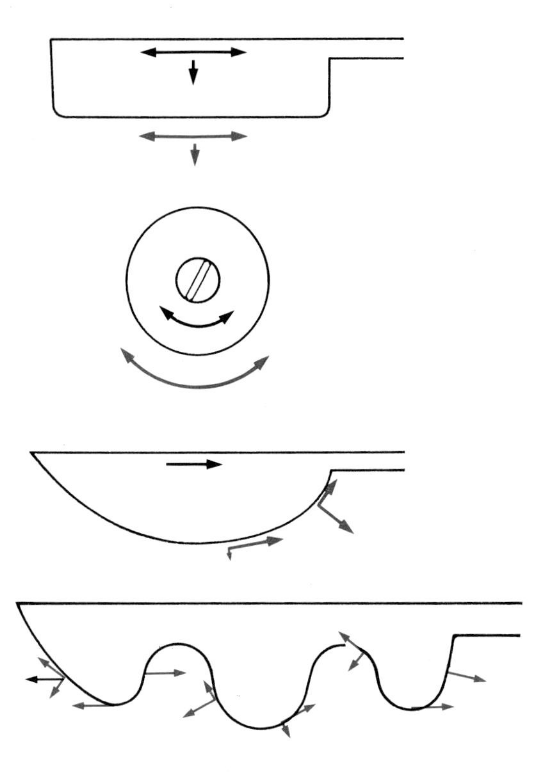

Fig. 49. **Attack angles of various blades.** A pure thrusting motion is possible only with a straight linear cutting edge, while a pure pull-through motion can be made with straight as well as circular edges. For all other edge shapes, every guidance motion creates a combination of both vectors, which is exploited to the maximum by the serrated edge

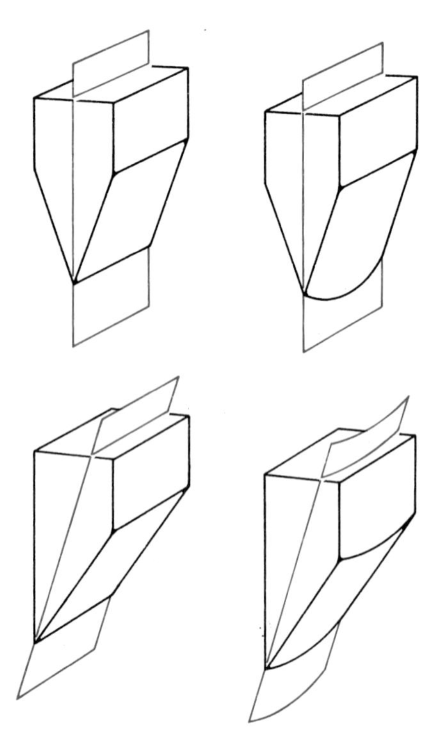

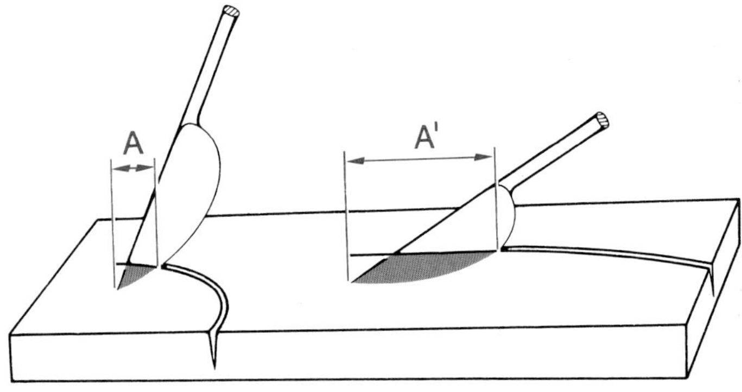

Fig. 51. **Blade position for making curved incisions.** To obtain cut surfaces which differ in shape from the preferential path, the lateral resistance must be minimized. *Left:* Upright blade position reduces lateral resistance and permits curvature of the incision. *Right:* Low blade position favors a straighter incision. *A* and *A'* length of blade immersed in tissue

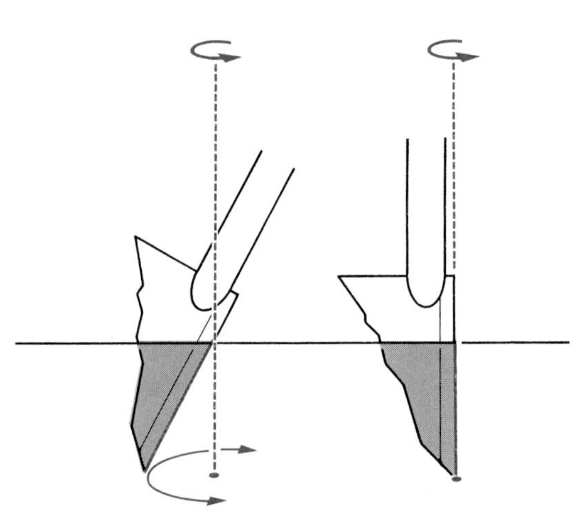

Fig. 52. **The axis of rotation for changes of direction.** If the cutting edge itself forms the axis of rotation, a smooth cut surface is produced *(right)*. But if the cutting edge is at an angle to the axis of rotation, each cutting point has a different radius of rotation, and the cut surfaces become irregular *(left)*

Fig. 50. **Preferential paths of linear blades**
Top row: Symmetrically-ground blades always have a plane preferential path regardless of the shape of the cutting edge.
Bottom row: Asymmetrically-ground blades have a plane preferential path only if the cutting edge is straight. This path is at an angle to the main carrier axis, however, and if the edge is guided along this axis, the lateral resistance is asymmetrical *(left)*. Asymmetrically-ground blades with a curved cutting edge differ from simple knives, since they have arcuate preferential paths and thus possess complicated cutting properties *(right)*

2.3.5 Blades with a Circular Cutting Edge (Trephines)

The preferential path of circular cutting edges is actually the *surface of a body of revolution*, i.e., a cylinder or a cone, depending on the shape of the ground edge (Fig. 53). Trephines with a *cylindrical* preferential path can be either rotated or advanced with symmetrical lateral resistance, while those with a *conical* preferential path create a symmetrical resistance only when cutting by rotation. When such an instrument is advanced,[33] the resistance becomes asymmetrical and the cut profile may deviate.

One result of the curved preferential path is that as the instrument penetrates deeper, the lateral resistance becomes so high that any lateral deviations of the cutting edge are hindered. However, the tissue may still shift and protrude upward through the trephine opening, so that the resulting cut surfaces no longer coincide exactly with the preferential path of the trephine (see Fig. 249).

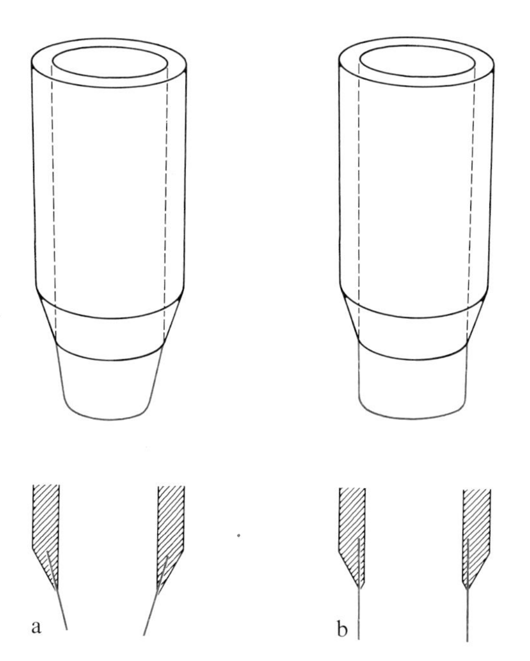

Fig. 53. **The trephine**

a If the cutting edge is ground only from the outside, the preferential path *(outlined in red)* is conical.

b If it is ground from both sides, the preferential path is cylindrical.
Note: the difference between the two forms of grinding decreases with the thickness of the blade

2.3.6 Scissors

The cutting properties of scissors are quite complex, in that the combination of two blades represents not just the sum of their individual cutting properties, but an entirely new instrument with its own unique characteristics (Figs. 54 and 55).

A scissors can cut in three different ways:
- by closing the blades
- by opening the blades
- with the tip of the blades.

Closure of the Scissors

As a scissors is closed, a *cutting point* forms which travels forward along the blades. At the same time, the tissue is squeezed and held fast between the blades (Fig. 56).[34]

The **cutting point** is formed as the two blade edges are pressed against each other during closure (Fig. 57). One vector component of the pressing force is created by the shearing stress associated with the scissors construction, the other by the closing movement itself. The *shearing stress* is created by the camber of the blades and is reinforced by a block on the opposite side of the joint.[35] This stress largely determines the cutting ability of the scissors, since a cutting point exists only if the force pressing the edges together is greater than the tissue resistance pushing them apart.[36] The second component which forms

[33] Advancement of such a trephine along its axis is no longer a simple thrusting movement, since the direction of advance forms an angle with the conical preferential path.

[34] Thus, scissors function neither by the "bite" mechanism whereby two linear cutting edges simultaneously come into contact for their full length, nor by the "punch" mechanism where a linear cutting edge is pressed against a base.

[35] In scissors which lack this block tension must be maintained by manual pressure. Such scissors are usually designed for right-handed use, but special left-handed models are available.

[36] The edge itself is "blunt" and serves mainly to ensure smooth blade motion. A certain roughness may even be desirable, since the friction will prevent tissue slippage and thus improve "sharpness" (extreme case: serrated coiffure scissors). Thus, visual inspection of the blade edges cannot assess the cutting ability of the scissors. This can be tested only functionally, i.e., by making trial cuts in a tissue-like material (e.g., soft, moist paper towels).

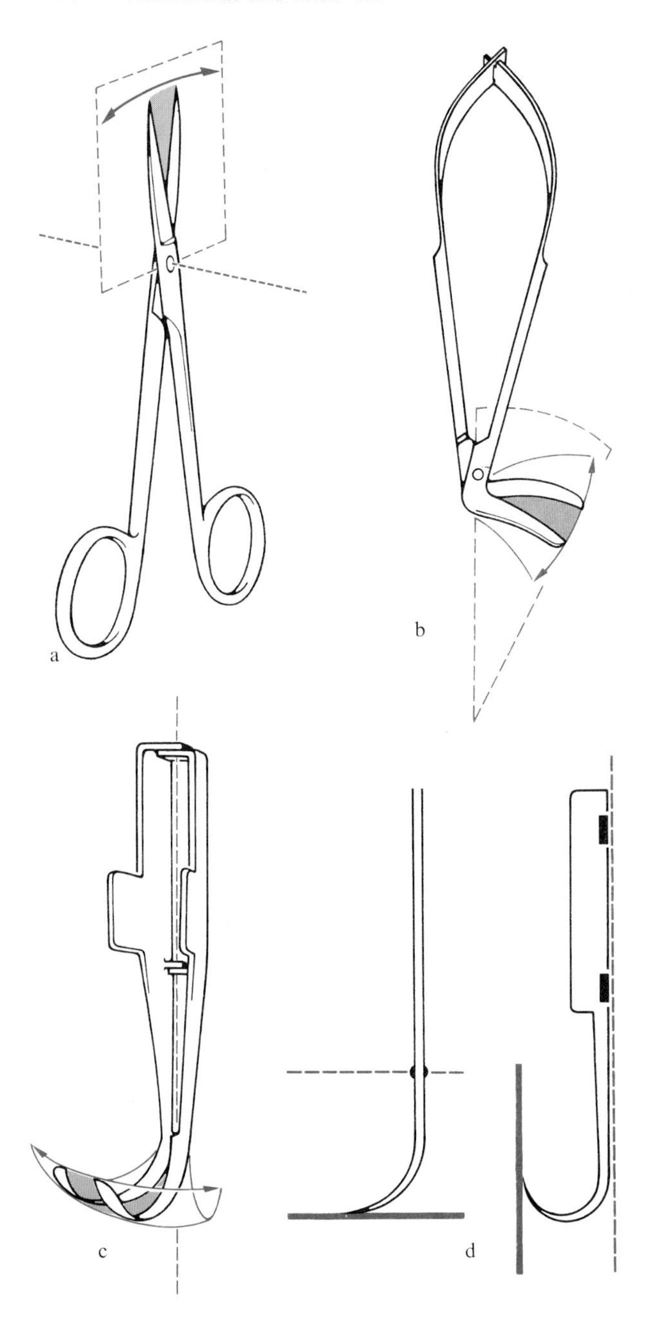

Fig. 54. **Types of scissors.** A scissors consists of two opposed blades connected by a joint (screw). The handles and blades can be combined in various ways. The position of the joint determines the maximum allowable blade curvature.
The guidance path, i.e., the surface over which the cutting edges are guided during the working motion, is determined and constrained by the construction of the instrument. *White areas outlined in red:* Guidance path of blades during opening. *Red area between the blades:* Guidance path during closure. *Arrow:* Guidance line of blade tips.

a "Straight" scissors with plane guidance path and ringed handles.

b "Angular" curved scissors with spring handle. The guidance path is the surface of a cone.

c Hinge-handled scissors with highly curved blades.

d Relation between blade curvature and joint position. The blade curvature is the maximum allowable when the tangent to the blade tip *(red line)* is parallel to the joint axis *(broken line)*. At higher curvatures the blade tips will come into contact before the scissors is completely closed. With a simple screw joint, the maximum allowable curvature is 90° *(left)*; with a hinge handle, 180° *(right)*

the shearing stress, the *closing movement*, is controlled by the manual pressure exerted by the surgeon and is also the "motor" for the forward motion of the cutting point (Fig. 60a).

As a *point cutting edge*, the scissors produces an *incision line* and can in principle divide only *two-dimensional* substrates. Thicker tissue layers must be pressed flat before cutting. However, the squeezing action of the blades increases the sectility of the tissue so that the

Fig. 55. **Shapes of blade tips**

	A	B	C
Shape of blade tips	sharp	semi-rounded	rounded
Ground edge extends to extremity of blade?	yes	yes	no
Action of blade tips when *thrust* into tissue			
– with blades open (preparatory to cutting by closure of scissors)	sharp	largely sharp	blunt
– with blades closed (preparatory to cutting by opening the scissors)	sharp	blunt	blunt
Cutting actions of tips during *working motion*			
– closure of scissors	sharp	sharp	blunt
– opening of scissors	sharp	blunt	blunt

Red points: ends of the ground edge; *small arrows:* "sharp" movements of the tips; *Broad arrows:* blunt movements

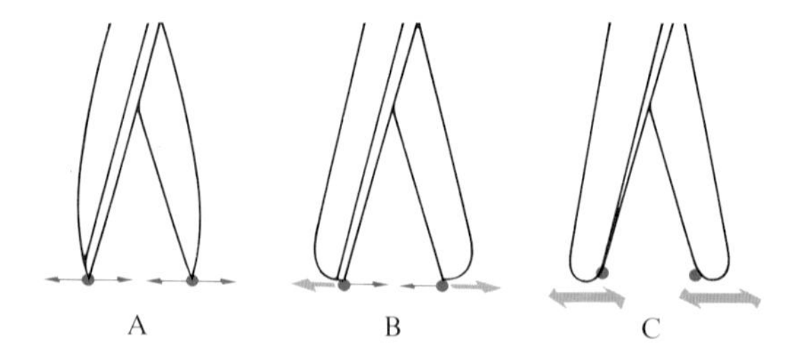

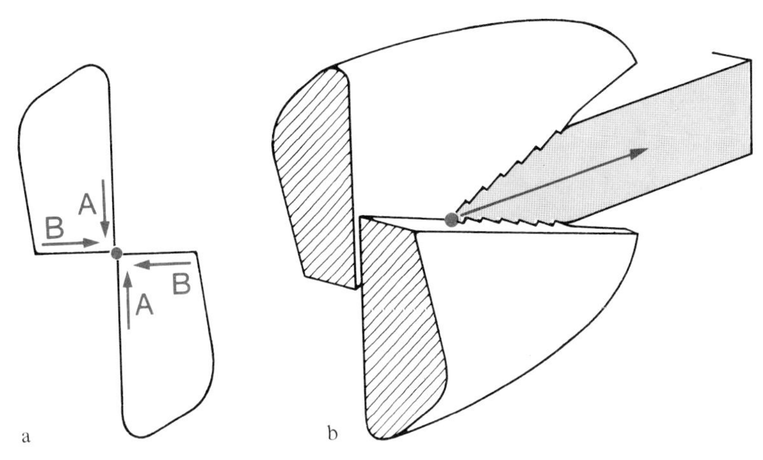

Fig. 56. **Principle of cutting during closure of scissors**

a A cutting point results from contact between the two ground edges and is formed by vector component *A* perpendicular to the joint axis (closing motion of scissors) and vector component *B* parallel to the joint axis (shearing stress).

b The cutting point moves forward, dividing the tissue fed to it by the closing blades (the material lying on the guidance path in the interblade area). At the same time, the tissue is held fast by the squeezing action of the blades (symbolized by barbs in the figure)

ground edges (which are blunt in themselves) will play a role additional to that of the cutting point. Due to the special functional properties of scissors, the preferential path of the edges and the guidance path cannot coincide, and so the result is always a complex cut profile with an S-shaped curvature[37] (Figs. 58, 59).

One of the principal advantages of scissors is that the squeezing action of the blades helps keep the tissue from shifting during cutting, and thus increases its sectility. A second advantage is the extraordinary freedom of movement, since the instrument acts as a *"point" cutting edge* which can be guided in any direction desired. By itself, the *working motion*[38] simply advances the cutting point along the blades, so that the resulting incision line corresponds exactly to the shape of the blades. By

[37] Remember: The preferential path of the blade is the bisector of the ground edges.

[38] Working motion: Moving the cutting point by simple closure with the scissors otherwise stationary, i.e., with a stable joint position.

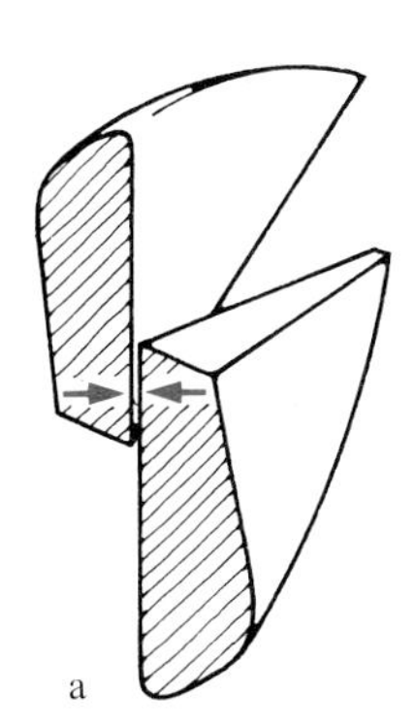

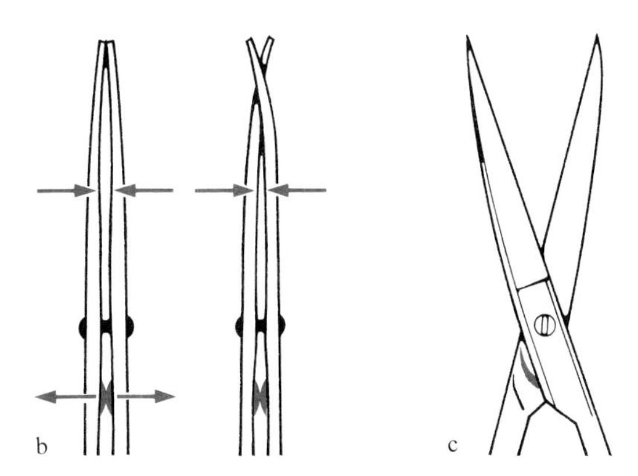

Fig. 57. **The creation of shearing stress**

a The stress presses the edges together from the sides.

b Spring tension is created by the camber of the blades. The lateral profile clearly shows that the blades come into contact only at a single point. A block *(red)* on the opposite side of the joint will help maintain the shearing stress. *Left:* Scissors closed. *Right:* Scissors half-open.

c Open scissors show position of block (*red*)

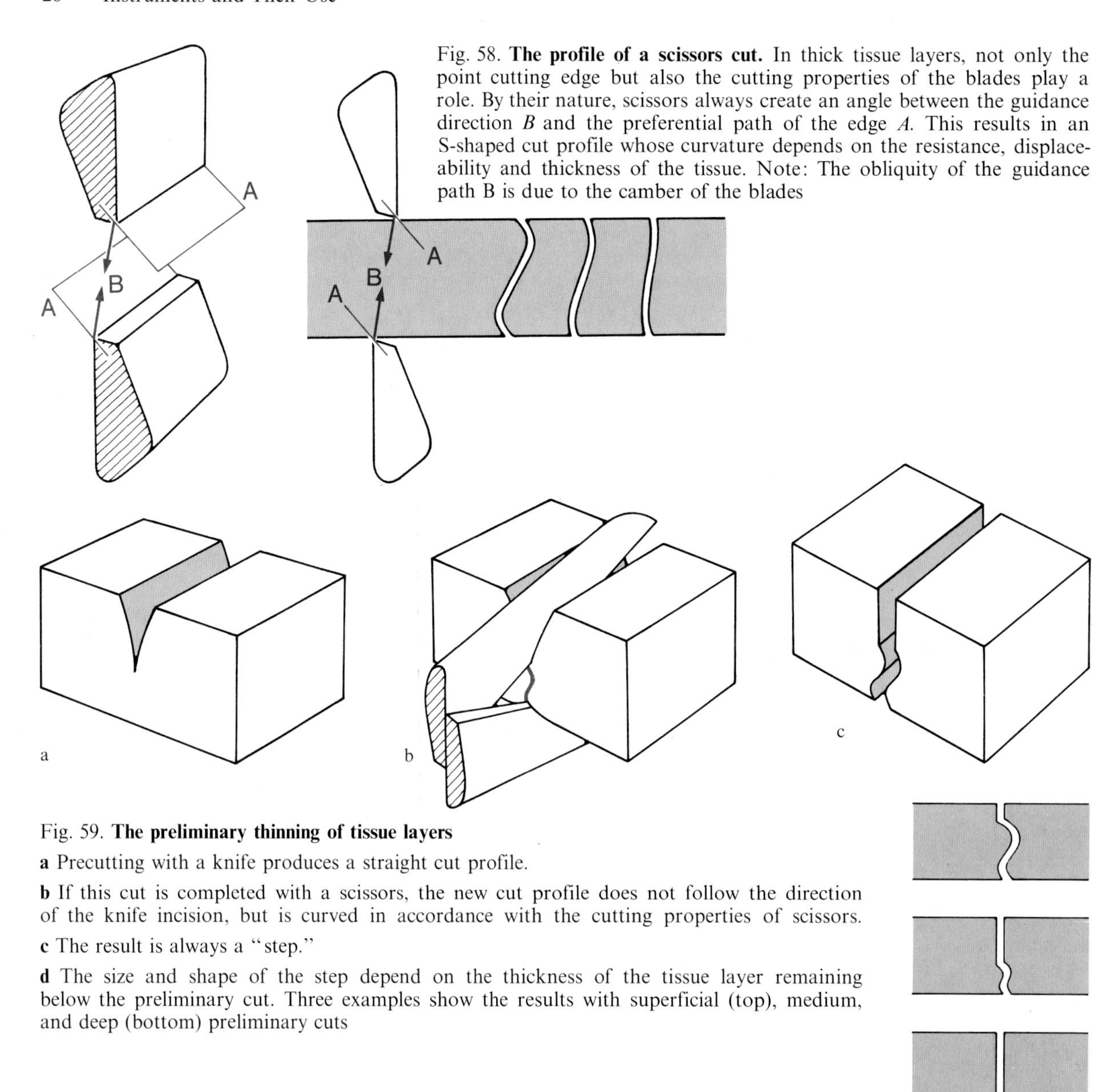

Fig. 58. **The profile of a scissors cut.** In thick tissue layers, not only the point cutting edge but also the cutting properties of the blades play a role. By their nature, scissors always create an angle between the guidance direction *B* and the preferential path of the edge *A*. This results in an S-shaped cut profile whose curvature depends on the resistance, displaceability and thickness of the tissue. Note: The obliquity of the guidance path B is due to the camber of the blades

Fig. 59. **The preliminary thinning of tissue layers**

a Precutting with a knife produces a straight cut profile.

b If this cut is completed with a scissors, the new cut profile does not follow the direction of the knife incision, but is curved in accordance with the cutting properties of scissors.

c The result is always a "step."

d The size and shape of the step depend on the thickness of the tissue layer remaining below the preliminary cut. Three examples show the results with superficial (top), medium, and deep (bottom) preliminary cuts

adding *guidance motions*,[39] the surgeon can produce cuts of any shape required, although the disadvantages of an asymmetrical lateral resistance will necessarily be present.

On the other hand, the use of scissors does present certain difficulties, since the **cutting conditions** change continuously as closure proceeds (Fig. 60). As the aperture angle decreases, the resistances increase.

The *working resistance*,[40] or the resistance to closure, varies with the amount of tissue between the blades, and this in turn increases steadily as closure proceeds (Fig. 60c). At the same time, mechanical advantage is lost as the lever arm lengthens, so increasing force must be exerted to close the scissors as closure progresses (Fig. 60e).

[39] Guidance motion: Moving the cutting point by advancing the scissors (i.e., by moving the joint).

[40] This working resistance is directed against the advance of the cutting point and against the sequeezing action of the blades, i.e., against movements with forward-directed vector components. It causes the tissue to shift toward the blade tip. So at high resistances the scissors must be thrust strongly forward, thereby pressing the tissue against the cutting point, in order to prevent undesired shortening of the cut.

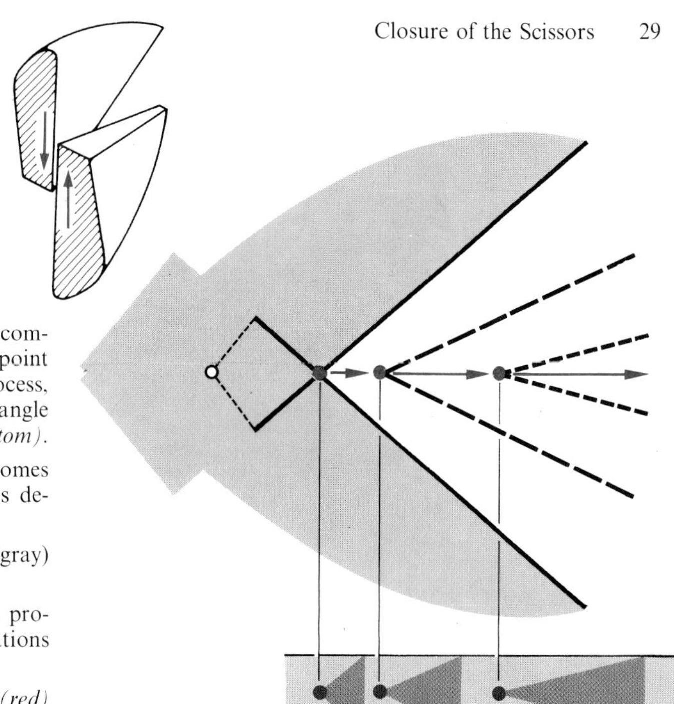

Fig. 60. **The process of scissors closure**

a The closing motion produces the second vector component needed to form the cutting point *(top)*. This point is simultaneously driven forward *(center)*. In the process, the aperture angle between the blades, and thus the angle of attack at the tissue, is gradually reduced *(bottom)*.

b As closure proceeds, the interblade area *(red)* becomes smaller, and the danger of inadvertant tissue lesions decreases.

c The amount of tissue lying between the blades (gray) increases, and with it the resistance to closure.

d The immersed blade area *(gray)* increases, with a proportional increase in lateral resistance. Lateral deviations of the blades become more difficult.

e The lever arm between the joint and cutting point *(red)* lengthens, and the transmissible force decreases

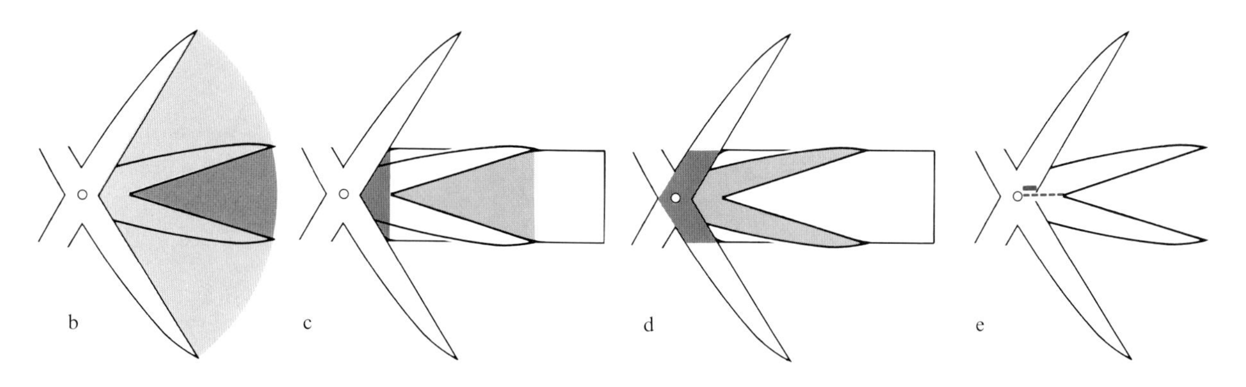

The *lateral resistance,* and thus the resistance to lateral swiveling of the scissors, is dependent on the area of blade pressed between the wound edges; this also increases as closure proceeds (Fig. 60d).

Now, since the displaceability of the tissue depends on the resistances present, the *curvature of the cut profile* changes as the blades close (Fig. 58). If the aperture angle is changed abruptly, an abrupt change of the profile also occurs. As a result, when cutting is done in *several steps* where the scissors are closed almost completely and then reapplied to the tissue with a larger blade aperture, the cut becomes jagged. This type of *serration effect* is a characteristic feature of scissors and so is unavoidable. On the other hand, *guidance-related* serrations are avoidable, i.e., those occurring during changes of direction (Fig. 61) or on complete closure of the blades (Fig. 62).

An important safety factor in the use of scissors is that the material in danger of being sectioned is confined to a well-defined area. This "danger zone" (the interblade area) is easily monitored. It is large with open scissors. But to prevent inadvertant lesions during cutting, the surgeon can keep this zone small by working with a small blade aperture[41] (Fig. 60b).

These considerations suggest some **rules** to be followed when working with scissors. The fewest problems arise when the shape of the blades corresponds to the intended shape of

[41] Example: Cutting tissue where the division of preplaced sutures must be avoided (e.g., iridectomies).

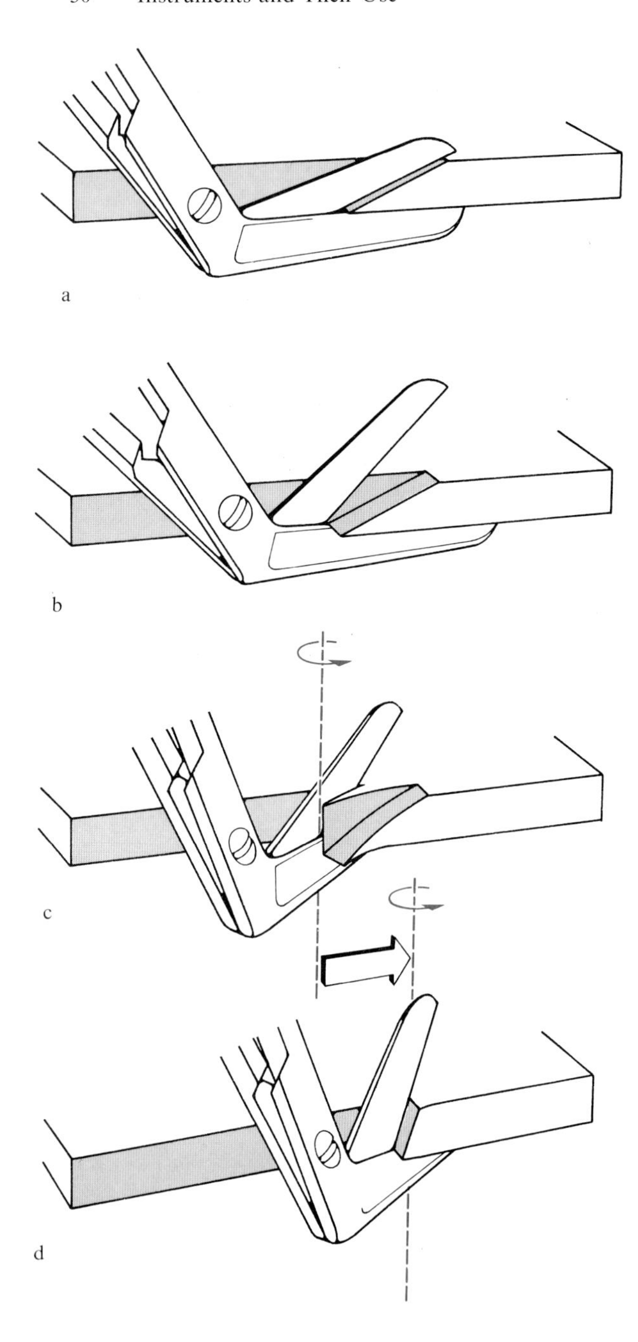

Fig. 61. **Reapplying the scissors when cutting in steps**

a Incomplete closure of the blades leaves a partially-divided wedge of tissue.

b When the scissors is reapplied, the angle of blade aperture is larger than the angle of the tissue wedge.

c If the guidance direction is altered when the scissors is reapplied, the partially-divided tissue wedge creates a serration.

d This serration can be avoided if, after the scissors is reapplied, the cut is first continued in the original direction (black arrow), and the scissors is not swiveled in the new direction until the tissue wedge is sectioned completely

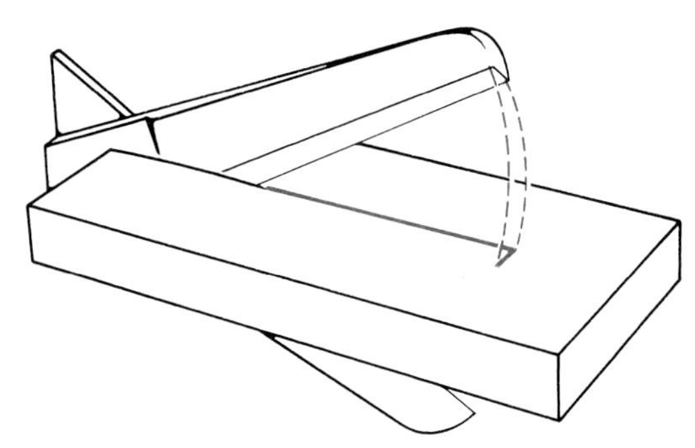

Fig. 62. **Serration on complete closure of scissors.** If the tip of the scissors penetrates completely into the tissue, its leading edge also acts as a cutting edge and produces a small lateral cut

the cut. The entire cut can be made *by the closing motion alone*. The attendant increase in lateral resistance is advantageous in that it acts to prevent deviations from the intended direction. The danger zone is confined to the area between the blades and so is easily watched.

If *additional guidance motions* are necessary, one can at least attempt to minimize the problems that result. The lateral resistance can be reduced by cutting with a large blade aperture. Of course this will make it more difficult to monitor the danger zone, especially during swiveling motions. But the difficulties of monitoring the interblade area can be minimized by performing the working and guidance motions *separately*, i.e., by keeping the joint stationary during closure, and by maintaining a constant blade aperture during swiveling motions.[42]

When cutting is done *in stages*, the danger of serration can be reduced by avoiding complete closure[43] and by making direction changes not at the moment the blades are reapplied, but only after the cut has been continued (Figs. 61, 62).

Since most of the *difficulties* in obtaining a high-precision cut with scissors are *related to the thickness* of the tissue layers to be cut, they can be reduced if the layers are first *made thinner* with another cutting instrument (Fig. 59). The deeper the preliminary cut, the lower the resistance that must be overcome by the scissors and the smaller their inherent disadvantages will be.

---

[42] See footnote 2, p. 3

[43] Many scissors are fitted with a mechanical stop to prevent complete closure.

Cutting by Opening the Scissors

When opened, scissors cut with the *back* of the blades and behave as *blunt instruments*. They can thus be used to perform dissections in preexisting spaces (see Fig. 168). The shape of the resulting "cut" depends mainly on the path of least tissue resistance. One will attempt, nevertheless, to adapt the guidance path of the blades (by the choice of blade shape and blade position) to the intended shape of the cut in order to avoid unintentional trauma to surrounding tissues.[44]

Cutting with the Blade Tips

Cutting with the blade tips may just involve the **final phase of "cutting by closure,"** in which the tissue is sectioned by the *cutting point*, and the blades are brought to full closure, thereby utilizing the outermost ends of the blades. This requires a scissors whose ground edges extend all the way to the tips (i.e., sharp or semi-rounded scissors, Fig. 55a, b). In addition, the effective sharpness of the instrument depends on the position in which it is held: The cutting point comes in direct contact with the targeted tissue fibers in any position with sharp-pointed scissors, but only in a perpendicular position with thicker-bladed scissors (Fig. 63).

But each blade tip also has the properties of an **individual instrument.** On the one hand, they can be **thrust** into tissue to place the blade in the starting position for cutting by either opening or closure: *Sharp tips* can force their way through the tissue in the guidance direction,[45] while *blunt tips* behave as spatulas

[44] Example: In enucleations, lesions of the orbital tissue are avoided if the blades are held snugly against the globe when opened.

[45] Example: "Pointed" scissors for penetrating after-cataract membranes or piercing the iris in basal iridencleisis.

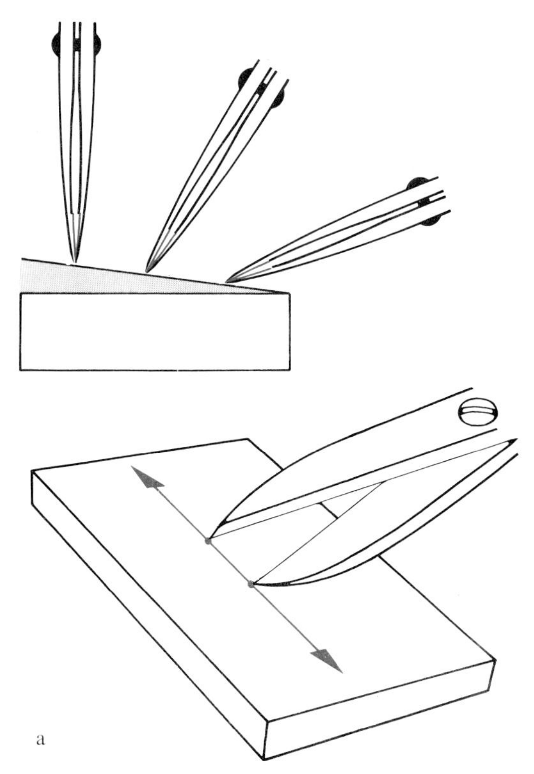

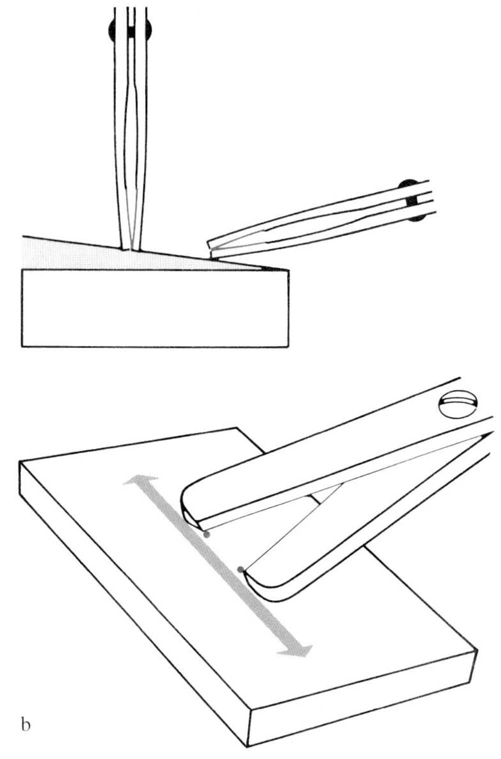

Fig. 63. **Cutting with the blade tips**

a When sharp-pointed scissors are used, the cutting edge comes into contact with the tissue fibers at any angle and can make a sharp cut in any position *(thin arrow)*.

b With tips of other shapes, the cutting point *(red)* is separated from the tissue surface by the thickness of the blade, and the tip behaves as a blunt instrument *(thick arrow)*. The fibers are sectioned directly by the cutting point only if the scissors is applied at right angles to the tissue surface and will not damage surrounding structures when the blades are introduced into cavities or spaces.[46] Blade tips may, on the other hand, be used with **lateral guidance motions** (motions of the blade tips during opening or closure of the scissors); they then behave as blunt or sharp instruments, depending on their shape and position (Fig. 55). *Sharp tips* act as point cutting edges regardless of their direction of motion or position. They produce linear incisions and differ from free point cutting edges (Figs. 43, 44) only in that their path is limited by the construction of the scissors. *Rounded tips* are blunt in any direction or position. The cutting ability of *semi-rounded tips* depends on the leading edge: The tip is blunt during opening, but sharp during closure (see Fig. 55).

[46] Example: Muscle scissors for advancing along the globe surface in the episcleral space, or corneal scissors for introduction into the anterior chamber.

1.3.7 Needles

Needles consist of a cutting component *(head)* which dissects the suture canal, a handle *(shaft)* by which the needle is held, and an *eye* through which the suture material is passed (Fig. 64).

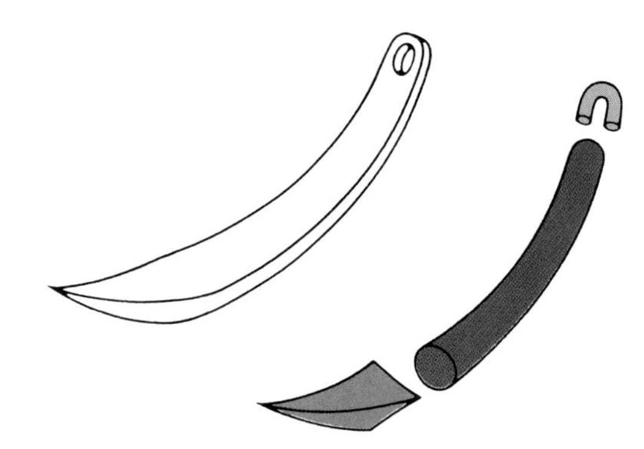

Fig. 64. **The parts of a needle.** A needle consists of a head (point shaped tip and lateral cutting edges), shaft and eye

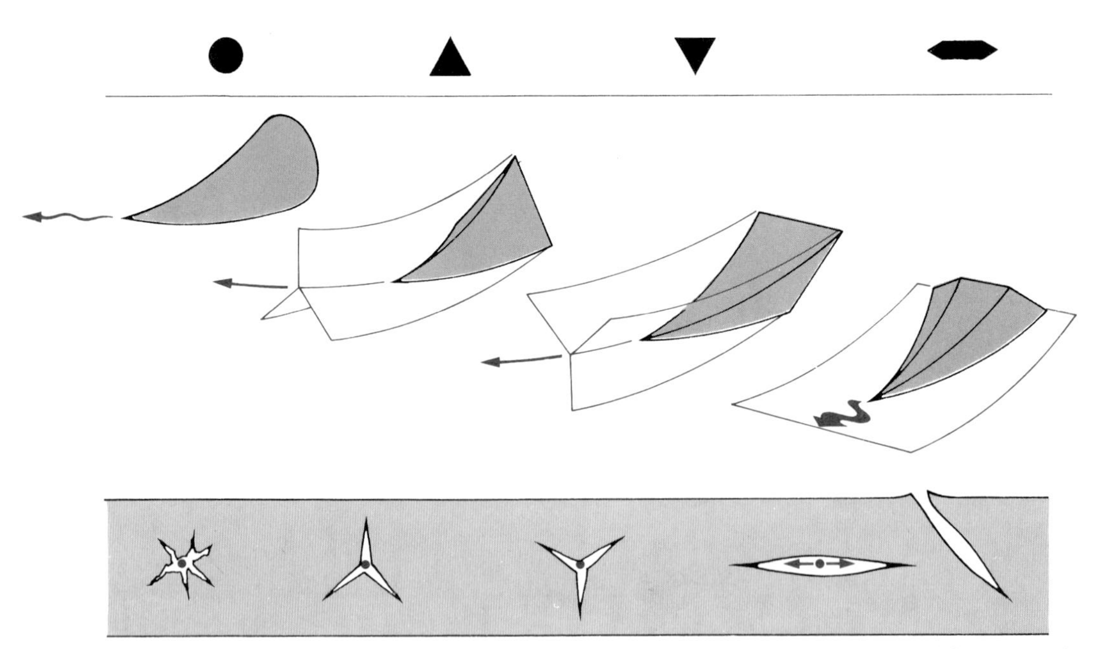

Fig. 65. **Shapes of needle heads.** The arrangement of the lateral cutting edges and their preferential paths determines the cross-sectional shape of the suture canal:
Round heads (left) pass through tissue by "blunt" dissection. The canal cross-section follows the course of spaces with low tissue resistance.
Three-edged heads (center) have three lateral preferential paths *(red outline)* and produce a canal with a Y-shaped cross-section. The center of the Y *(red)* corresponds to the path of the tip and thus to the surgeon's intensions. The cross-section of the canal extends from this point either more superficially *(center left)* or more deeply *(center right)*, depending on the position of the vertical edge. The three-dimensional arrangement of the preferential paths stabilizes needle guidance, since the lateral resistances will act to prevent any deviations.
Two-edged heads (right) produce a slit-shaped canal whose central axis corresponds to the path of the needle tip. Lateral deviations are quite possible, since the preferential paths of the two cutting edges are congruent. For this reasond the needle may cut the surface at the tissue unless held and guided strictly parallel to it *(right)*

The **cross-section of the suture canal** depends on the *arrangement of the cutting edges,* each of which makes its own cut (Fig. 65). Thus, a *three-edge* head makes three cuts, each in the direction of the associated preferential path. A *two-edge* head makes two cuts in the same plane. A *round-bodied* (edgeless) needle tears a canal through the tissue.

Needles with heads larger in cross-section than the parts that follow produce a large-diameter canal and lower the resistance to passage of the shaft and thread.

The **longitudinal profile of the suture canal** corresponds to the *path of the needle tip* (Fig. 67a). Being a geometric point, the needle tip can in theory be guided in any direction. In reality, however, its mobility is limited by lateral resistance, which varies with the configuration of the preferential paths of the lateral edges (Fig. 65) and with the shape of the shaft.

The lateral resistance is lowest when the path of the needle tip precisely follows the curvature of the shaft, i.e., when the needle shape is congruent with the planned suture canal. In practice, this desire for congruence is opposed by the requirement that the shaft be longer than the suture canal so that it can be easily grasped by the needle holder when passed in and out (Fig. 66). Incongruence, however, is not an enormous disadvantage, since it does not affect the shape of the suture canal, which depends entirely on the guidance of the tip (Fig. 67).[47] When the shaft is pulled through the canal, the effect is merely an increase of the lateral resistance, thereby deforming either the tissue or needle. This places correspondingly higher demands on needle stability: The greater the incongruence between the needle and stitch canal, the higher is the tissue resistance, and the more stable the needle must be.

[47] Thus, after the point emerges, formation of the canal is complete and can no longer be influenced by passage of the shaft. At this point the surgeon's task is merely to bring the needle smoothly out of the canal. Any attempt at corrective maneuvers will only deform the tissue or needle.

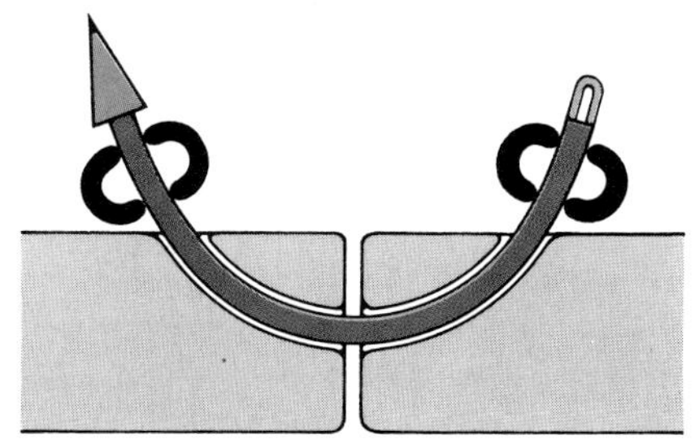

Fig. 66. **Length of the shaft.** To preserve the delicate head and eye, the needle is held only by its shaft, or "handle." Thus, the shaft must be long enough to be accessible to the needle holder *(black)* during both insertion and removal

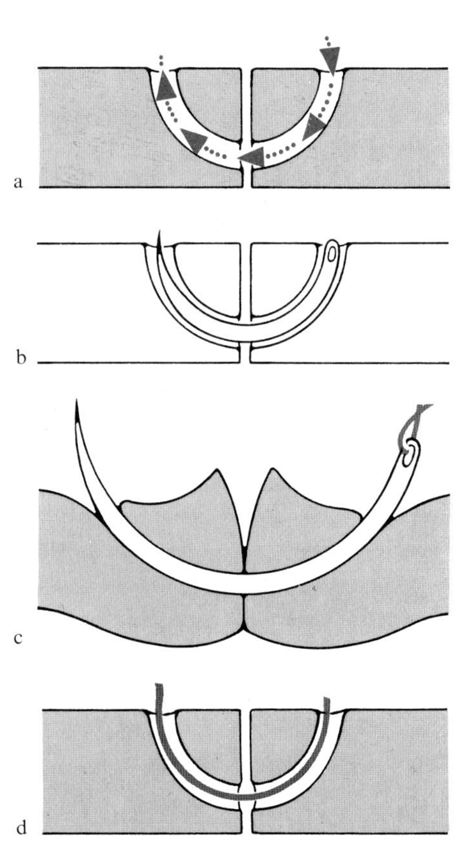

Fig. 67. **Shape of the suture canal and needle shape**

a The shape of the suture canal depends on the path of the needle tip.

b If a $^1/_2$-circle needle is congruent with the suture canal, it cannot be withdrawn

c A needle must be longer than the planned suture canal. Despite its larger radius, it will still be able to cut this canal if the tip is guided correctly; but the shaft will deform the surrounding tissue.

d After removal of the needle, the deformed tissue returns to its original shape; the canal assumes the shape desired

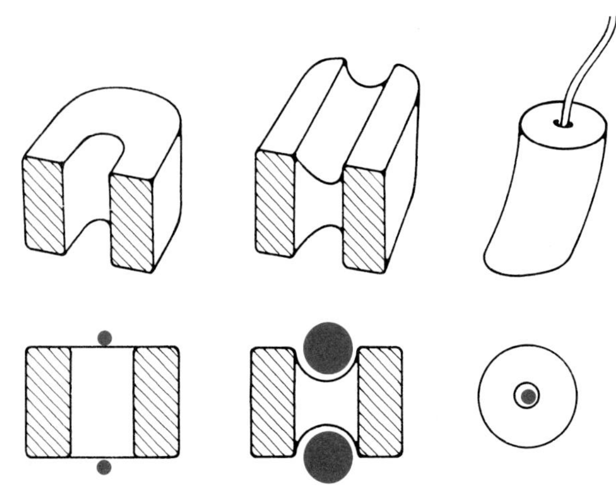

Fig. 68. **The needle eye and thread diameter**
A *simple eye (left)* is suitable for thin threads which add little to the total cross-section *(bottom)*.
A *recessed eye (center)* reduces the total cross-section when thick threads are used.
In *atraumatic sutures (right)*, the thread is fused into the end of an eyeless needle

Requirements as to the shape of the **eye** depend on the thickness of the suture material (Fig. 68), since the addition of the thread diameter must not significantly increase the total cross-section. The extremely fine threads used in ophthalmic surgery pose no problem in this regard. Thus, the advantage of "atraumatic sutures" lies more in their convenience (no threading) than in a true technical superiority.

2.4 The Uniting of Tissues

The uniting of tissues by biological processes is comparable to gluing with a slow-setting adhesive. It is the task of the surgeon to secure firm apposition of the wound edges until the "glue" has set.[48]

The surgical joining of tissue thus has two main goals: 1) Compression of the wound edges, and 2) their secure splinting in this position. The means to this end is the suture, which consists of an intramural segment and a free overlying segment. The *splinting* function is performed solely by the intramural segment (splinted zone); both segments may contribute to *compression* (Fig. 71).

Sutures which only splint the wound **(apposition sutures)** are adequate if compression is produced by other forces[49] (Fig. 69). Any suture form provides satisfactory apposition, as long as the loop of thread is exactly the length of the suture canal and fills it completely (Fig. 89a).

Conditions are different if the suture itself must produce the compression (Fig. 70). To maintain pressure between the wound edges, a **compression suture** must be tightened until the compliance of the enclosed tissue is exhausted (Fig. 72). This is accomplished by shortening the suture. *But while tightened loop*

[48] The requirements of the surgical joining technique are thus determined by the speed of the "setting" process. If an artificial quick-setting glue is available, it is sufficient to press the wound edges together briefly with a forceps. But if one has to rely on scar formation, techniques must be chosen in which the apposing instrument is retained for a sufficiently long period in the tissue. Long-lasting sutures are especially important when the healing tendency is poor, i.e., in tissue which is poorly perfused whether due to its anatomical structure (avascular tissue of the eye), surgical trauma (diathermy, overtightened sutures), or the presence of obstructions (foreign material embedded in the wound, etc.).

[49] Endogenous forces (e.g., intraocular pressure, lid pressure) or external aids (e.g., contact lenses).

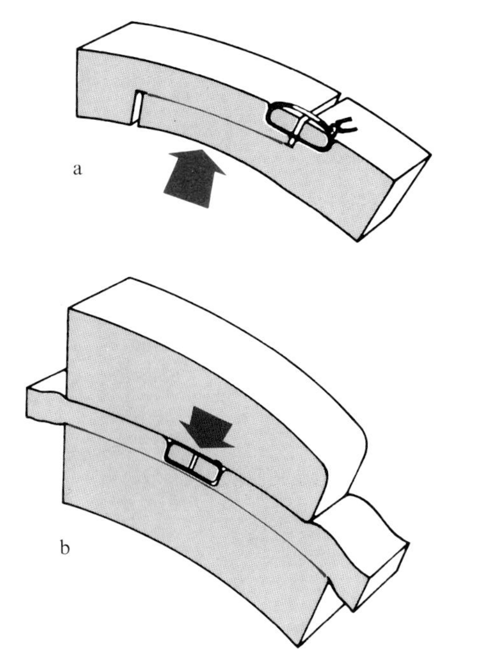

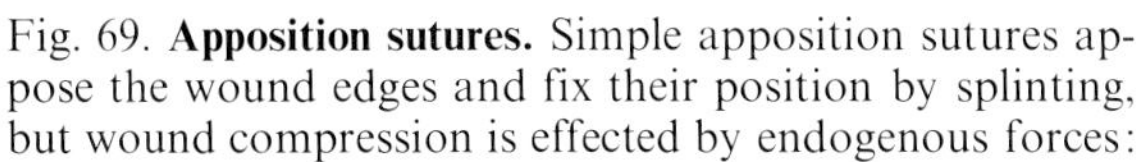
Fig. 69. **Apposition sutures.** Simple apposition sutures appose the wound edges and fix their position by splinting, but wound compression is effected by endogenous forces:

a *Intraocular pressure* presses the lamellae of a step incision together.

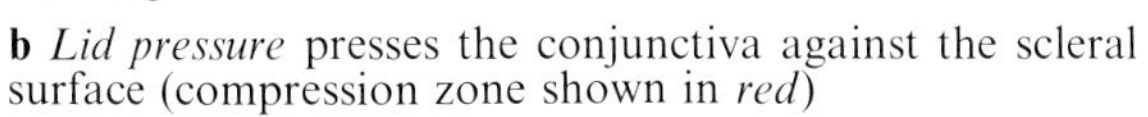
b *Lid pressure* presses the conjunctiva against the scleral surface (compression zone shown in *red*)

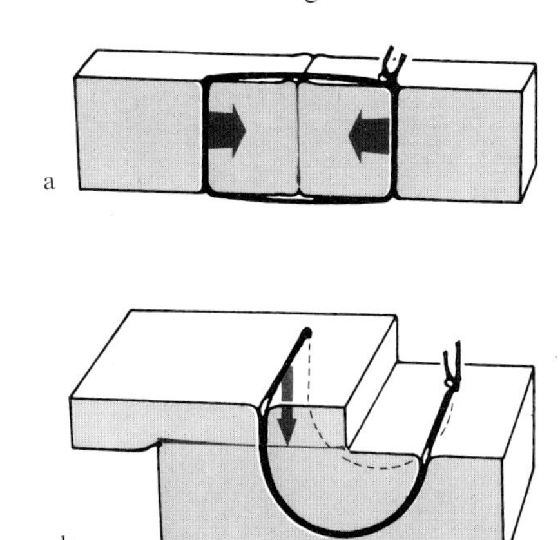

Fig. 70. **Compression sutures.** The compression is effected by the suture itself.

a A *loop suture* presses the edges of the wound together.

b A *mattress suture* is used to stitch a thin tissue layer onto a firm sublayer (Compression zone shown in *red*)

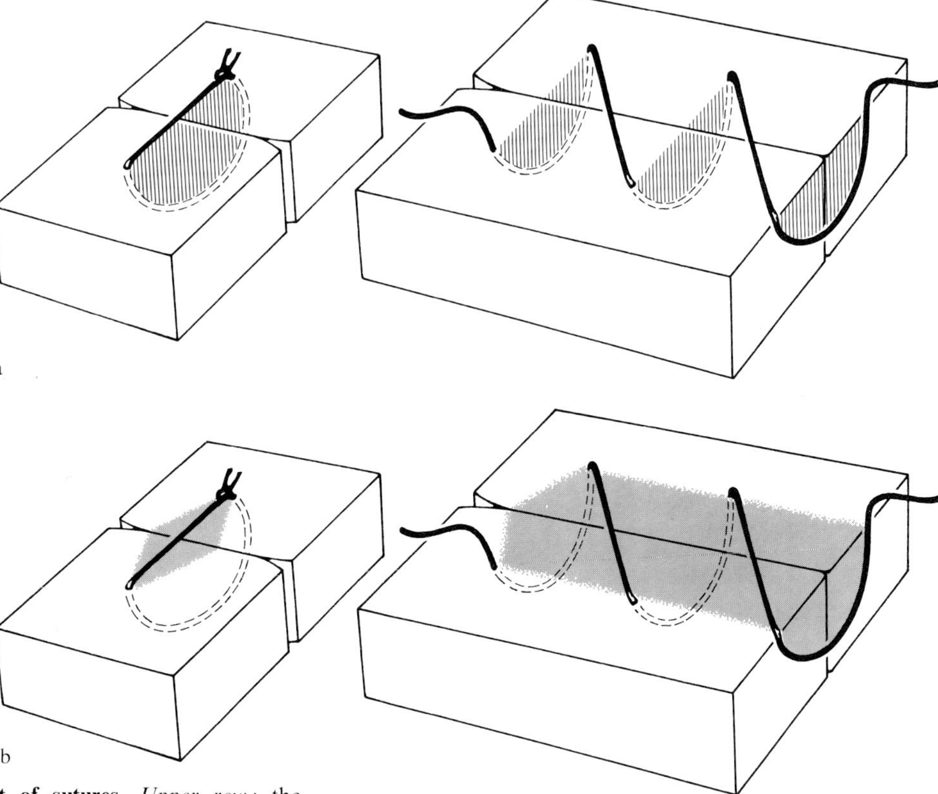

Fig. 71. **Active component of sutures.** *Upper row:* the compressed zone is shown in *pink*. *Lower row:* the splinted zone is *hatched*.

a *Loop sutures:* The zone of maximum compression and the splinted zone are in the same plane.

b *Running sutures:* The compression zone extends for the length of the suture, but only the intramural portions are splinted

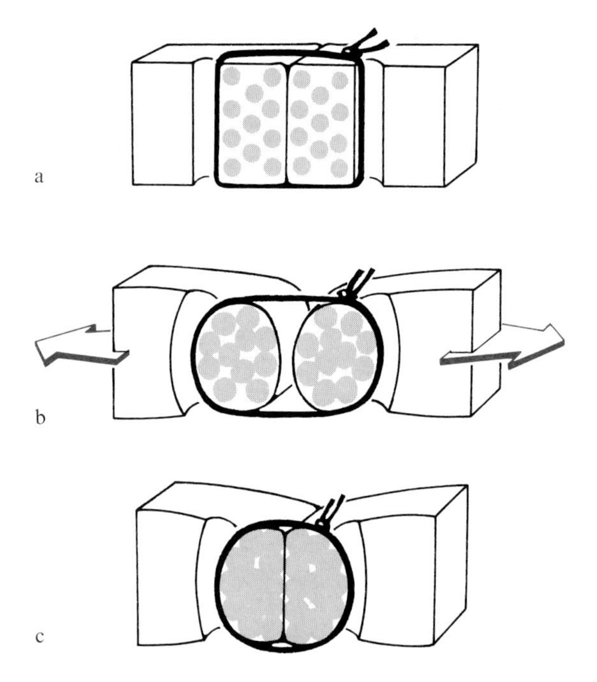

Fig. 72. **Mode of action of compression sutures**

a If the suture is exactly the length of the suture canal (and the overlying tissue segment), it gives satisfactory apposition.

b Traction exerted on the wound edges may then open the wound, inasmuch as the tissue enclosed by the loop can be compressed.

c The compression suture is effective when it compresses the enclosed tissue from the outset to the extent that it can no longer yield to external forces

sutures tend to assume a circular shape, running sutures tend toward the shape of a straight line (**"rule of suture tightening,"** Fig. 73). The tissue surrounding the suture is also forced into this shape, and so compression always deforms the entire wound area. The nature of the expected deformation can be deduced from the rule of suture tightening. Since this deformation is unavoidable with compression sutures, it must be incorporated into the operating plan in advance when such sutures are used. Whenever possible, however, compression sutures should be avoided and incisions employed which utilize other forces to effect wound compression (Fig. 69).

But even when simple apposition sutures are applied, suture shortening can play a role. It is true that here all suture forms are suitable, but only as long as the sutures are not placed under tension. If in the postoperative period the sutures are stressed by external forces (Fig. 72b), they become deformed, at least as long as the forces persist. Hence, the *deformation tendency* of the tissue according to the tightening rule must be taken into account whatever suture type is selected.

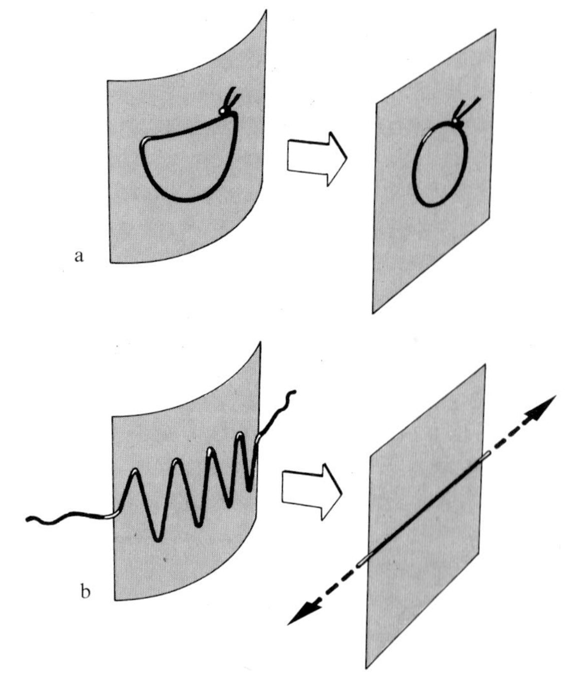

Fig. 73. **The rule of suture tightening**

a A loop suture tends to assume a circular shape when tightened.

b A running suture tends toward the shape of a straight line. *Note:* Both forms tend to lie in one plane

2.4.1 Loop Sutures

With loop sutures, the compression action is greatest in the *suture plane between the needle entrance and exit* and gradually diminishes in a lateral direction (Fig. 74). The efficacy of a suture depends on the **"zone of adequate compression,"** or the zone in which the wound

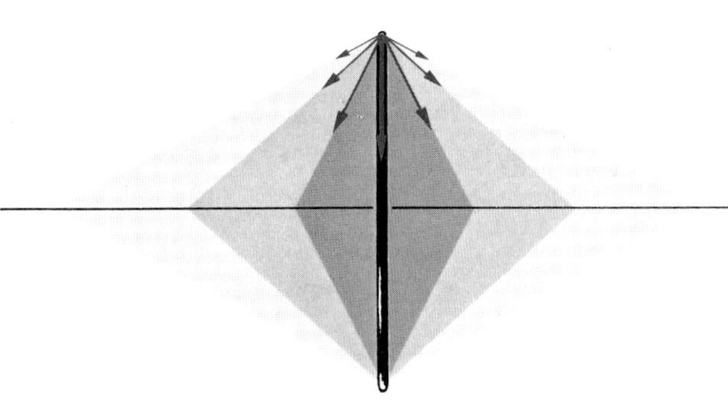

Fig. 74. **Compressive action of a loop suture.** The compressive action diminishes in a lateral direction from the "zone of maximum compression" along the line between the needle entrance and exit

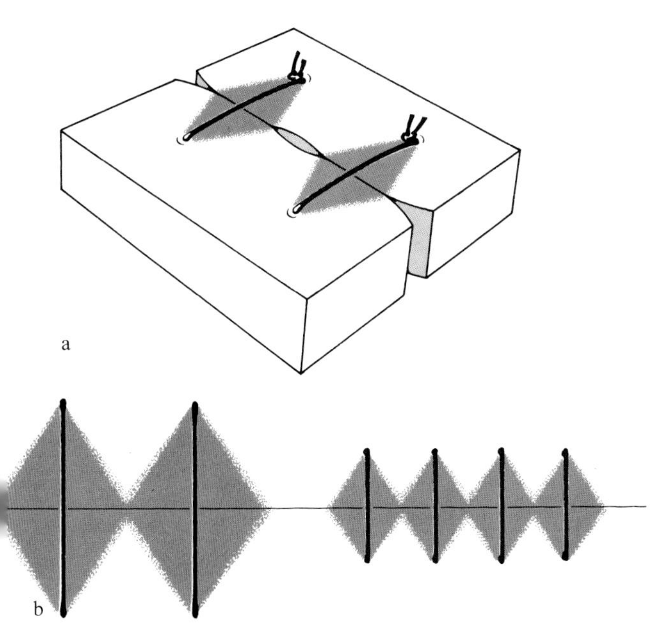

Fig. 75. **Adequate spacing of loop sutures**

a The wound edges are still compressed on both sides of the sutures in the "zones of adequate compression" *(pink)*. Between these zones, the wound is open.

b To ensure continuity of closure, the sutures should be spaced so that the "zones of adequate compression" are in contact. Long sutures (i.e., those with large loops) have broader zones of adequate compression and can be spaced farther apart *(left)* than short sutures *(right)*

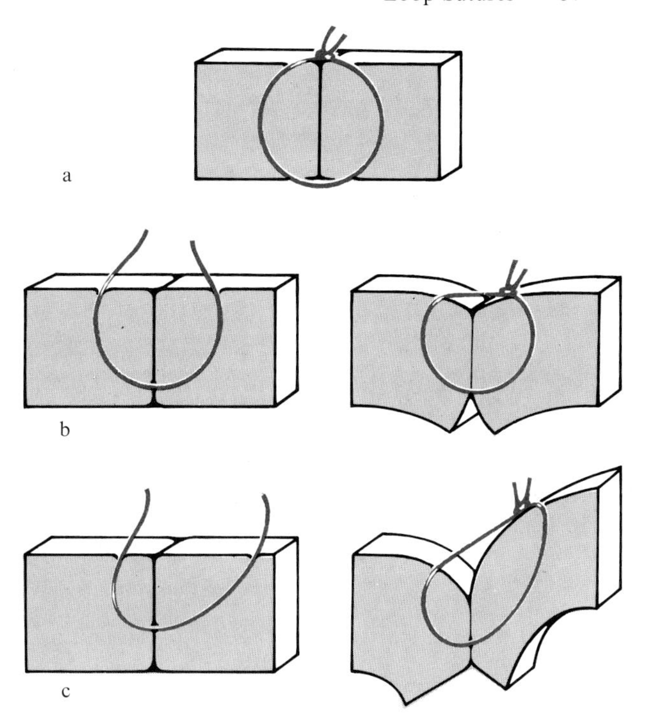

Fig. 76. **Tissue deformation on tightening of loop sutures.** Concomitant tissue shift when the suture assumes a circular shape.

a The theoretically ideal suture has a circular shape from the outset and causes only slight tissue deformation when the loop is tightened.

b Semicircular sutures *(left)* shorten the distances in the enclosed tissue, thereby causing the outside portions of the wound to gape (right).

c Asymmetrically-placed sutures *(left)* compress the tissue on each side of the wound to a different degree and thus create a "step"

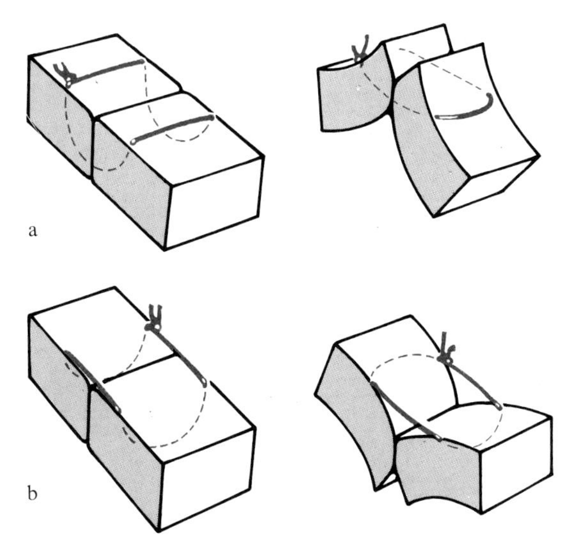

Fig. 77. **Tissue deformation on tightening of mattress sutures.** Concomitant tissue shift in the everting (**a**) and the inverting (**b**) mattress suture when the loop comes to lie in one plane.

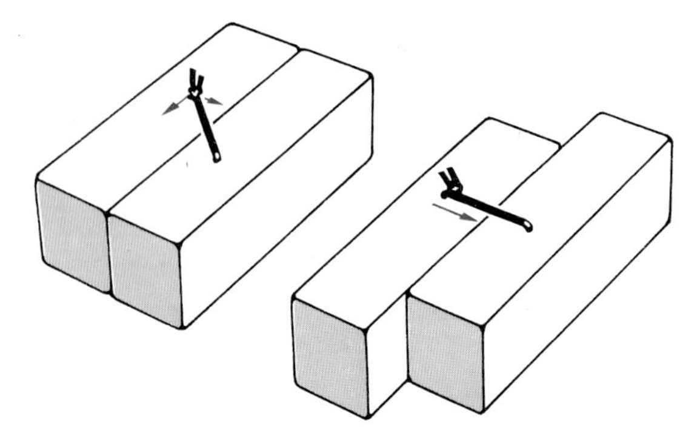

Fig. 78. **Shifting of wound edges on tightening of suture.** In sutures placed at an angle to the wound line, the tension vector has a component parallel to the wound *(left)*, with the result that as the suture is tightened, the wound edges will shift laterally until the suture is perpendicular to them *(right)*

is held so securely closed that it can withstand counteracting forces. Compressive wound closure is achieved when the "zones of adequate compression" are in contact with one another (Fig. 75). The extent of these zones is dependent on the *diameter of the suture loops* and *their degree of shortening*. An increase of the spacing between sutures requires either lengthening of the suture or tightening of the loops.

The tissue deformation that occurs in any suture when the loop is tightened leads to the *inversion* or *eversion* of the wound edges, in accordance with the rule of suture tightening (Figs. 76, 77).

If loop sutures are placed at right angles to the wound line, they exert only a compressive action. In obliquely placed sutures, on the other hand, the tension vector has a component parallel to the wound line, and the edges of the wound will shift laterally (Fig. 78) when the suture is tightened.

2.4.2 Simple Running Sutures

Running sutures distribute tension *uniformly* over the area which they include (Fig. 79a, b). The tension cannot be arbitrarily varied at selected points along the suture, nor can the suture withstand forces applied *locally* (Fig. 79c).

Simple running sutures always have force components that are parallel to the wound edges, and so tightening the suture always causes a **lateral shifting of the wound edges** (Fig. 80). This shifting is complete when the wound-parallel vector components have equal magnitudes in both directions; in theory, this occurs when the stitch shape is that of an isosceles triangle (Fig. 80, S_2). In reality, however, even then there is a tendency for the would edges to shift laterally, because the vectors encounter unequal resistances in each di-

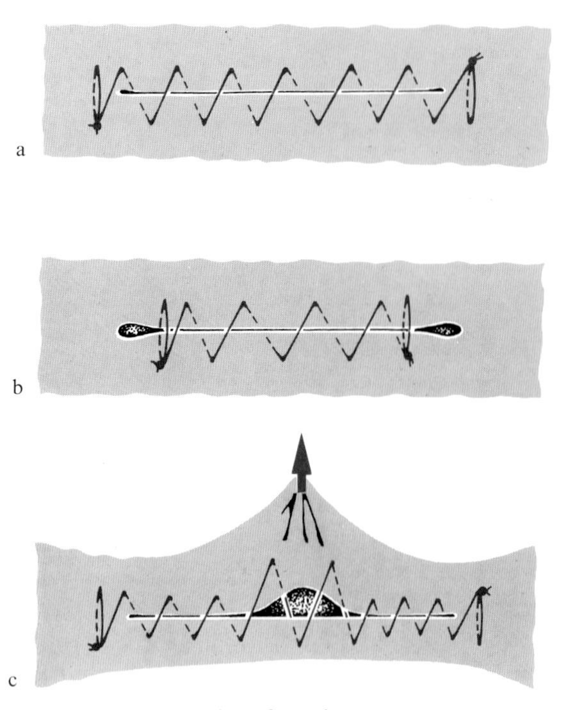

Fig. 79. **Compressive action of running suture**

a The suture tension is distributed evenly over the area it includes.

b If the ends of the wound are not included (i.e., if the suture does not begin in healthy tissue), they will not be compressed.

c If localized forces are applied, the wound may open at the site of application as tension in the vicinity is equalized

Fig. 80. **Various forms of running suture.** Unlike the loop suture, the splinting (intramural) segment *(broken line)* and the overlying segment *(solid line)* are in different planes. Lateral shifting is favored by the wound-parallel component *(V)* of the tension vectors in the direction of the *overlying* segments, since the resistance is lower in this direction. This component is greatest in the "typical" running suture S_1 and is completely absent in the inverse running suture S_3.

Type of running suture (rs)	S_1 "typical" rs	S_2 symmetrical rs	S_3 "inverse" rs
Lateral shifting (Magnitude of vector component in direction of overlying suture segments)	++	(+)	0
Quality of splinting (Continuity of splinted zones)	–	+	++
Technical difficulties in placing the suture (Length of intramural segment and its angle to the wound line)	(+)	+	++

The splinted zones are *hatched*; their projection at the wound line is *shaded pink*

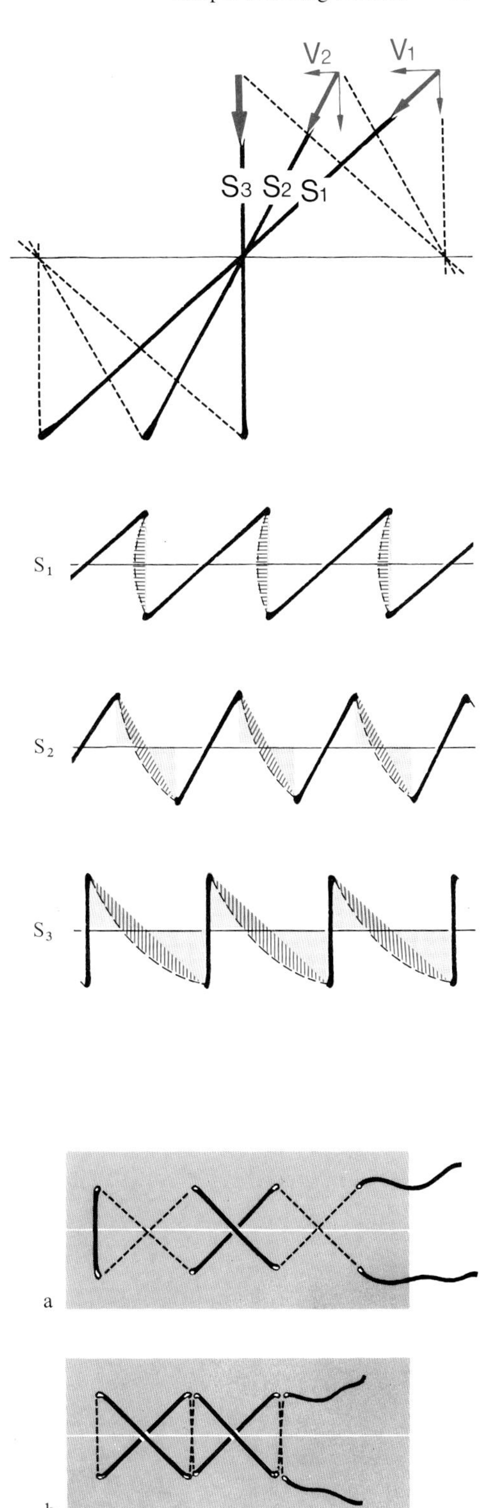

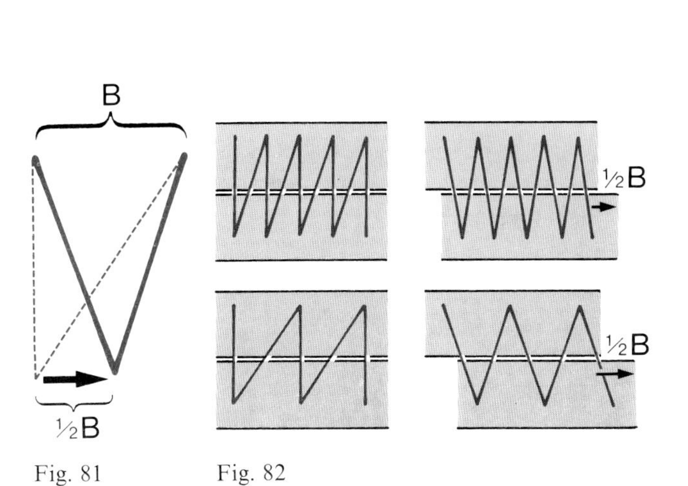

Fig. 81 Fig. 82

Fig. 81. **Lateral shift and stitch width.** In the simple running suture, the lateral shift to a symmetrical stitch form is equal to half the width of the base B of the stitch *(left)*

Fig. 82. **Reduction of lateral shift.** The shift is smaller for narrow stitches *(top right)* than for wide stitches *(bottom right)*

Fig. 83

Fig. 83. **Neutralization of lateral shift by countersuture**

a Bootlace suture with oblique intramural segments.

b Bootlace suture with perpendicular intramural segments. The same suture canal can sometimes be used for suturing in both directions

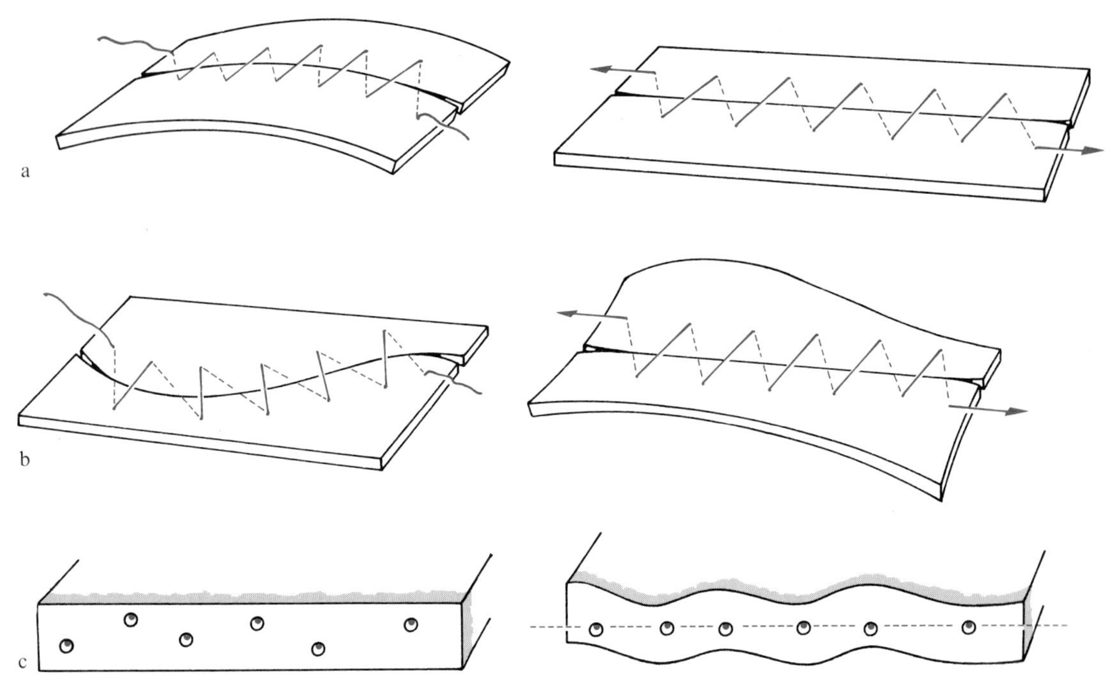

Fig. 84. **Tissue shift with running suture**. Application of the rule of suture tightening.

a Arched surfaces are flattened.

b A curved wound line is straightened, accompanied by torsion of the surrounding tissue.

c The suture tends to occupy a single plane when tightened, and the surrounding tissue is correspondingly raised or depressed. If not all the suture canals cross the wound edge at the same level, the tissue surface becomes irregular

rection: In the direction of the *overlying* suture segments the resistance is lower than in the direction of the *intramural* segments, and therefore the wound-parallel vector components have a greater effect. In practice, lateral shifting is minimal when the overlying segments are perpendicular to the wound line (Fig. 80, S_3).

The *distance* by which the wound edges may shift laterally is dependent on the distance between the needle exit points, or the *stitch width* (Fig. 81).

The lateral shifting of simple running sutures can easily be reduced by selecting appropriate stitch forms (e.g., *inverse running suture*), by *decreasing the stitch width*[50] (Fig. 82), and finally by placing a *countersuture* ("bootlace suture") to equalize tension (Fig. 83).

Much more difficult to cope with are the **concomitant deformations of the wound area** that occur when a tightened suture tends toward the shape of a *straight line* (Fig. 84). These deformations limit the range of application of the simple running suture, especially when a compression suture is required. The ideal wound shape for closure by running suture is a circle (Fig. 85). In this case lateral shifting is unimportant, and the level (plane) of the suture is unchanged when the suture is pulled tight.

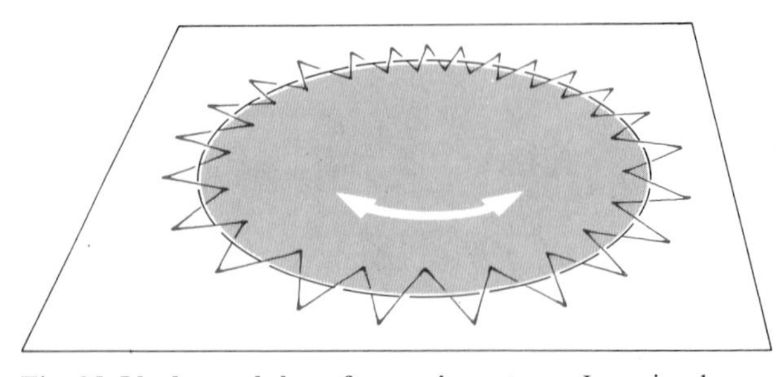

Fig. 85. **Ideal wound shape for running sutures.** In a circular wound, the simple running suture is ideal because the wound already lies in one plane, and lateral shifting is of no consequence

[50] See also Fig. 92.

2.4.3 Continuous Chain Sutures

In the continuous chain suture the thread is passed through the previous loop before the needle is reinserted.

On the one hand, such sutures possess the properties of *loop sutures,* in that the overlying and intramural segments fall in the same plane; on the other hand, they are like *running sutures* in that they distribute tension evenly, since the individual loops are fixed only by the relatively slight friction of the linking segments.

Continuous chain sutures (Fig. 86) can be used like loop sutures to appose and compress wound edges (with the possibility of subsequent tension regulation), or for stitching one tissue layer onto another[51] (with a continuous compression zone produced by the overlying suture segments).

As a continuous chain suture is tightened, no lateral shifting of the wound edges occurs. The shortening of the suture causes a *tightening of the linking segments,* which, as they tend toward linearity, are forced onto the shortest path connecting the two ends of the suture. This tendency can be utilized to regulate the position of the linking segments by choosing an appropriate obliquity of the suture (Fig. 87). The shifting tendency of the linking segments can be avoided by means of *meander sutures.* In their simple form they have discontinuous overlying segments. In the reverse meander suture there is a continuous overlying zone, whose position is fixed and not altered by suture tension (Fig. 88).

[51] Example: Conjunctival flaps onto the cornea or sclera (see also Fig. 182).

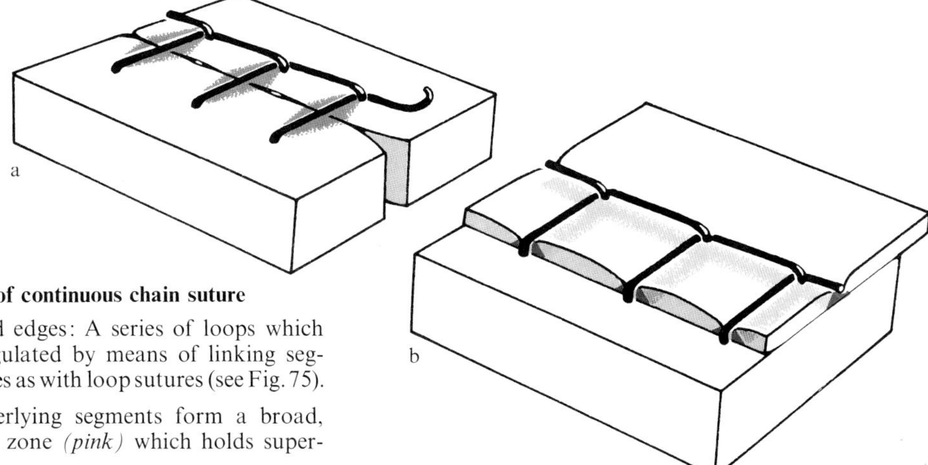

Fig. 86. **Mode of action of continuous chain suture**

a *Compression* of wound edges: A series of loops which allows tension to be regulated by means of linking segments. Compression zones as with loop sutures (see Fig. 75).

b *Stitching-on:* The overlying segments form a broad, continuous compression zone *(pink)* which holds superposed layers together

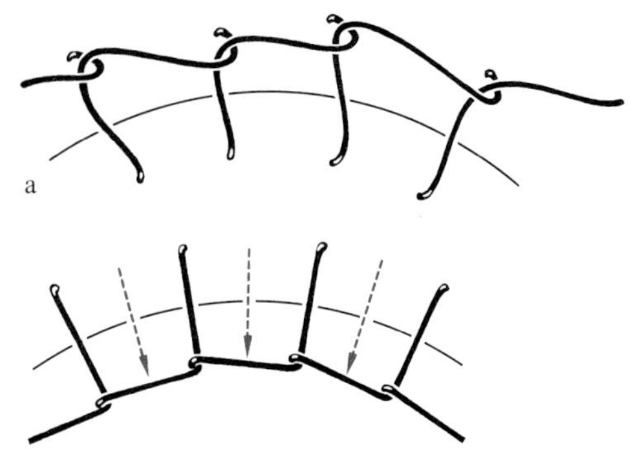

a

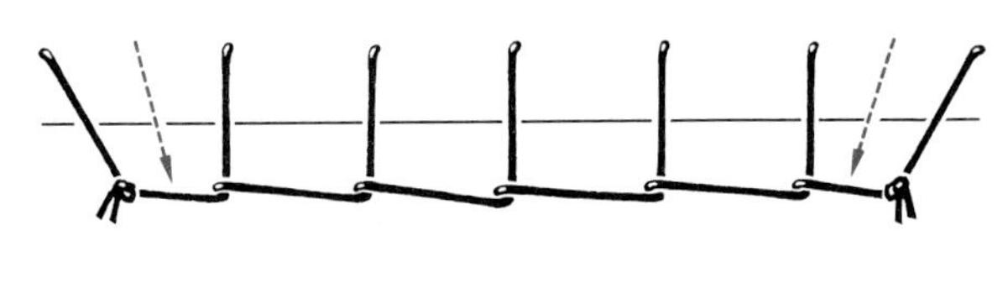

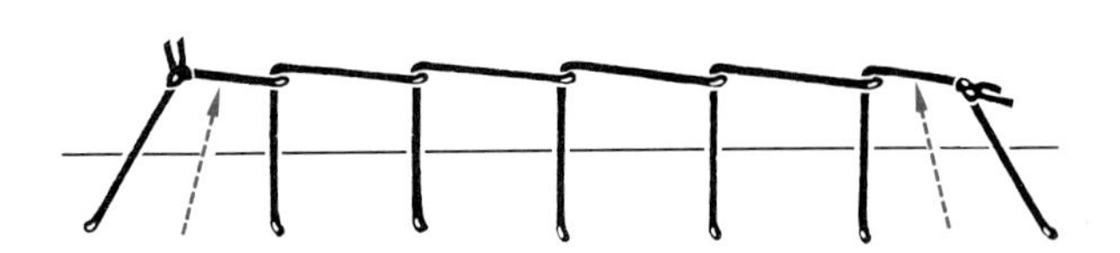

b

Fig. 87. **Behavior of continuous chain suture on tightening.** When the suture is tightened, the linking segments are shifted onto the shortest connecting path.

a On curved wound lines *(left)*, the linking segments are drawn toward the center of curvature *(right)*.

b On straight wound lines, the position of the linking segments can be controlled by angling the ends of the suture to make either the upper or lower connecting line shorter

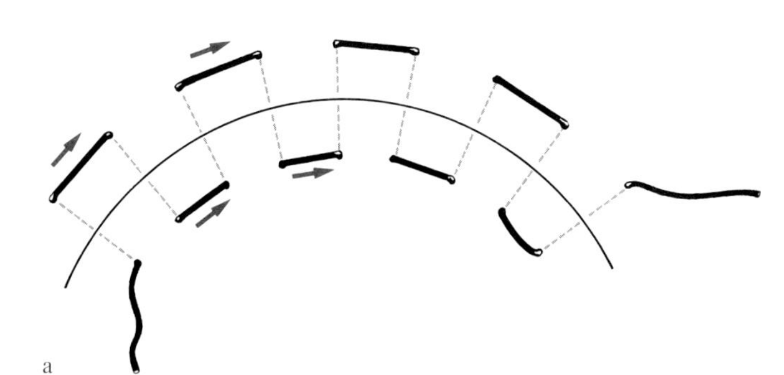

a

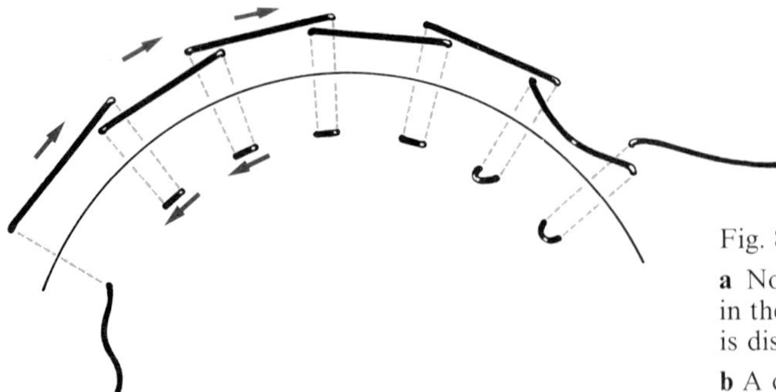

b

Fig. 88. **Meander sutures**

a No shifting of the overlying linking segments occurs in the simple meander suture. The zone of these segments is discontinuous.

b A continous zone of non-shifting overlying linking segments is obtained by a reversing meander suture

2.4.4 Relationship of Suture and Suture Canal

A suture can perform its splinting function only if it fills the suture canal completely (Fig. 89a). This condition is seldom met in ophthalmic surgery, because the suture material is considerably thinner than the needles employed, and thus thinner than the suture canal. As a result, the *threads may shift* in the canal, and the *wound edges may shift* relative to the splinting (Fig. 89b).

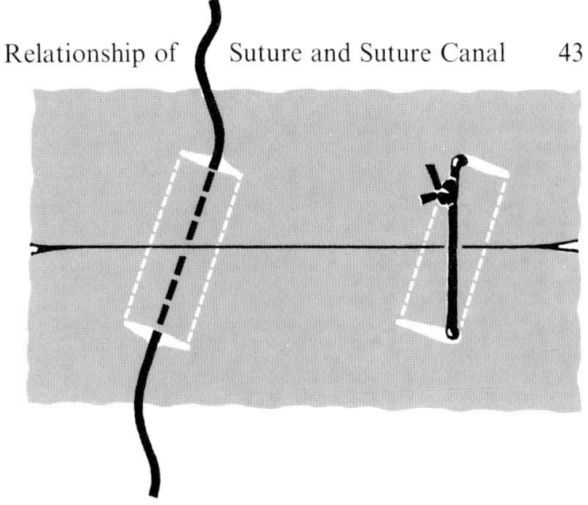

Fig. 91. **Shifting of thin threads in an oblique suture canal.** If the axis of the suture canal is diagonal to the wound line, wound-parallel vector components develop on the thread which persist until it is perpendicular to the wound. If the suture canal is wide enough, the thread may shift with no concomitant shifting of the wound edges (see Fig. 78).

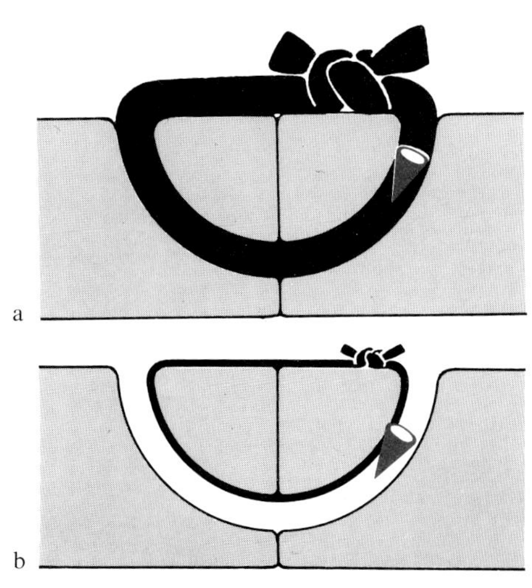

Fig. 89. **Disparity in the diameters of the thread and suture canal**

a A suture acts as a splint if the thread diameter is as large as the lumen of the suture canal. The thread axis then equals the path of the needle tip *(red)* and coincides with its guidance direction (as determined by the surgeon's intentions).

b If the thread is much thinner than the lumen, it is shifted onto the shortest connecting path

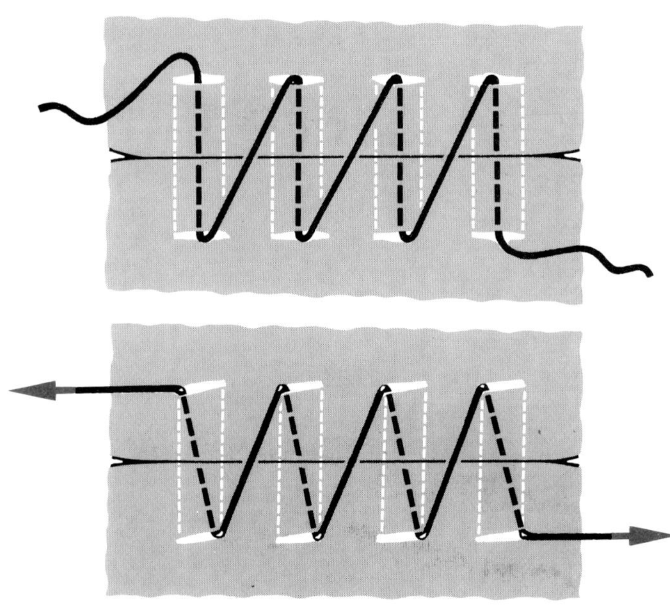

Fig. 92. **Shifting of thin threads in a running suture.** In the simple running suture *(top)*, tension can be equalized simply by the shifting of the thread in its canal *(bottom)*, thereby avoiding any lateral shifting of the wound edges

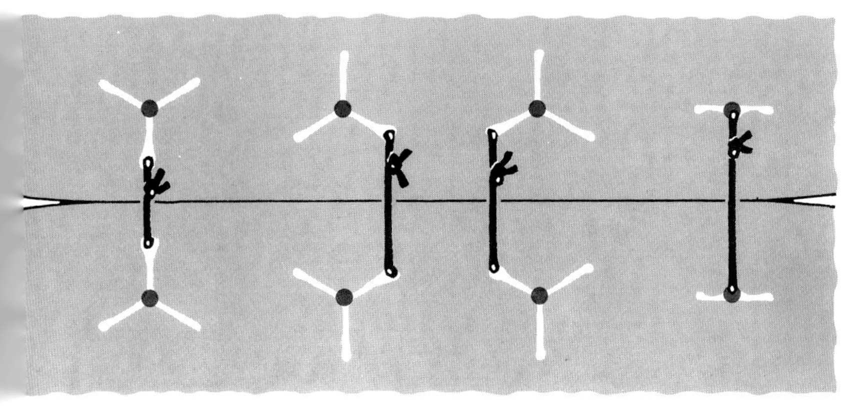

Fig. 90. **Shifting of thin threads in the suture canal.** The path of the shortest connection within the canal varies with the canal cross-section. In the canal cut by a triangular needle, the thread shifts away from the path of the needle tip *(red)* either closer to the wound margin *(left)* or into one of the side limbs *(center)*. In a slit-shaped canal *(right)*, the thread remains in the center only if the canal is precisely perpendicular to the wound line

As soon as a thin thread is pulled tight in a wide suture canal, it assumes a position which may be different from that which the surgeon intended and defined by his guidance actions. It moves onto the *shortest connecting path,* which may lie closer to the surface, wound margin or adjacent suture, depending on the cross-section of the canal (Fig. 90). The final thread position is especially difficult to predict if the suture canal is oblique, but can be estimated beforehand by a tensile test (Fig. 95) and corrected to some degree by regulating the thread tension.

Shifting of the thread within the suture canal allows the thread to be shortened with no consequent tissue deformation and can thus correct certain deficiencies of canal placement (Figs. 91, 92). However, due to the discrepancy between the intentions of the operator (guidance of needle tip) and the result (position of thread axis), there is always a risk of imprecise apposition in such cases. When thin threads are used, therefore, their shifting tendency must be anticipated and allowed for when selecting the needle (which determines the canal cross-section).

It can be assumed that the splinting action of thin threads will improve in most cases *during the course of wound healing,* as the suture canal gradually cicatrizes and its cross-section approaches that of the thread. A

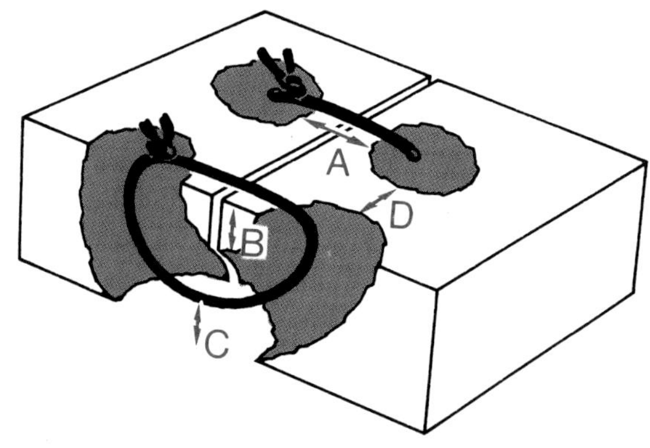

Fig. 93. **Effect of the inflammatory canal on suture spacing.** The development of the inflammatory canal reduces the length of the intact tissue bridges to the wound margin *(A)*, the outer surface *(B)*, the inner surface *(D)* and adjacent sutures *(D)*. For sutures which evoke inflammatory reactions, larger values must be chosen for A, B, C and D than when non-irritating suture materials are used

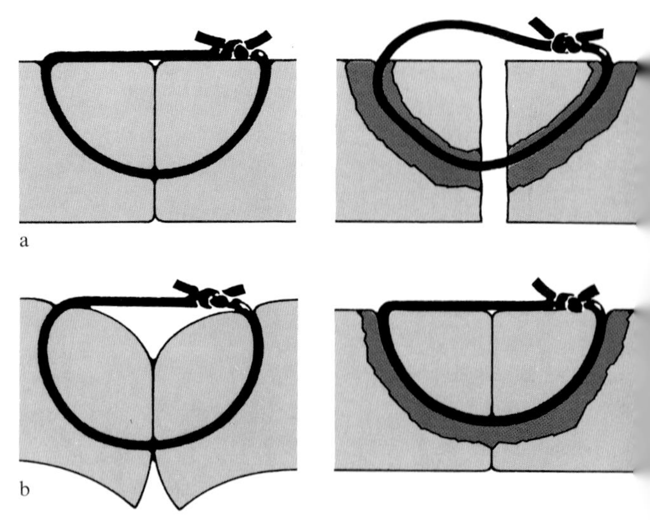

Fig. 94. **Effect of the inflammatory canal on wound apposition**

a Threads correctly placed initially *(left)* are loosened by dilatation of the suture canal in the postoperative period, and the wound opens *(right)*.

b The wound deformation caused by overtightened threads *(left)* is relieved by the loosening effect of the inflammatory canal *(right)*: "self-adaptation of sutures"

Table 1

	A Wire	B Twine	C Sheathed twine
Surface	smooth	rough	smooth
Flexibility	low	high	high
Distensibility	depends on material	good	depends on material and thickness of sheath
Tissue-compatibility	good	fair	good

It can generally be assumed that the suture materials available commercially have good compatibility. Of course there are slight differences, the general rule being that for a given material, the thinner, smoother and more flexible the thread, the better its compatibility

process with the opposite effect may also occur, however: The canal may dilate as the result of an inflammatory response which varies in intensity with the tissue compatibility of the suture material (Table 1), and an "**inflammatory canal**" may gradually form about the thread (Fig. 93). If wound adhesion is still inadequate at this point, the wound may reopen (Fig. 94a). However, the inflammatory canal can also favorably influence the course of healing in that it *adjusts the suture tension* by loosening overtight threads (e.g., compression sutures) and thus reverses the tissue deformations caused by them (Fig. 94b).

The possible formation of an inflammatory canal should always be allowed for in the operating plan, since it influences the selection of suture material. Sutures placed close to the wound edges, tissue surface or adjacent sutures require a material which is as *nonirritating* as possible.[52] On the other hand, sutures which must produce initial tissue deformation may be made from a mildly irritating material[53] so that later the tissue reaction and consequent loosening effect will correct the deformation.

[52] Example: Plastic monofilament.
[53] Example: Twisted, braided or glued silk.

2.4.5 Knots

The *holding strength* of knots depends largely on the *friction* created within the tightened loops. The quality of the suture material plays an important role, therefore: its surface roughness, compressibility and flexibility. The less friction created by the material, the greater the contact area that must be established by the knotting technique. While a simple double knot is adequate for suture materials with high friction[53] (Fig. 97a), several loops must be made in materials which are relatively smooth and inflexible,[52] with the thread passed several times through each loop (Fig. 96).

The first loop, called the *apposing loop,* performs the actual suturing function: It fixes the edges of the wound in the correct position. All additional loops serve only to *secure* the apposing loop.

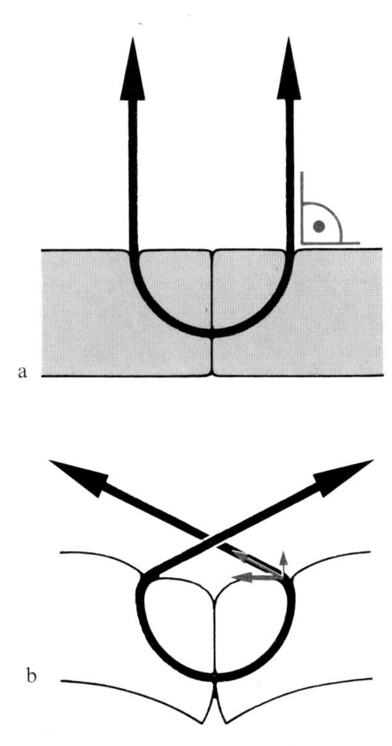

Fig. 95. **Tightening the thread in the suture canal**

a The distance between the points of entry and exit is not affected if the thread is pulled vertically upward from the surface when tightened.

b If the threads are pulled together during tightening, vectors are formed in the direction of the wound edge which draw the points closer together

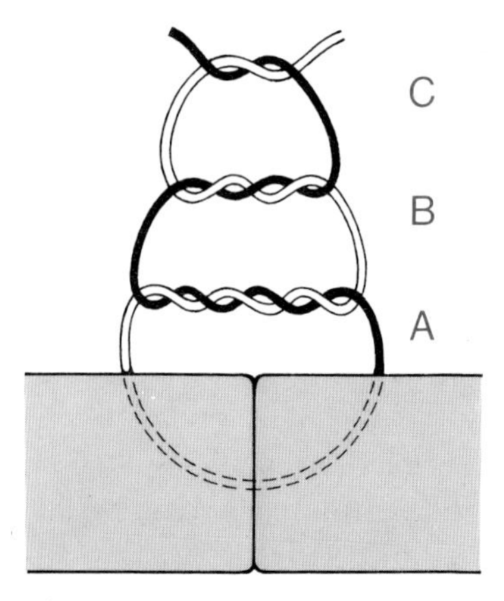

Fig. 96. **The reinforced knot**

A apposing loop; *B, C* securing loops.
A The friction which fixes the position of the apposing loop until the securing loops are tied can be increased by looping the thread several times (here: three).
B If the first securing loop were much shorter than the apposing loop, it would deform it, and in elastic suture materials the resulting forces could reopen the knot. To achieve approximately equal lengths, the suture is also passed repeatedly (here: twice) through the securing loop.
C For stiff material, the first securing loop can be reinforced by a second

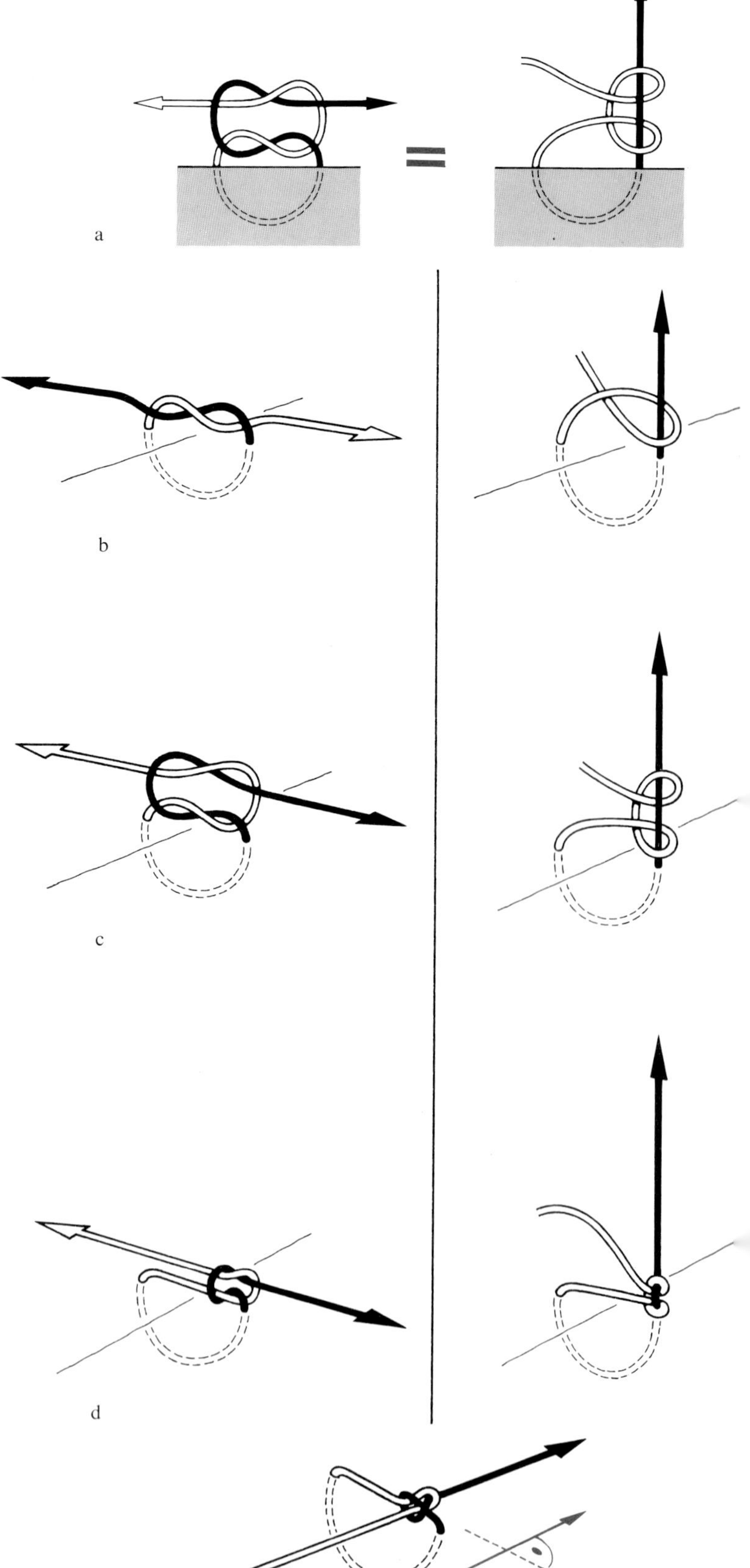

Fig. 97. **The square knot and slip knot**

a Starting from the same loop arrangement, a simultaneous horizontal pull on both ends of the thread produces a square knot *(left column)*, while a vertical pull on only one end forms a slip knot *(right column)*.

b Applying the apposing loop: The square knot *(left)* is already in the correct position, while the slip knot *(right)* is still loose.

c Applying the securing loop.

d Establishing the knot position.

e Tightening the securing loop: at right angles to the suture plane so that suture tension will not be affected further

In **square knots,** the apposing loop is first placed in its definitive position and held there during the securing maneuver (Fig. 97, *left*). In **slip knots,** the apposing and securing loops are first placed loosely and then drawn together into the correct position (Fig. 97, *right*). Both knots can be tied from the same initial loop arrangement, and only the *direction of traction* on the threads determines which type of knot will result.

The knot preferred in a given case will depend largely on the frictional properties of the suture material. *Rough threads* favor square knots, because their high friction holds the apposing loop in place. They make poor slip knots, because the knots may close before they are in the correct position. In contrast, *smooth threads* are easily tied into slip knots but are not good for square knots because the apposing loop tends to loosen before the securing loop is tied. The friction can be increased by passing the thread repeatedly through the loops, but of course a rather bulky knot is the result (Fig. 96).

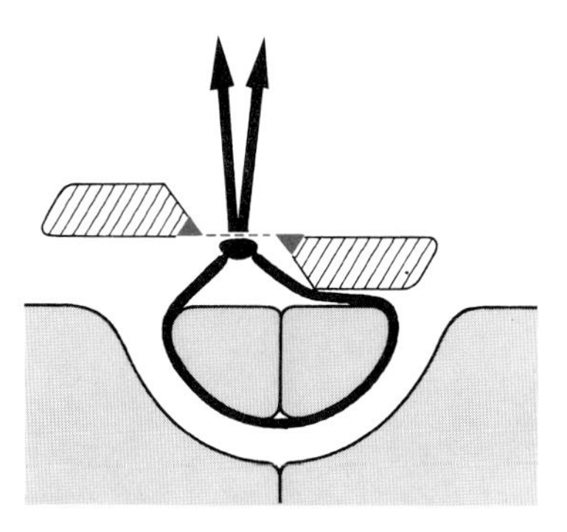

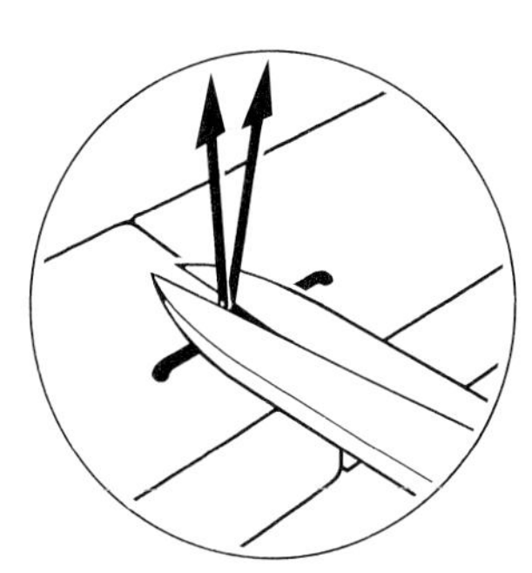

Fig. 98. **Cutting the ends of the thread close to the knot with a scissors.** The knot must be pulled up against the cutting point, the degree of traction depending on the thickness of the blades. Since the knot is hidden from view, accurate guidance is difficult and there is a danger of severing the loop or leaving the ends too long

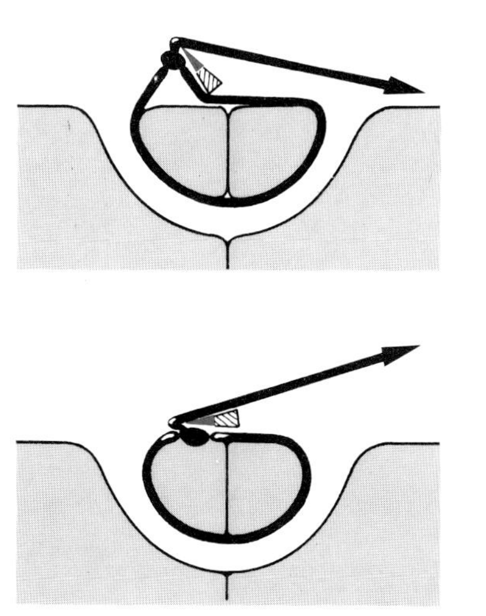

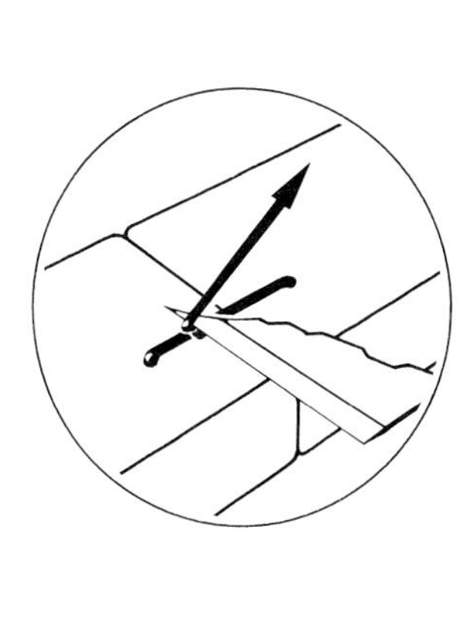

Fig. 99. **Cutting the ends of the thread close to the knot with a razor blade tip**

Top: If loop tension allows the thread to be pulled upward a bit, the blade edge can be raised to improve visibility. The knot is pulled up against the cutting edge, the thread is stretched over it and, with the blade stationary, is snapped off with a quick tug.

Bottom: To cut the end without raising the loop, the blade is laid flat over the knot, its cutting edge flush with the edge of the knot. Then the end of the thread is drawn back and snapped off with a quick tug. The lack of visibility is no great hindrance because once the topographic relationship is established between the cutting edge and edge of the knot, it remains unchanged

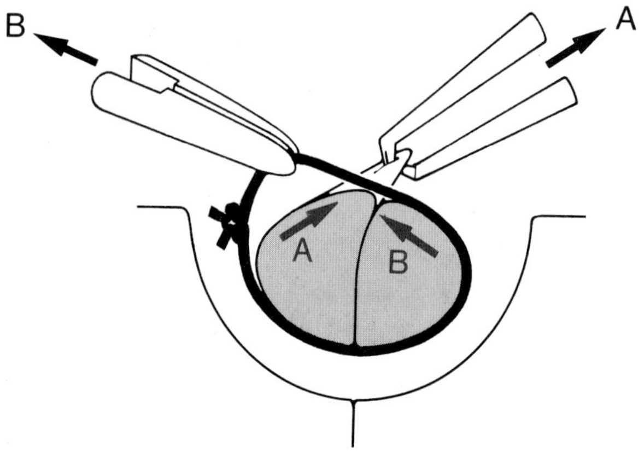

Fig. 100. **Slipping the knot into the suture canal.** To enable the knot to slip over the step at the entrance to the canal, the tissue encompassed by the loop is compressed briefly. This is done on the " knot " edge of the wound by applying countertraction with forceps (*A*), and on the other edge by traction on the thread itself (*B*)

When the knot is tied, care must be taken to apply all forces so that the position of the wound edges is not altered. By applying the *rule of vector separation,* one attempts to eliminate any vector components directed toward the wound line: The tightening of the thread in the suture canal is separate from the knotting maneuver (Fig. 95); the direction of traction on the securing loops is at right angles to that on the apposing loops (Fig. 97e).

Knots have an irritating action which can be reduced by pulling the knot into the suture canal (Fig. 100), provided the size of the knot is smaller than the lumen of the canal, and the ends of the thread are clipped sufficiently close to the knot (Figs. 98, 99).

3 The Application of Thermal Energy

3.1 The Application of Heat

Heat damages tissue by the *coagulation* of protein and the *shrinkage* of collagen. The surgeon's task is to inflict the correct degree of tissue damage so as to achieve the desired effect without causing undesired secondary injuries.[54]

The effect of heat on tissue is basically a function of *temperature*. A sufficient amount of energy must be delivered to the target site to heat it to the temperature required. This heat is either produced outside the tissue and carried to it via a heat conductor, or is generated within the tissue itself (Fig. 101).

The main problem in both methods is control. This is made difficult by the fact that the critical parameters of heat transport vary during heat application; these are *thermal conduction* and *thermal convection*.[55] For this reason, regulating the heat input according to *heat-production measurements* (cautery or cryoprobe temperature, voltage of diathermy current) is unreliable. Thus, control is possible only by observing tissue changes and therefore very difficult in cases where the effect can be seen neither directly nor by ophthalmoscope.

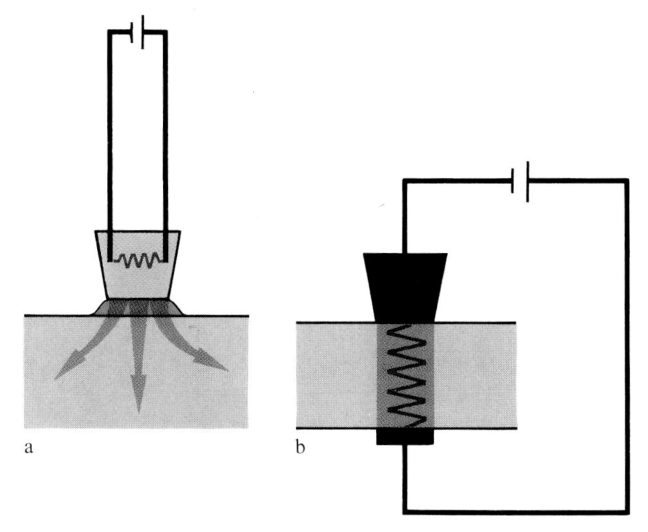

Fig. 101. **Methods of heating tissue**

a Transmitting heat to the tissue: Heat produced outside the tissue is transmitted to the site of action. The critical factors are thermal conductivity and heat capacity.

b Generating heat in the tissue (diathermy): The heat is generated at the site of action. The critical factors are the electrical properties of the tissue

3.1.1 Heat from an External Source

Heat is transported to and removed from tissues in a heat transfer chain (Fig. 102) which consists of *heat production, transfer resistance* and *elimination*. The process can be controlled by varying any of these elements.

Heat production: The necessary energy is supplied either by *large* quantities of heat with a predetermined, *precisely-regulated* temperature (large-capacity cautery, Fig. 103), or by *small* quantities of heat with a *higher* temperature (small-capacity cautery, Fig. 104). Constraints are placed on the capacity of the cautery by the dimensions of the ocular structures, and on its temperature by the danger of over-effect (Fig. 105a). For this reason the

---

[54] In *hemostasis* (shrinkage of vascular walls and coagulation of their contents), for example, the surrounding tissues should not undergo shrinkage to the extent that the wound edges are deformed and reapposition is difficult. Deep effects must be avoided, and internal eye structures must be spared. On the other hand, deep effects are the operative goal when *aseptic inflammatory foci* are induced as a stimulus for scar formation (retinal detachment surgery, obliteration of the ciliary body in glaucoma surgery). Here, shrinkage of the sclera should not be so severe that the intraocular pressure is unduly raised. However, scleral shrinkage is necessary to produce *wound dehiscence* in fistulating glaucoma operations. To achieve the actual *division of tissue*, carbonizing temperatures are employed.

[55] *Conduction* is a material constant which, in tissues, depends essentially on moisture content; it is reduced by drying. *Convection* is the transfer of heat by fluids in motion. In homogenous tissues, it depends mainly on blood flow, i.e., it is diminished by compression or coagulation of the vessels. Convection at surfaces is accomplished by free-moving fluid layers.

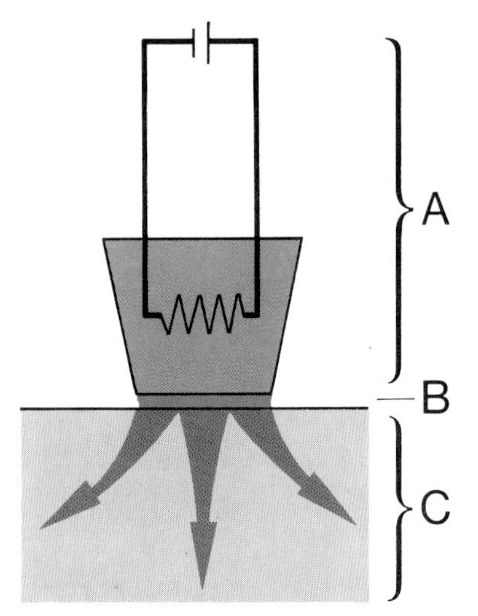

Fig. 102. **The heat transfer chain.** *A* Heat source. *B* Transfer resistance (tissue surface). *C* Dissipation and elimination (tissue)

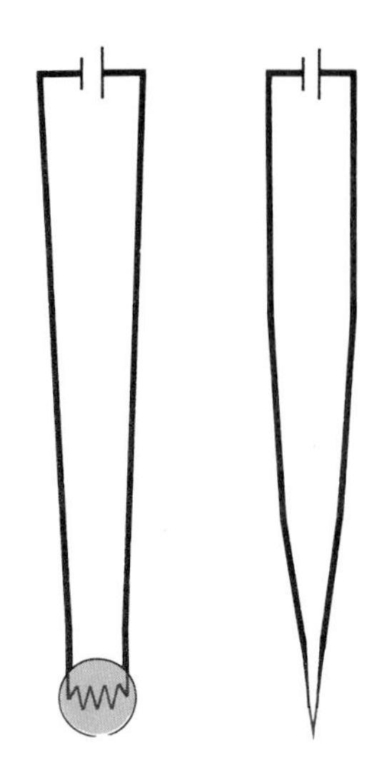

Fig. 103 Fig. 104

Fig. 103. **Large-capacity heat transmitter (spherical cautery).** Large dimensions = large capacity. This cautery requires a correspondingly longer reheating time (in air) after its heat is transmitted to the tissue

Fig. 104. **Small-capacity heat transmitter (wire loop).** Small dimensions = small capacity, high temperature. Control is extremely difficult. Small-capacity cautery is best suited for surface coagulation

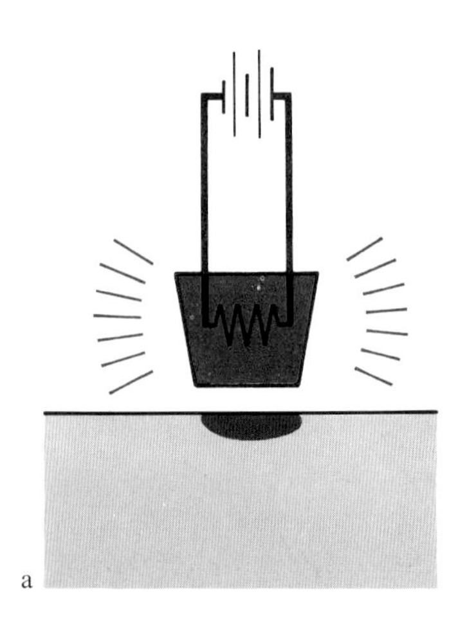

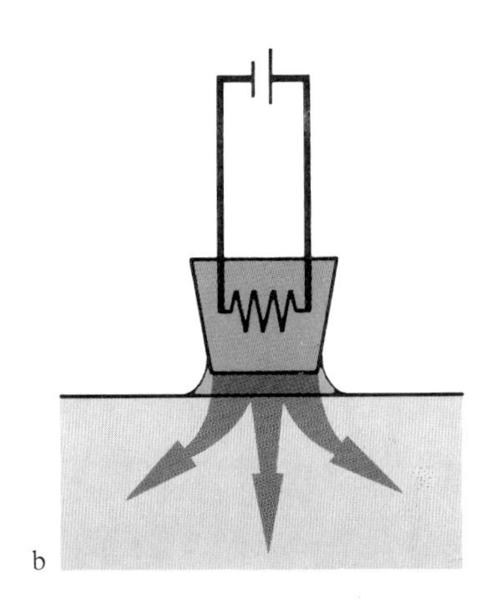

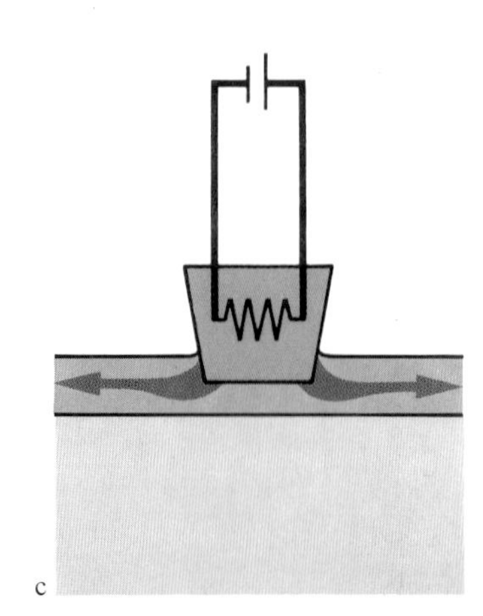

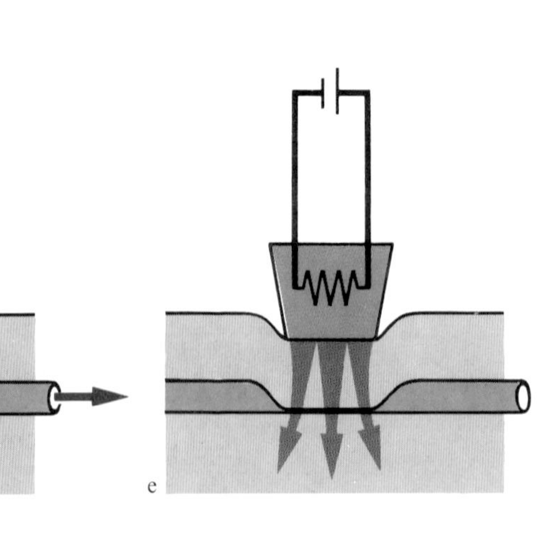

Fig. 105. **Means of controlling heat transmission**

a Increasing the cautery temperature (in air). On contact with the tissue, drying increases the transfer resistance, with the risk of thermal overeffect.

b Moistening the surface improves heat transfer to the tissue.

c Dissipating the heat by large amounts of liquid on the tissue surface.

d Eliminating the heat from the tissue via the bloodstream.

e Interrupting the blood flow (by compression) increases the thermal effect by reducing heat loss

process is more easily controlled by influencing the next two elements of the transfer chain.[56]

The **transfer resistance** is a function of *moisture content.* If the tissue surface is dry (Fig. 105a), the heat cannot penetrate to deeper levels, and coagulation is superficial (which further increases the resistance: danger of over-effect). Moist surfaces have a lower resistance and are therefore prerequisite for deep penetration (Fig. 105b). If there is a continuous liquid film, however, it dissipates the heat and thus lessens the effect of the procedure (Fig. 105c).

The **elimination of heat** in the tissue (Fig. 105d) can be most easily influenced by varying the *blood flow* through the area. By exerting firm pressure on the applicator, the surgeon can compress the vessels and thus increase the coagulative effect (Fig. 105e).

Care must be taken in practice that the *quantity of heat* introduced is commensurate with the *volume of tissue to be heated.* The volume is small in highly localized surface coagulation (Fig. 106a), somewhat larger in the treatment of larger areas by dynamic surface coagulation (Fig. 106b), and largest in deep coagulation, when a continuous heat influx is necessary to offset dissipation (Fig. 106c). Quantities of heat suitable for a large tissue volume would overheat a smaller zone. Due to their different heat requirements, the various modes of application must not be intermixed without correspondingly adjusting the level of heat input (cautery temperature).

[56] The effect of a high-temperature cautery can be controlled to some extent by regulating the contact time, i.e., by "daubing" the tissue with the applicator ("digital" instead of "analog" application).

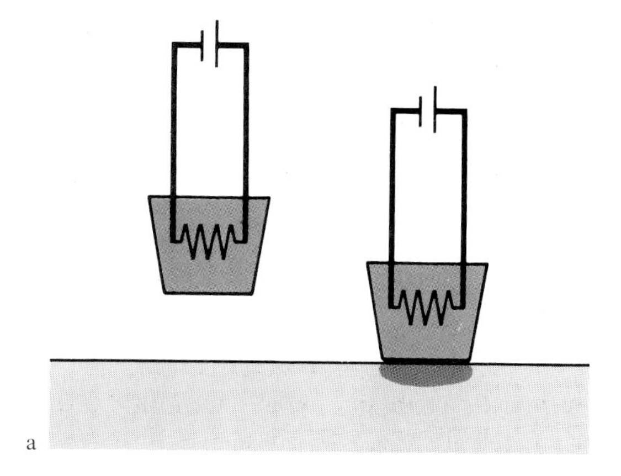

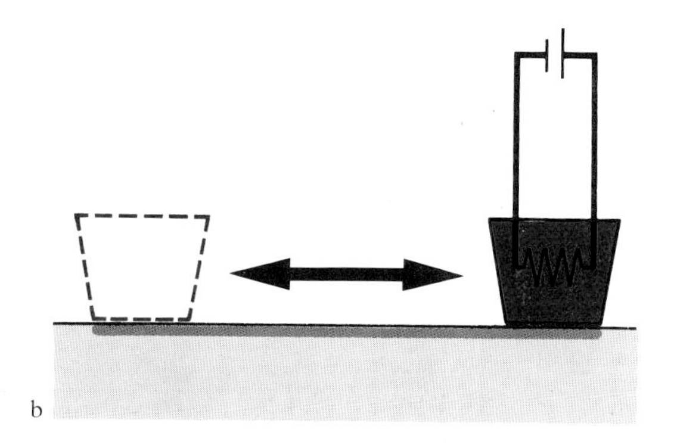

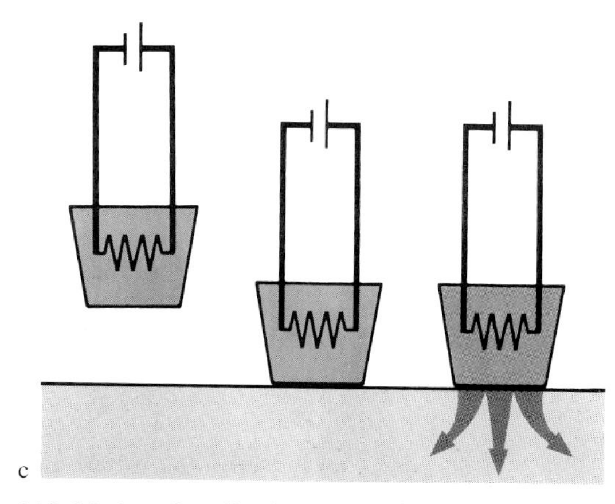

Fig. 106. **Modes of application of heat transmitters**

a *Surface coagulation (static):* The applicator is preheated and applied warm to the tissue. All heat is transmitted in a circumscribed area; transmission is controlled by regulating the temperature.

b *Surface coagulation (dynamic):* The preheated applicator is moved back and forth on the tissue surface. Larger quantities of heat (= higher temperatures) are required than in static coagulation. Heat transmission is controlled by the speed of applicator movement.

c *Deep coagulation:* The applicator is applied cold to the tissue, then heated. Heat begins to flow into the tissue during heatup. A long time is required for the onset of action. Large quantities of heat are needed, and the effect is difficult to assess

3.1.2 Production of Heat in the Tissue: Diathermy

Heat production depends on the properties of the electric circuit comprised of the *voltage source, indifferent electrode, electrical resistance* of the tissue, and *active electrode*. The **voltage source** delivers alternating current in a frequency range suitable for the generation of heat. The **indifferent electrode** is made as large as possible in order to minimize the current density there (Fig. 107).

The **electrical resistance** depends to some degree on the diameter and spacing of the electrodes, but mainly on the *electrolyte content* of the tissue and is therefore variable during coagulation.

The **shape of the active electrode** determines the distribution of current density in the tissue (Fig. 108). As the *contact area* increases, the current density rises at deeper levels, but higher voltages are also required. If the same electrode is applied "at a point" in one instance and over a larger area in another (Fig. 109), the voltage must be adjusted accordingly.

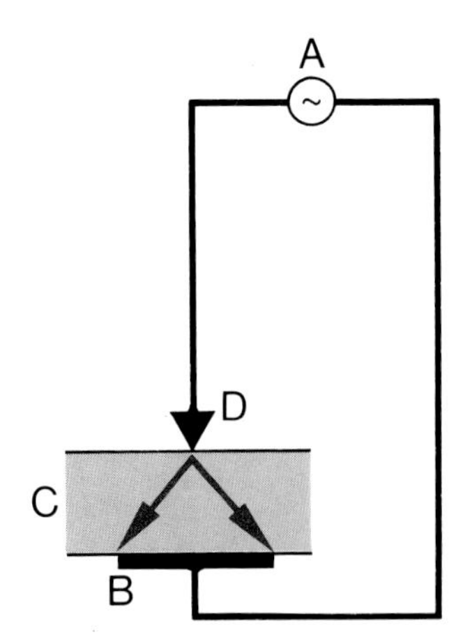

Fig. 107. **Electric circuit for generating heat in tissues.** *A* Voltage source. *B* Indifferent electrode. *C* Tissue resistance. *D* Active electrode

Thus, the generation of heat in deeper parts can be promoted by a moist surface and broad electrodes. Heat production can be confined to the tissue surface by drying the contact area and using slender electrodes, although deep effects also may occur in such cases and are not apparent superficially.

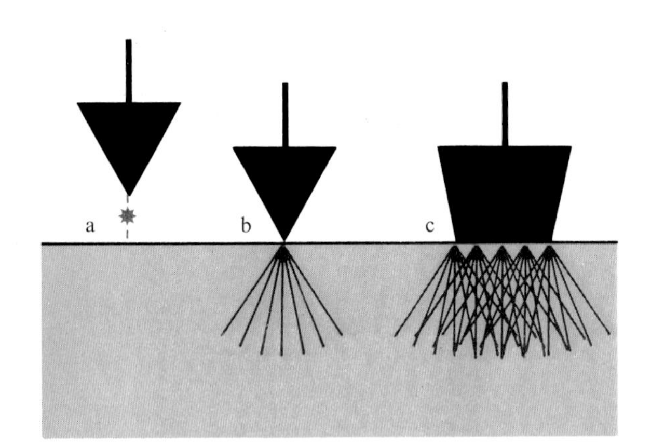

Fig. 108. **Shape of the active electrode**

a If a high voltage is applied prior to tissue contact, a spark will form (danger of tissue destruction).

b Point electrodes concentrate their energy at the site of application (surface).

c Broad electrodes produce a high current density also at deeper levels

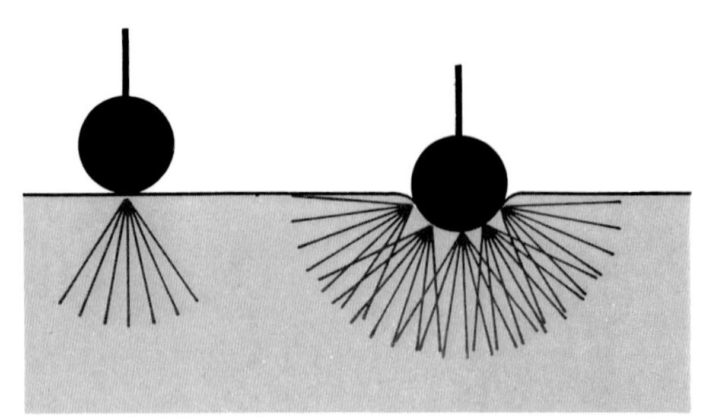

Fig. 109. **Spherical electrodes.** Spheres can act as point or broad electrodes, depending on the area of contact. The voltage must be adjusted for the mode of contact employed

3.1.3 Bipolar Diathermy

In bipolar diathermy, a voltage is produced between *two* slender, identically shaped *active electrodes* (forceps blades) which either grasp the tissue to be coagulated or are immersed in a liquid film on the tissue surface[57] (Fig. 110).

If the electrodes are applied **directly to the tissue** (Fig. 111), control is difficult. As soon as the intervening tissue shrinks, the blade spacing (which determines heat production) decreases; also, the resistance is altered by dessication. At the moment the desired effect appears, there is already a danger of over-effect.

On the other hand, if the electrodes are immersed in an **electrolyte-containing liquid**

[57] Caution: If the forceps tips touch while the voltage is on, a short-circuit will occur and the tips will fuse.

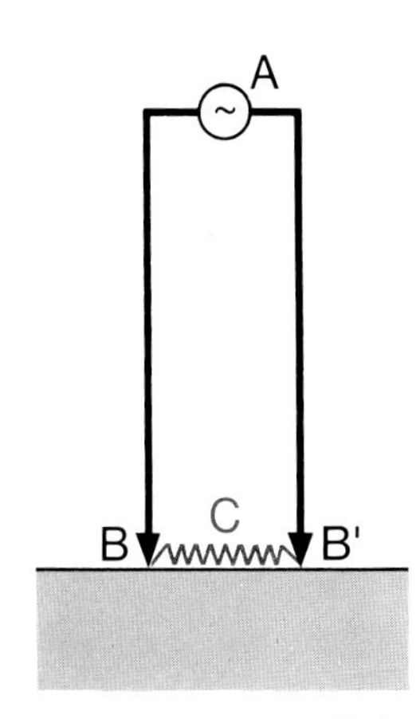

Fig. 110. **The electric circuit in bipolar diathermy.** *A* Voltage source. *B* Active electrodes. *C* Heat-producing resistance

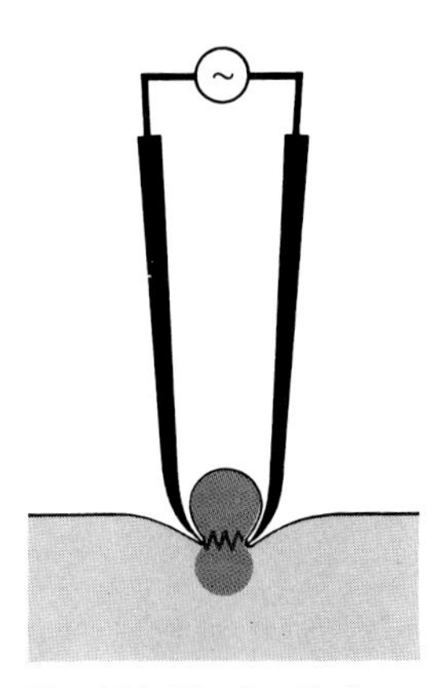

Fig. 111. **Bipolar diathermy in the tissue.** The tissue grasped between the forceps blades is heated

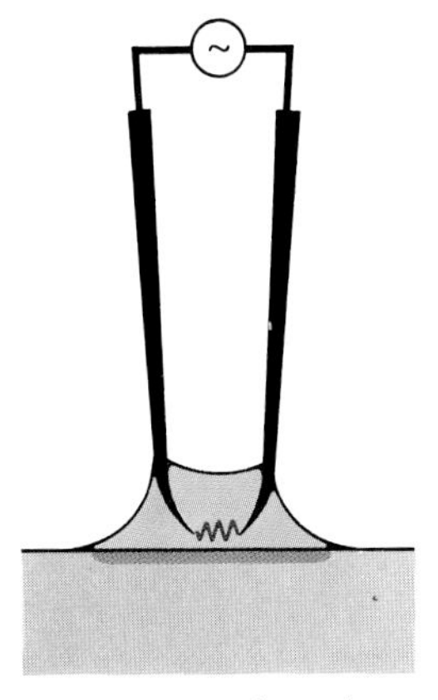

Fig. 112. **Bipolar diathermy in a liquid film.** An electrolyte-containing liquid is heated and forms a heat-transfer medium

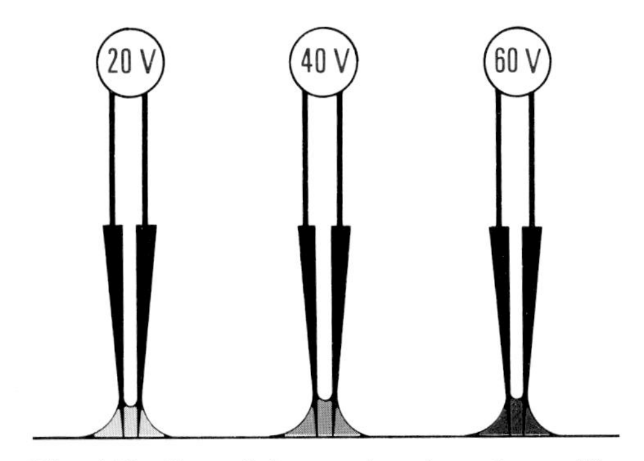

Fig. 113. **Control by varying the voltage.** The electrode spacing is kept constant

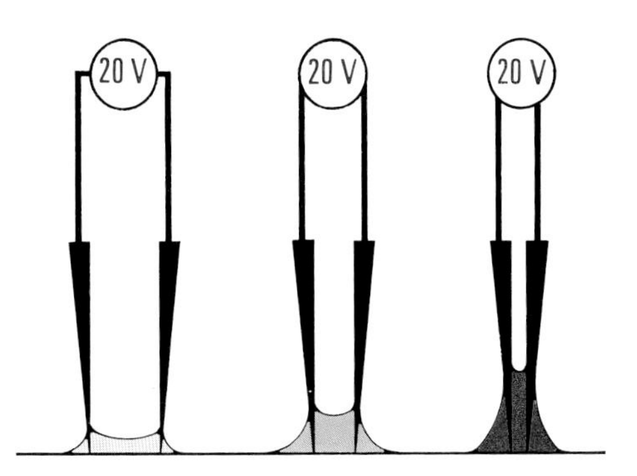

Fig. 114. **Control by varying the spacing.** The voltage remains constant

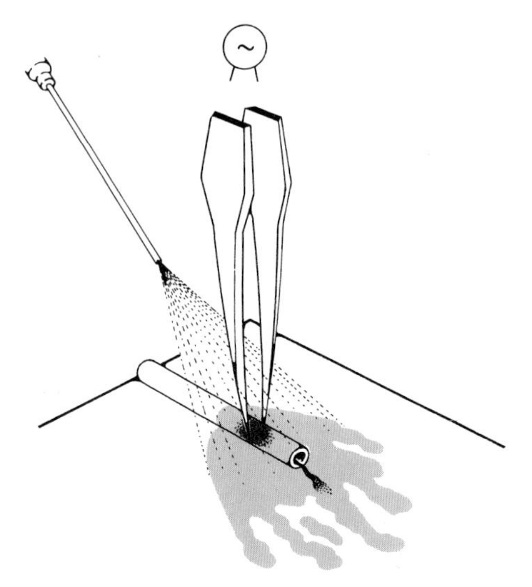

Fig. 115. **Control by heat dissipation.** Irrigating the surface during the coagulation of a bleeding vessel prevents the (relatively large) quantity of heat from penetrating to deeper layers

film (such as physiological saline), and the liquid is heated, an ideal *heat-transfer medium* is produced (Fig. 112). Its temperature is limited by its boiling point, which is easily held constant, and its transfer resistance remains constantly low.

Control is accomplished by *varying the voltage* (Fig. 113), *varying the electrode spacing* (Fig. 114) and *varying heat transfer* by *irrigation* (Fig. 115).

3.2 The Application of Cold

Freezing is a means of producing *tissue damage* without the coagulation necrosis or connective-tissue shrinkage that accompany heating.[58] Moreover, the ice ball formed acts as a *mechanical grasping instrument* in that it is continuous with the freezing instrument and the tissue structures and thus forms a firm adhesion between them. But unlike mechanical instruments, the cryoprobe exerts no pressure on the tissue and thus causes no deformation.[59] Since cold transmission is essentially heat transmission in reverse, the same rules apply.

The **cold source** is a cryoprobe (Fig. 116), which may be cooled by evaporation (the change from a solid or liquid to a gas) or the rapid expansion of gases (Joule-Thomson effect). Different cryoprobes differ mainly in their means of control and the associated technical costs. Control by lowering the *cryoprobe temperature* is effective only with regard to the *speed* of the process; it has little effect on the size of the ice mass, since this is itself an insulator which hinders further cold transfer at a certain layer thickness.

[58] Examples: Cell destruction, induction of aseptic foci of inflammation, but not hemostasis.
[59] Sample indications: Lens capsule, epithelial cysts.

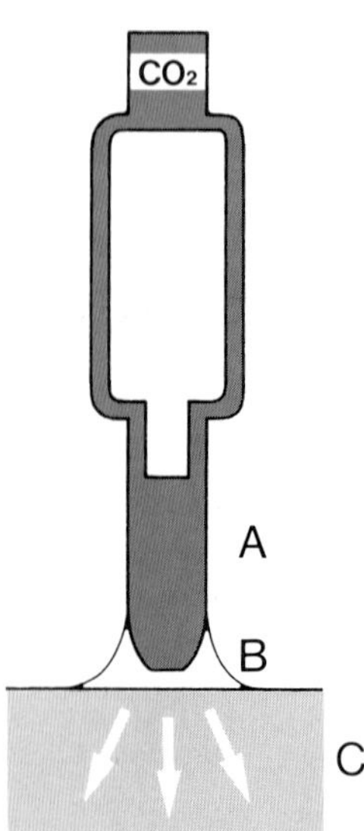

Fig. 116. **The cold transfer chain.** *A* Cold source (cryoprobe). *B* Transfer resistance. *C* Dissipation and elimination in the tissue

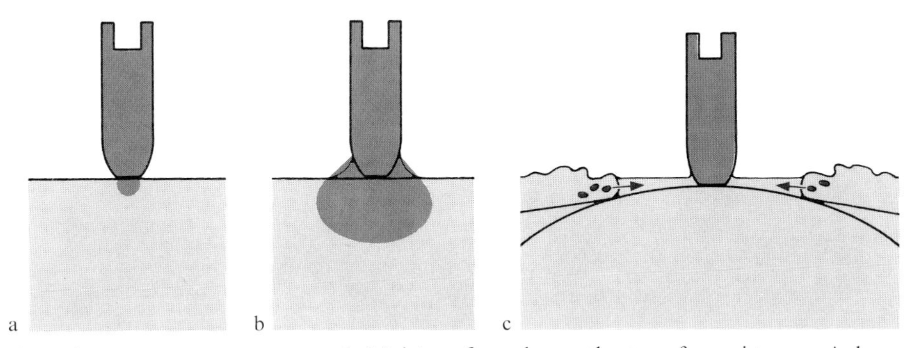

Fig. 117. **Control of the transfer resistance**

a A dry surface has a high resistance, and little ice forms in the tissue.

b Moist surfaces lower the transfer resistance: A large ice ball forms which attaches the cryoprobe to the tissue.

c A liquid film conveys heat from the environment; no freezing occurs

The **resistance to cold transfer** is determined by the same factors which govern heat transfer (Fig. 117).

Ice formation in tissues depends on their *moisture content* (conduction and convection) and *electrolyte content* (freezing point). It is tissue-specific and may therefore proceed at different rates in adjacent tissues. If ice formation is observed in a particular tissue layer, the analogous freezing of other parts cannot be inferred.[60] These differences in freezing tendency can be tactically utilized as a means of grasping a solid body in a liquid medium.[61]

In the practical application of cold (Fig. 118), the deepest penetration is achieved when the instrument is in contact with the tissue before it is activated. If the cryoprobe has already been cooled in the air, a layer of ice forms about the applicator which acts as an insulator and interferes with cold transmission. As a result, the coagulative effects are entirely superficial, and adhesion is poor.

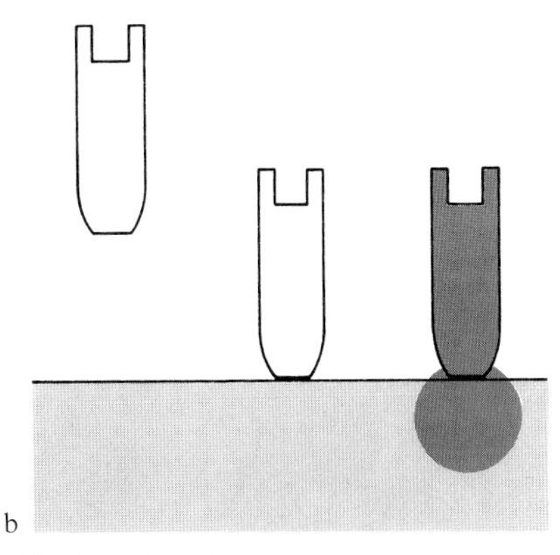

Fig. 118. **The application of cold**

a A cryoprobe cooled in air acquires an ice film which acts as an insulator to hinder cold transmission to the tissue.

b If the cryoprobe is not cooled until in contact with the tissue, the temperature falls continuously. The depth of penetration is greater, but more time is required for ice formation

[60] Examples: Ice formation in the relatively dry lens capsule does not necessarily mean that ice has also formed in the interior of a water-rich lens (intumescent cataract, morgagnian cataract). Also, the size of the frozen zone on the surface of the sclera gives no information on the size of the frozen uvea or retina (due to the vascular heat-conduction of the choroid).

[61] Example: Dislocated lens in the fluid vitreous.

4 The Application of Light Energy

In **photocoagulation,** heat is produced by the action of concentrated light waves. The energy chain consists of the *light source,* the *light path* through the optical system, and *dissipation of heat* to the environment.

The "transmission resistance" is low in transparent media, but high in the tissue to be treated (absorption).

Energy input is easily controlled by the diameter of the light spot, the intensity of the light, and the duration of exposure. The various resistances are easily assessed (tissue transparency), and the effect is visible.[62]. In conventional light sources and low energy lasers the energy has no effect on transparent media and is merely transported through them; its effects occur only in light-absorbing tissues. **High-power lasers** which emit high energies in very short pulses[63] produce mechanical as well as thermal effects. They can be used to divide tissues by the removal of material,[64] provided the presence of the resulting debris in the tissues is acceptable.

One consequence of the tremendous power density of such lasers is that tissue destruction takes place even in media which appear transparent to the observer, and thus have a low "transfer resistance." To keep the light path clear, therefore, the beam must be spread in order to reduce its power density.

The laser light is brought to focus at the intended site of action, the absorption of energy increasing to enormous values with increasing power density (nonlinear effects, optical breakdown). Microexplosions occur which damage the tissue not only thermally but also, and most severely, by shock waves. The destructive effect is determined not only by the energy of each individual pulse, but also by the sequence characteristic, i.e., the temporal sequence of pulses of constant or varying intensity.

5 The Utilization of Chemical Effects (Electrolysis)

Direct current flowing between an active and indifferent electrode produces not only heat, but a *chemical action* as well: the dissociation of electrolytes with the release of gas. In the process, alkali radicals induce a *colliquative necrosis* which occurs without significant tissue shrinkage. Acid radicals, by contrast, cause a *coagulation necrosis* with tissue shrinkage.

[62] Example: Excessive heat generates steam bubbles.
[63] Such as giant pulsed lasers which emit in the nano-or picosecond range.
[64] See p. 14.

II The Significance of the Pressure Chambers of the Eye

1 General

The strategy of ocular surgery is on the one hand *tissue strategy*, dealing with the division, displacement and uniting of tissues. On the other hand it is what one might call *space strategy*, dealing with the creation and maintenance of spaces between tissues for purposes of pressure equalization and fluid circulation.

Now, one of the distinctive features of eye surgery is that the operations are performed on *pressure chambers*. As a result, surgical measures may have effects at a distance from the actual operative site. Problems may mount, unnoticed by the surgeon, and suddenly become manifest at a later time. If the operator is familiar with the properties of the parts that behave as pressure chambers, he will be able to recognize the problems as they arise and take appropriate countermeasures. This is especially important with regard to preventing the most annoying complications, that is, undesired protrusions of tissue from the eye.[1]

The pressure chambers of the eye have elastic walls and are filled with fluid, and so they are subject to *Pascal's law*. When a chamber is deformed until the smallest surface area per unit volume is attained, the wall tension will increase and, with it, the internal pressure of the chamber. Since the fluid in the chamber is incompressible, the wall tension is always equal *over the entire surface*. Consequently it does not matter, as far as pressure is concerned, at which point on the chamber a force is applied. This means that every surgical measure has both *local* and *general* effects on the pressure chamber involved.

[1] Example: Prolapse of the vitreous, iris, etc.

2 The Pressure Chambers of the Eye

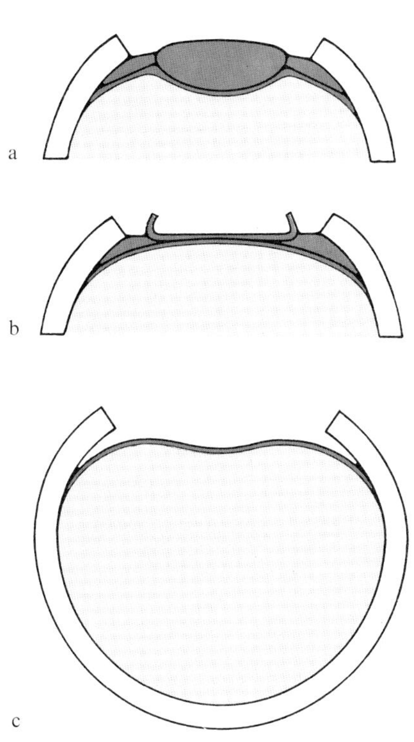

Fig. 120. **The vitreous chamber.** The pressure chamber deviates from a spherical shape by the volume of the anterior chamber or the anterior chamber and lens. The structure of its anterior wall, the diaphragm, is variable.

a The lenticulo-zonular membrane consists of the distensible zonular fibers and the relatively rigid lens. It is the most resistant part of the diaphragm.

b After the anterior lens capsule is opened, the diaphragm consists of the zonulo-capsular membrane, which contains no more rigid parts.

c If the zonulo-capsular membrane is breached, only the delicate hyaloid membrane remains

The **entire globe** is a pressure chamber, a sphere with a wall of relatively uniform stability (Fig. 119). This globe is subdivided by a diaphragm into two other pressure chambers: the *anterior chamber* and the *vitreous chamber*.

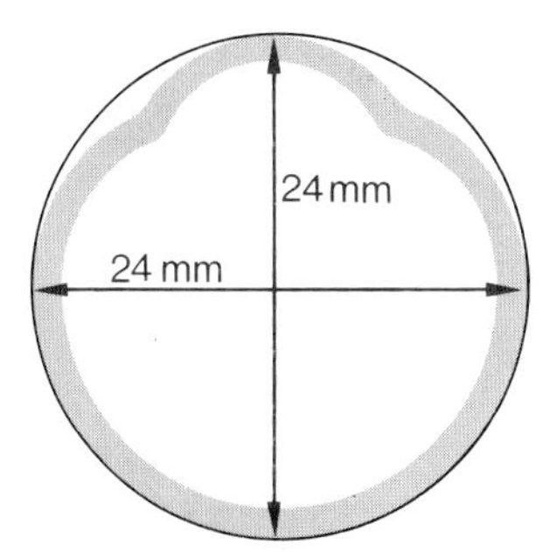

Fig. 119. **The eyeball.** The pressure chamber of the entire globe is approximately spherical. The stability of its wall, comprised of the cornea and sclera, is fairly homogenous

If the anterior chamber is opened (i.e., destroyed as a pressure chamber), one chamber still remains in the eye. This "**vitreous chamber**" differs from the eyeball as a whole in its *shape* and the *properties of its wall.* The anterior portion of this wall is formed by the *diaphragm,* which is less resistant than the sclera and consists of several membranes (Fig. 120). If one of these membranes is punctured during the course of an operation, it is no longer part of the pressure-chamber system, and the wall is weakened. The innermost membrane is the delicate *hyaloid membrane* of the vitreous body. If this membrane is ruptured, the pressure chamber is destroyed (Fig. 121).

Note: The *iris* is perforated by the pupil and so is actually *not* a part of the diaphragm. However, due to its opacity it is an important indicator of the behavior of the transparent membranes.

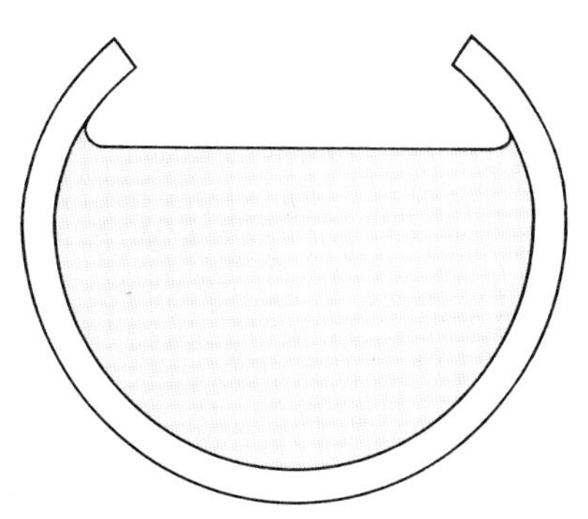

Fig. 121. **Destruction of the vitreous chamber.** If the anterior hyaloid is destroyed, the fluid of the vitreous body loses its membranous containment

3 Effects of Pressure Changes

The pressure in a pressure chamber is measured by determining the wall tension either by deformations of the wall itself or by a counterpressure exerted from the outside (measuring instrument).

In the pressure chamber of the **entire globe,** the tension of the homogenous wall can be estimated by palpation of the eye, or measured with an impression or applanation tonometer (Fig. 122a).

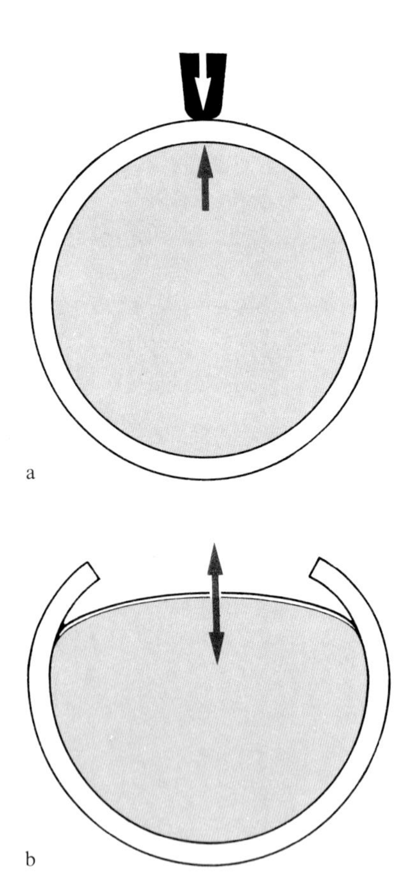

Fig. 122. **Determining the pressure in the pressure chambers**

a The pressure in the entire globe can be measured by applying an external counterpressure.

b The pressure difference between the anterior and vitreous chambers can be estimated from the position of the diaphragm

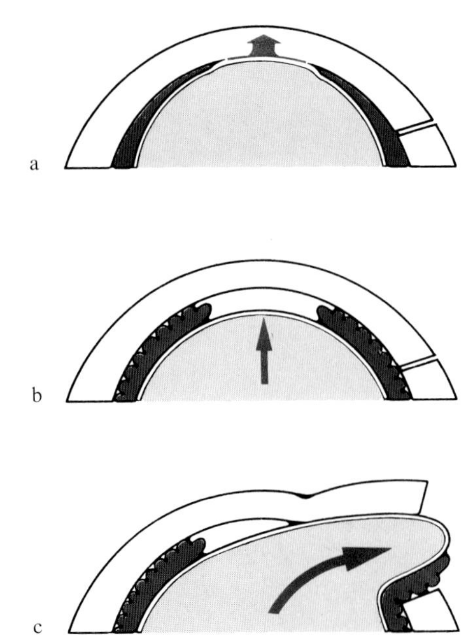

Fig. 123. **Positive pressure in the vitreous chamber after the anterior chamber is opened.**

a *Negative pressure* in the anterior chamber: The diaphragm is pulled forward by capillary attraction; the trabeculae of the iris are pressed flat against the posterior corneal surface, and normal iris relief is lost.

b A *pressure increase* in the vitreous space: The anterior chamber is drained, but some aqueous fluid remains in front of the diaphragm. The iris relief is maintained, because a pressure increase sufficient to flatten the iris would lead to the situation in **c**.

c *Positive pressure in the vitreous chamber* overcomes the elastic counterpressure of the cornea. The wound opens, the vitreous prolapses

In the **vitreous chamber,** pressure is estimated from the deformation of the more distensible part of the wall, the diaphragm. This is displaced either outward or inward from its normal position if a pressure difference develops between the anterior and vitreous chambers (Fig. 122b).

After the anterior chamber is opened the *position of the diaphragm* is an important criterion for assessing the situation: The diaphragm remains in its *original position* only if the pressure in the vitreous chamber does not exceed atmospheric.

If the diaphragm moves outward, the pressure in the vitreous chamber is elevated (Fig. 123b). The diaphragm will protrude even through the cornea if the elastic counterpressure there is insufficient (Fig. 123c).

On the other hand, if the pressure difference is caused by capillary attraction of the diaa

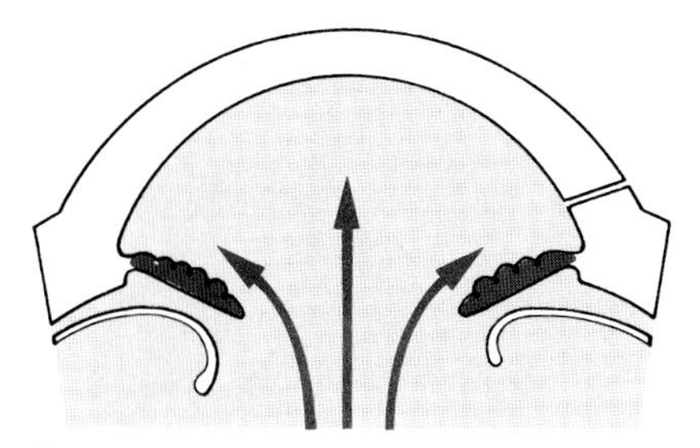

b

Fig. 124. **Equalization of pressure between the chambers ("reposition of the diaphragm")**

a Production of a *counterpressure in the anterior chamber.* A sufficient resistance to outflow from the pressure chamber must be created (e.g., by wound closure).

b *Pressure decrease in the vitreous body:* Vitreous transfer due to perforation of the diaphragm

phragm to the posterior surface of the cornea (Fig. 123a), it stems from a negative pressure in the anterior chamber. The vitreous pressure is not elevated in such a case, as evidenced by the immediate recession of the diaphragm when fluid reaches the wound edges and (due to the negative pressure) is drawn into the anterior chamber.

If the diaphragm recedes, pressure in the vitreous chamber is lower. If this is not due to a pressure increase in the anterior chamber, it must be the result of a pressure decrease in the vitreous chamber (Fig. 124), which can occur only through its destruction. Thus, spontaneous recession is a sign of vitreous loss due to perforation of the diaphragm.

4 Deformations of the Eye and Their Effects on the Pressure Chambers

Deformations of the pressure chambers are the cause of intentional[2] or unintentional[3] protrusions of tissue from the eye.

Any deformation of the **entire globe** will lead to a pressure increase if the wall of the eyeball is intact, or to the prolapse of solid or liquid material if the wall is perforated. The point at which the deforming forces are applied is immaterial (Fig. 125).

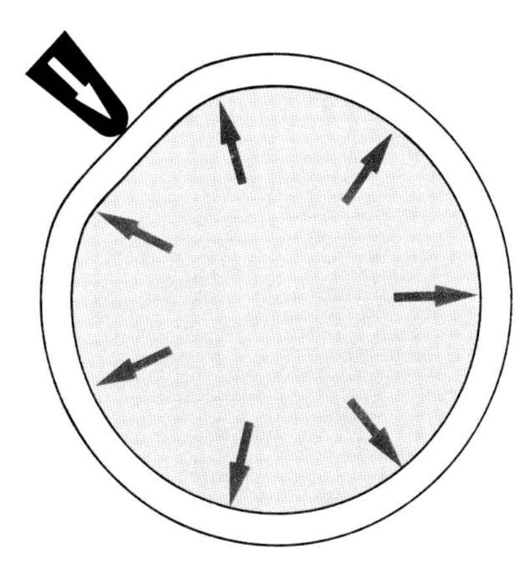

Fig. 125. **Deformation of the globe.** A sphere has the smallest possible surface area per unit volume. Any alteration of its shape will either increase the wall tension or reduce the volume. It does not matter where the deforming forces are applied (Pascal's law)

In the case of the **vitreous chamber,** however, the point of application is an important factor (Fig. 126). Deformations at the level of the *diaphragm attachment* produce extensive shifts of material and lead rapidly to the protrusion of tissue from the eye. Deformations *below the attachment* primarily raise the chamber pressure but may also lead to prolapse through stretching of the diaphragm.[4]

The two mechanisms of prolapse differ in that the former can be a "pressureless," purely geometric prolapse with a chance that

---

[2] Example: Lens expression.

[3] Example: Vitreous prolapse.

[4] Iris prolapse is based on different mechanisms, since the iris is not part of the diaphragm. A prolapsing iris first flattens against the wall of the globe, and then protrudes as pressure increases (Fig. 276c). Prolapse thus depends on the pressure in the entire globe and can therefore be produced even by deformations above the diaphragm (Fig. 126a).

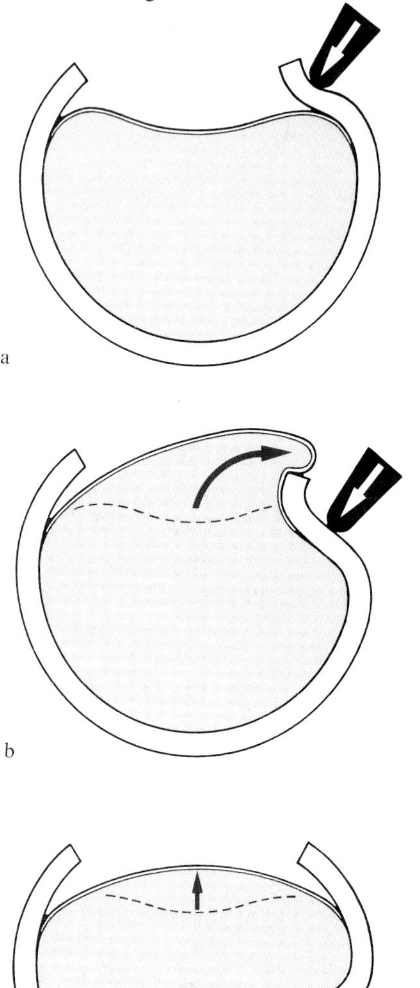

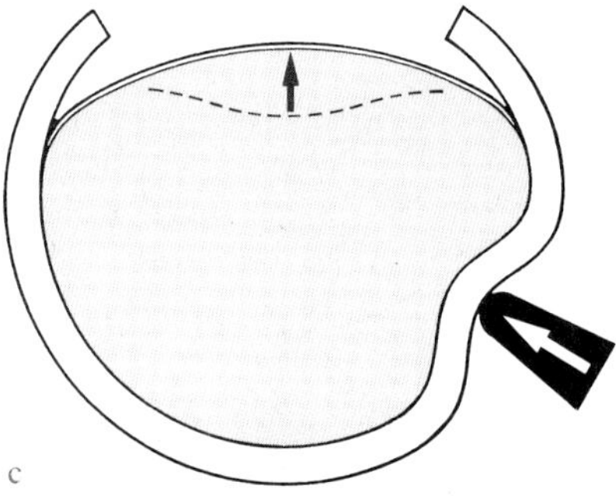

Fig. 126. **Deformations of the vitreous chamber.** The effects of a deforming force depend on its point of application.

a Deformation of the globe *above* the diaphragm does not affect the pressure chamber.

b Deformations at the diaphragm attachment relieve stress on the membranes and lead to a considerable "pressureless" shifting of substance.

c Deformations *below* the diaphragm lead to a pressure elevation in the vitreous chamber, increase the tension on the diaphragm and cause it to bulge

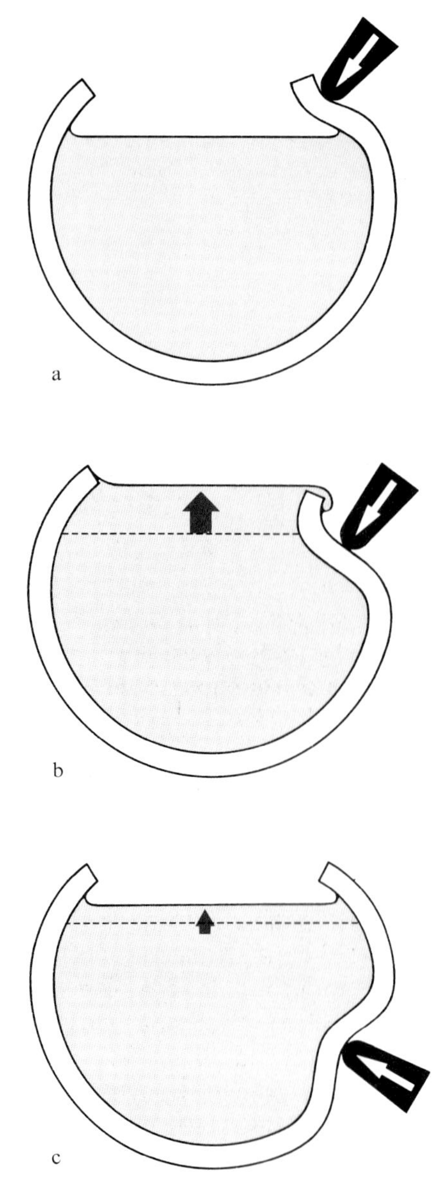

Fig. 127. **Deformation effects in the breached pressure chamber.** The effect depends on the site of the deformation.

a Deformations of the globe above the fluid level do not alter this level.

b Deformations at the fluid level reduce its surface area. The rise of the fluid face is large in relation to the volume displaced.

c Deformations below the fluid level do not alter its surface area and therefore cause a smaller rise than in **b**

the diaphragm has remained intact and that the condition can be reversed by eliminating its cause. In the latter, the prolapse is *pressure-induced,* and there is a considerable danger of rupture of the anterior hyaloid membrane.

If the pressure chamber of the vitreous is *destroyed,* the pressure can no longer increase, and a deformation causes only a shifting of vitreous substance. For a given volume of shift, the rise of the fluid level is greatest when the deformation reduces the surface area of the fluid (Fig. 127). Here, too, the effects of a deforming force depend upon its point of application.

5 The Origin of Deformations

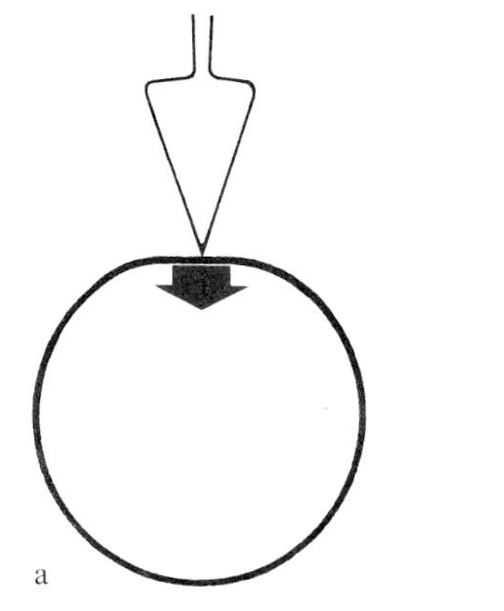

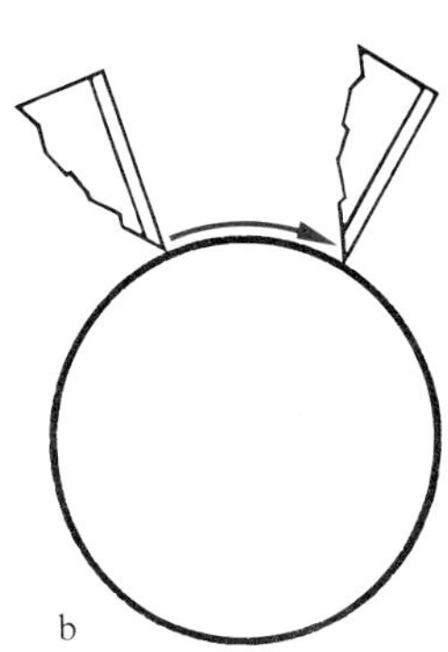

Fig. 129. **Effects of deforming forces on the fixated globe**

a Vector components in a perpendicular direction (toward the globe center): maximum deformation of the pressure chamber

b Vector components in a tangential direction (parallel to the globe surface): minimum deformation

Forces applied to the globe partially *deform* it and partially *displace* it. Which effect is predominant depends on the resistance of the globe wall to deformation and the resistance of the orbital contents to displacements of the globe. The smaller the latter resistance, or the greater the *passive mobility of the globe*, the less it will be deformed by a force.

The **inward mobility** of the globe is limited mainly by the resistance of the *orbital cushion* (Fig. 128a). Its **outward mobility** is limited by the extensibility of the *eye muscles* (as well as any obstructions such as lid retractors, rigid lid margins, etc.) (Fig. 128b). In **movements of the globe about its center of rotation,** like the rotation of a spheroidal joint in its socket, all the anatomical conditions are geared toward *maximum* mobility; hence the resistance is minimal (Fig. 128c).

All events which restrict the passive mobility of the globe[5] increase the risk of deformation by the action of unplanned forces. At the same time, forces which are intended to act directly on the tissue are fully utilized only if the globe is rendered immobile. Thus, unrestricted passive mobility is desirable as a *long-term safety strategy* during most of the operation, but will be abolished *for short intervals* by fixation when a particular manipulation requires it.

When the globe is fixed, only the **direction of application of a force** determines whether the pressure chambers will be deformed (Fig. 129): The deformation is maximal under a *perpendicular* force, and minimal under *tangential* forces.

[5] Example: An increase of orbital tissue resistance due to infiltration or hemorrhage (Fig. 128a); muscular tension (Fig. 128b, c).

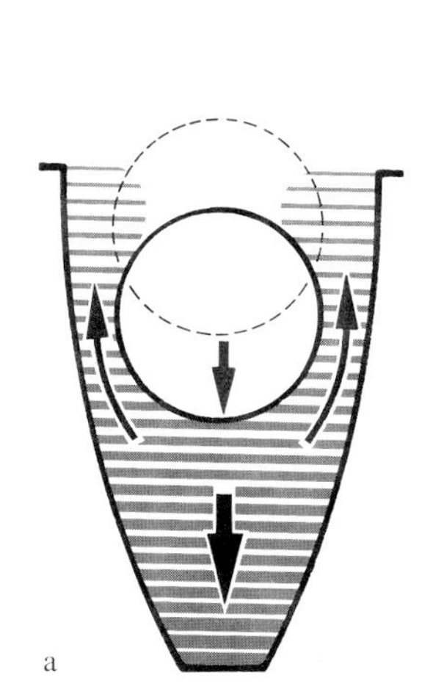

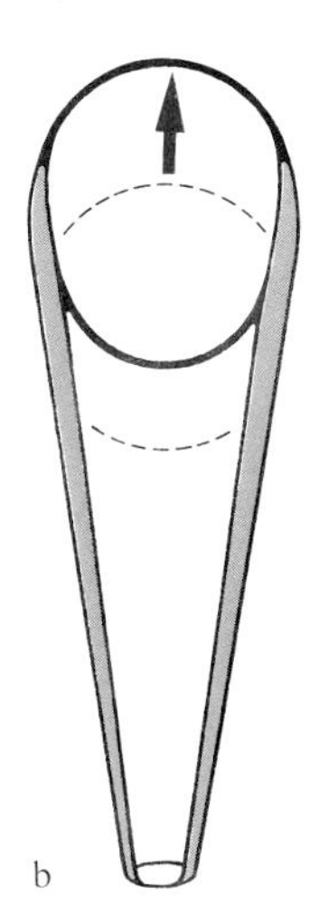

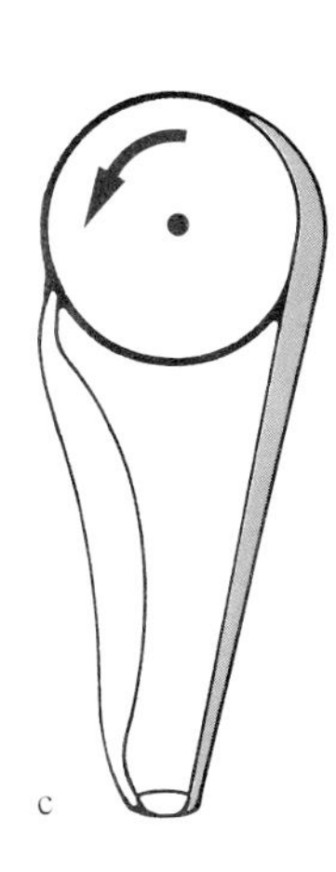

Fig. 128. **Passive mobility of the globe**

a The resistance to inward movements of the globe depends on the compliance of the orbital cushion

b Resistance to outward movements of the globe. The ocular muscles are stretched by outward traction; if stretched sufficiently, they will even indent the globe wall

c Resistance to movements about the center of rotation. Rotary movements meet little resistance and are restricted only in case of a high muscle tone

6 Margin of Deformation

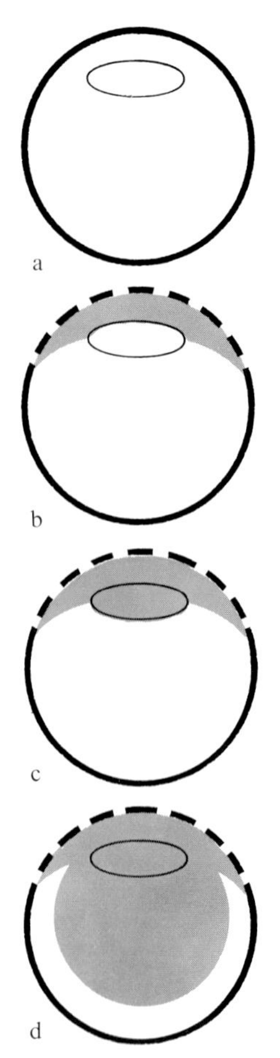

Fig. 130. **Margin of deformation**

a Goal of surgical strategy: Integrity of the entire globe. No loss of tissue or fluid is acceptable. The margin of deformation is determined by the ratio of wall strength to intraocular pressure

b Goal: Integrity of the vitreous chamber. Aqueous loss is now acceptable. The margin of deformation (*pink*) equals the volume of the aqueous chamber.

c Goal: Integrity of the vitrous chamber, but lens extraction is planned. The margin of deformation is increased, now equaling the volume of the lens and anterior chamber.

d If vitreous loss is acceptable, the margin of deformation corresponds to practically the intire internal volume of the eye

Since deformations of the globe are unavoidable during surgery, it must be determined how great the deformations may be without jeopardizing the operative result. The magnitude of the deformation-induced displacement of tissue which can still be tolerated is called the *margin of deformation*. Its extent depends upon the operative goal (Fig. 130). For example, no loss of substance is acceptable if the pressure chamber of **the entire globe** must remain intact. In this case the margin of deformation is determined by the *wall strength* and the *intraocular pressure*. If the integrity of **the vitreous chamber** is the goal, the loss of aqueous fluid is acceptable, and the margin of deformation equals the *volume of the anterior chamber*. If removal of the lens is also planned, the margin of deformation is increased by the lens volume. Finally, if **vitreous loss** is acceptable, the margin of deformation equals almost the entire contents of the globe.

The margin of deformation available to the surgeon will in each case determine the necessary precision of the surgical manipulations. A large margin is an important safety factor and gives the surgeon freedom in his choice of methods. Every attempt will be made to *increase the margin of deformation*, therefore.

If the integrity of the *entire globe* is required[6], this is ensured by increasing the wall strength (by secure wound closure) or by reducing the intraocular pressure (limiting aqueous production[7] or reducing the globe volume[8]). As for the *vitreous chamber*, the margin of deformation can be increased by reducing the vitreous volume (reducing aqueous production has no effect!).

In contrast, a small margin of deformation limits the operative possibilities by proscribing many techniques. If one of the events described in the previous chapters produces a deformation and thus "uses up" a portion of the original margin, a smaller margin of deformation is left for further manipulations.

Thus, the margin of deformation can vary during the course of an operation. If the surgeon is to apply his measures correctly and modify them as needed[9], he must constantly monitor the situation to determine the margin of deformation available at any given time. A sudden *decrease in the margin of deformation*[10] is an important **warning sign.** If it cannot be ascribed to the surgical manipulations themselves, then it is due to endogenous deforming forces[11] which must be quickly identified and brought under control.

[6] Such problems are encountered in the postoperative phase following intraocular surgery and are to be considered in all potentially deforming measures involved in postoperative care, as well as in globe-deforming operations following prior surgery (e.g., retinal detachment surgery after cataract extraction).

[7] Example: Carboanhydrase inhibitors.

[8] Example: Osmotically active substances, bulbar massage.

[9] Example: Switching from an intrabulbar to extrabulbar iridectomy, or from extraction to expression during a lens delivery.

[10] Rise of intraocular pressure or bulging of the diaphragm.

[11] Example: Muscular tension, expulsive hemorrhage.

7 The Prevention of Deformations

The eye cannot be completely protected from external forces, as this would require its complete mechanical encasement. Partial corsets can be used to protect the areas most exposed to danger. But partial corsets are themselves a source of deformation if they are tilted by external forces, the resulting displacement of tissue depending on the dimensions of the system (Fig. 131).

Localized wound areas can be protected from deformation by specially-shaped corsets (Fig. 131 d). To protect the **entire vitreous chamber,** measures must be limited to protecting those *areas* whose deformation is most hazardous, from those *forces* which are most likely to cause such deformations. This can be achieved with stabilizing rings affixed at the muscular insertions, which are incidentally also at the level of the diaphragm attachment (Fig. 132). Of course such rings cannot prevent indentation of the globe by the eye muscles more posteriorly at points where the globe diameter exceeds the ring diameter (Fig. 133). To protect the equatorial region as well, an additional corset is required.

In all efforts at mechanical protection, the investment of time and labor must be weighed against the expected gain. These efforts will be dictated mainly by the degree to which deformations can be tolerated[12].

[12] This is especially true for equatorial rings (Fig. 133b, c). Their disadvantages include the technical difficulties of fixation as well as the increased deforming action of the larger system size. On the other hand, forces applied in the equatorial region produce relatively slight effects (Figs. 126c, 127c) which can be adequately absorbed by a moderately large margin of deformation.

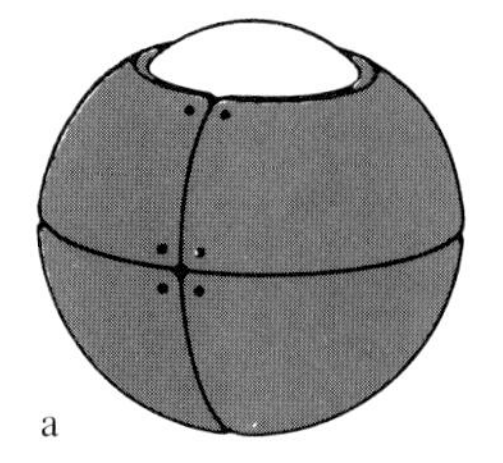

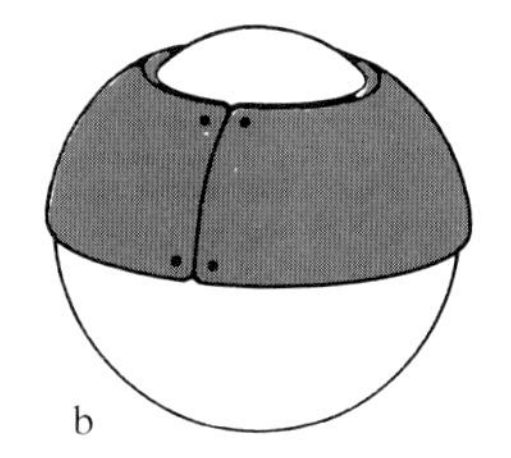

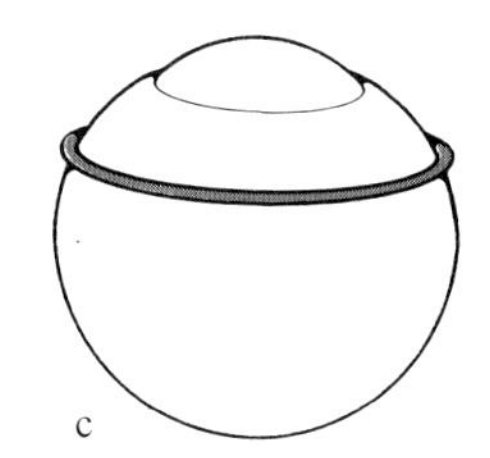

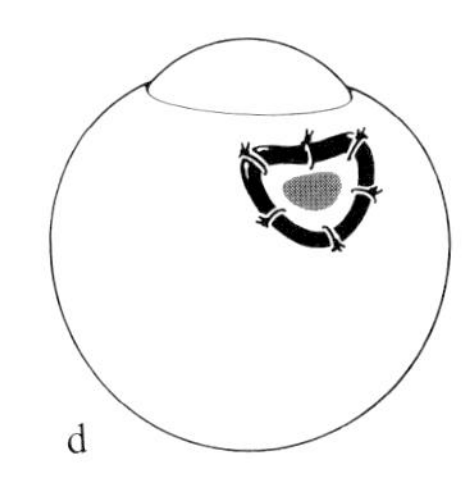

Fig. 131. **Corset systems**

a Complete protection could be achieved only by the complete mechanical encasement of the eyeball and is therefore unfeasible.

b Partial corsets can themselves produce deformations with a resulting displacement that depends on the width of the system.

c Reducing the width ultimately leads to an annular system.

d Local deformation of a circumscribed wound area is prevented by a corset which follows the wound contour

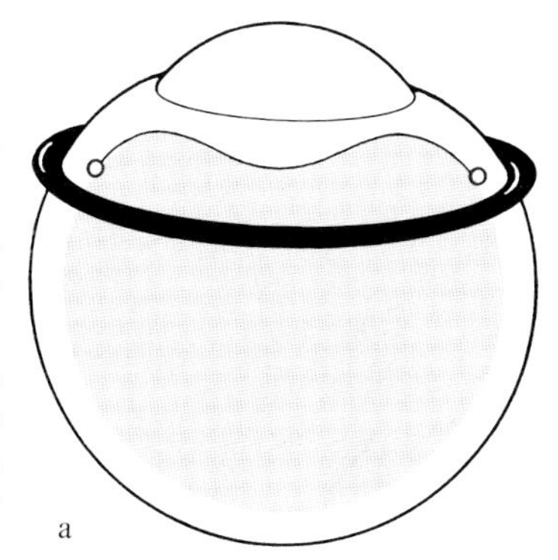

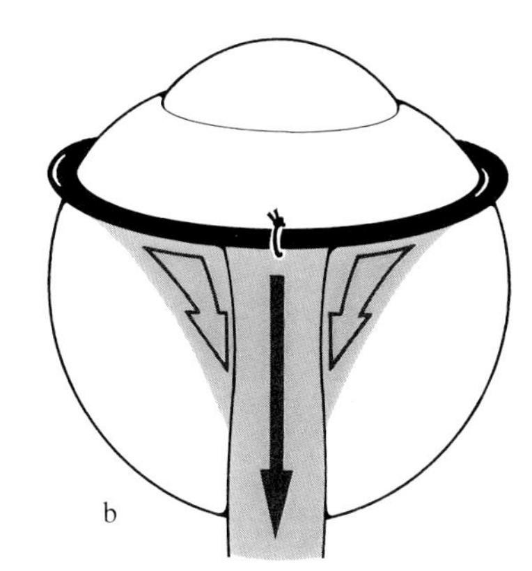

Fig. 132. **Stabilization of the vitreous chamber**

a A ring, fixed at the level of the diaphragm attachment, protects against those deformations which cause the greatest shift of intraocular tissue (see also Figs. 126b, 127b).

b If the ring is sutured in place at the insertions of the muscles, their force is distributed over a larger and more stable area, and thus their deforming action is reduced (see also Figs. 128b and c)

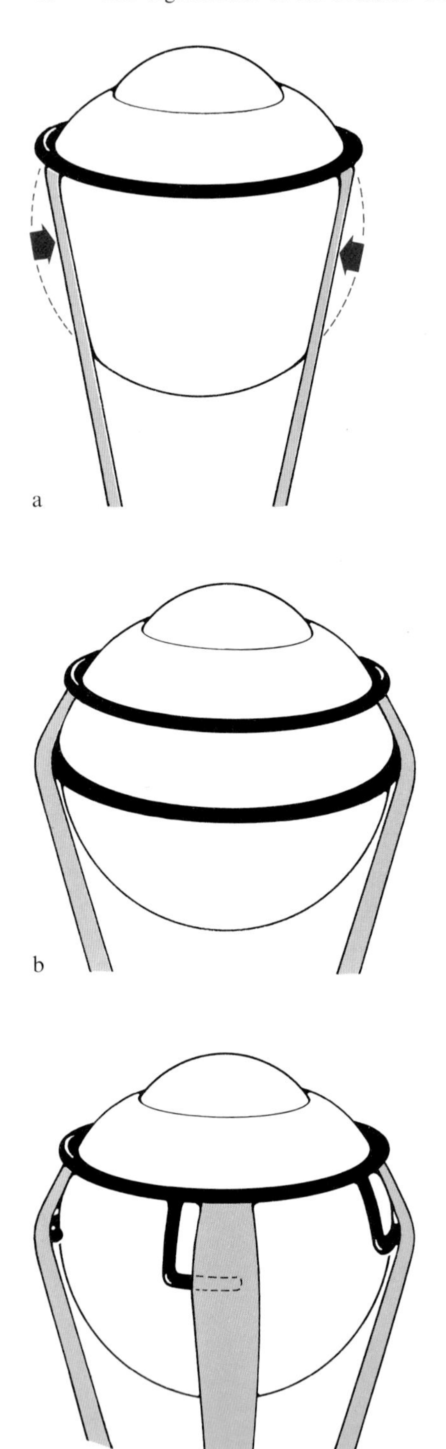

Fig. 133. **Protection of the equatorial region.**

a Indentation of the equatorial region by ocular muscle contraction.

b Such deformations can be reduced by an additional ring attached at the equator.

c If the corset systems are interconnected by bridges to facilitate insertion below the muscles, the system area is increased (analogous to Fig. 131 b)

8 Safety Strategy

From our analysis of the effects of forces on the pressure chambers of the eye, we can derive general guidelines for the development of a "safety strategy".

The **prime safety factors** are *unrestricted passive mobility of the globe* and a *large margin of deformation.*

Thus, increasing both factors is the goal of all preoperative measures, sedation, anesthesia, and medication to lower the vitreous pressure. They are also important during preparation of the operative field, the selection of lid retractors, the indications for canthotomy, etc. Direct protection of the globe (by corsets) is possible only to a limited degree and is effective only if an adequate margin of deformation is present.

Once the operation has begun, safety can be maintained by placing minimal demands on the available safety margins during manipulations. This is done by:

- limiting movements of the globe to *rotation about its center,*
- selecting operative methods in which perpendicular vectors are avoided and instruments are applied *parallel to the globe surface.*

III Preparation of the Operative Field

1 General

Preparation of the operative field must be undertaken with the greatest care, for errors in this phase jeopardize the course of the operation and are often impossible to correct later on.

Before the operation actually begins, a check is made to determine whether the goals of the preparatory phase have been achieved:

- loss of pain sensation
- immotility of the extraocular muscles
- unrestricted passive ocular mobility:
  - no exophthalmos through orbital infiltration
  - no contact of eyeball with lid margin or lid retractor
- no deformation of the eyeball (reduced margin of deformation), i.e., no increase of intraocular pressure.

2 Disinfection

No means are known for effecting total sterilization of the operative field. For this reason, intraocular surgery cannot be undertaken if a *manifest germ reservoir*[1] is present, and must be postponed until this reservoir has been cured.

The **palpebral skin** and the **cilia**[2] are treated with topical disinfectants. The palpebral glands should be redisinfected at the end of the preparatory phase, since germs may have been extruded by insertion of the lid retractors, etc. Additional protection is afforded by applying *impermeable adhesive drapes* to the skin out to the margins of the lids. These drapes should be as compliant as the palpebral skin so that they create no tension when the lids are retracted.

The **conjunctiva** may be treated only with mild disinfectants, which should be applied by copious flushing to penetrate all folds up into the fornix.

Since the operative field is not completely sterile despite all measures, any intraocular manipulation poses a risk of infection which can be reduced only if strict limits are placed on the indications for such measures, and unnecessary incisions, irrigations, etc. are avoided. Fluid accumulated in the conjunctival sac must be continuously removed lest it enter the interior of the eye through a wound. Instrument parts which are introduced into the eye should not come in contact with the fingers, lids, cilia or conjunctiva.

As a general rule, the risk of contamination increases with the *duration of the operation.*

3 Anesthesia

Ocular anesthesia has two goals: to abolish *sensory* innervation and thus produce insensibility, and to paralyze *motor* innervation to prevent muscular contractions and increase passive ocular mobility by reducing the myogenic tone.

None of the ordinary techniques satisfies all the requirements of an ideal anesthesia (Table 2), but this is not necessary in every operation. The most suitable techniques can be selected according to the type of operation planned and can often be combined to achieve an optimal effect.[3]

3.1 Instillation Anesthesia

The ocular structures most sensitive to pain are the integument (conjunctiva and cornea) and the anterior uvea (iris and ciliary body).

Topical anesthetics such as oxybuprocaine and lidocaine are used to anesthetize the conjunctiva and cornea. **Deep-acting anesthetics** such as cocaine can produce anesthesia for most intraocular operations. Instillation anesthetics are thus adequate for procedures in which unrestricted muscular motility does not jeopardize the operative goal.

---

[1] Example: Infectious skin diseases, dacryocystitis, conjunctivitis.

[2] Resection of the cilia yields only a slight advantage compared with the patient's postoperative discomfort, since the main source of microorganisms is not so much the cilia themselves as the hair follicles and their glands.

[3] For example, the dangers in the final phase of general anesthesia can be avoided if the palpebral and ocular muscles have been immobilized by infiltration anesthesia. In the case of large perforation wounds, it may be advisable to mitigate the consequences of deformations during administration (in both injection and general anesthesia) by increasing the margin of deformation by preplacing a few apposition sutures under instillation anesthesia.

3.2 Injection Anesthesia

Injection anesthesia can produce insensibility through infiltration of the ciliary ganglion, immobilize the eye through infiltration of the ocular muscles, and prevent lid closure by paralysis of the orbicularis muscle.

Adequate margins of safety[4] are essential for injection anesthesia, since infiltration of the tissues by the injected substance itself or a hematoma can reduce passive ocular mobility and may even decrease the margin of deformation in some cases. This is also true if reinjection is necessary to prolong the anesthesia. The range and duration of action of the anesthetic can be influenced by the presence of *additives*.[5]

3.3 Akinesia of the Orbicularis Muscle

Akinesia of the orbicularis muscle is induced to prevent closure of the lids.

Direct infiltration of the muscle is associated with a swelling of the lid which may interfere with the course of the operation. Conduction anesthesia of the facial nerve does not affect the operative field (Fig. 134). **Preauricular**

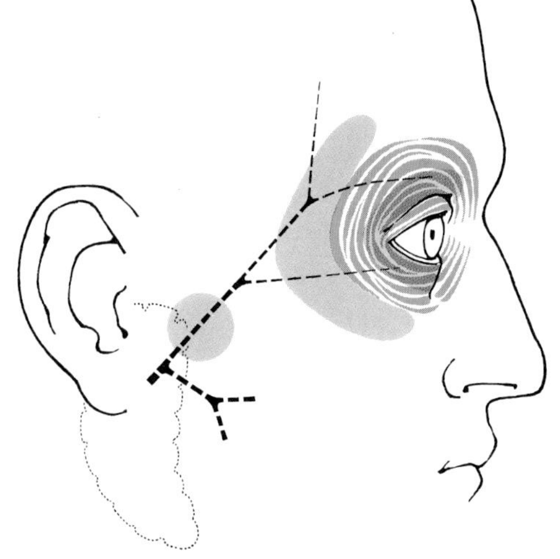

Fig. 134. **Means of producing akinesia of the orbicularis muscle**

From right to left: Direct infiltration of the orbicularis muscle. Parorbital conduction anesthesia. Preauricular conduction anesthesia

[4] Intact or securely-sutured globe wall.

[5] *Hyaluronidase* promotes the diffusion of the anesthetic in the tissue through the depolymerization of hyaluronic acid in the interstitium (but has no effect on proteins, i.e., on the capillary walls, sclera, fibrin or blood coagula). The action of hyaluronidase can be enhanced by mechanical pressure on the injected area (compression, massage). The duration of action of the anesthetic is shortened by the increased diffusion.
Vasoconstrictors (epinephrine, octapressin) prolong the action of the anesthetic. They inhibit the absorption of the agent and lower its general toxicity. The risk of hemorrhage is reduced, but the critical blood flow to some tissues (e.g., the optic nerve) may also be diminished. Vasoconstricting agents may have generalized effects as a result of absorption, so any contraindications to such additives must be considered prior to operation.

Table 2. **Comparison of various anesthetic techniques.** The colored squares show where the practical techniques satisfy the requirements of an ideal anesthesia.

	Insen-sibility	Akinesia	Effect on passive mobility of the globe		Effect on margin of deformation	
			Increase	Decrease	Danger of decrease during initial phase	during final phase
Ideal anesthesia	+	+	+	–	–	–
Instillation anesthesia	+	–	–	–	–	–
Retrobulbar anesthesia	+	+	+ by relaxation of muscles	+ infiltration of orbital tissue (dose dependent)	+ infiltration of orbital tissue (dose dependent)	–
General anesthesia	+	+	+ with good muscle relaxation	(+) without relaxation	(+) in case of technical difficulties: (defense, agitation, vomiting)	(+)

akinesia (Fig. 135A) requires only a small injection of anesthetic. It blocks all the zygomaticotemporal fibers but may also block the descending branches, which can cause transitory oral paralysis. **Parorbital akinesia** (Fig. 135B) infiltrates the nerve over the bony orbital rim. Infiltration of the fibers leading to the outermost parts of the orbicularis is important, since they are particularly active in lid closure.

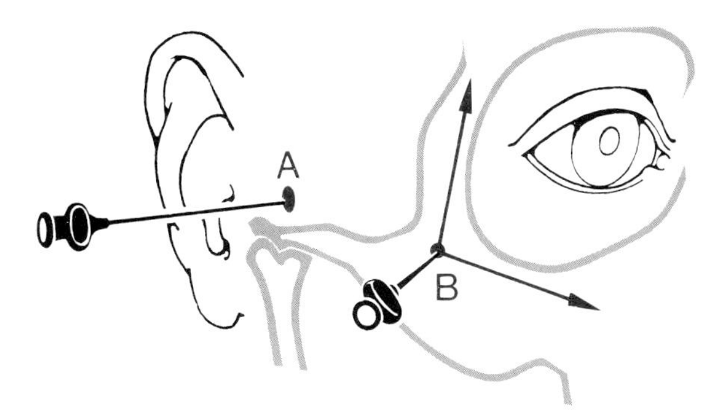

Fig. 135. **Injection sites for producing conduction akinesia**

A Preauricular injection: about 1 cm^3 is injected at a depth of 1 cm anterior to the tragus, i.e., anterior to the mandibular tubercle (which can be located by palpation when mouth is opened and closed).

B Parorbital injection: puncture is made over the highest point of the zygomatic arch, which affords access in all directions. Needle is inserted upward and nasally along the bony orbital margin. The needle is withdrawn to the tip before changing direction in order to avoid traumatizing slewing movements within the tissue

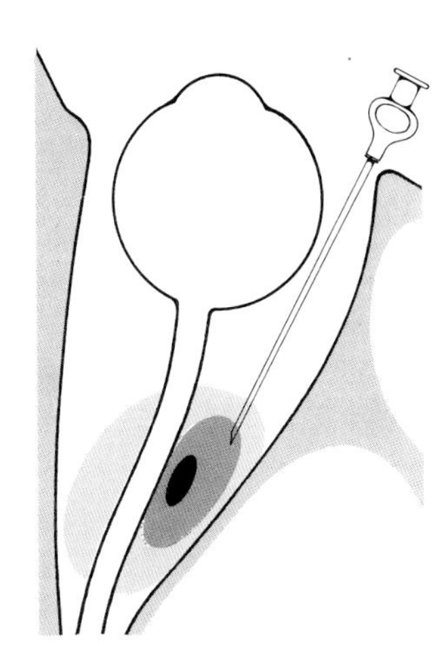

Fig. 136. **Retrobulbar infiltration.** To avoid optic nerve injury, the needle should be kept in the temporal half of the orbit and should penetrate no farther than 1.5 cm behind the globe

3.4 Retrobulbar Anesthesia

Retrobulbar anesthesia is done to block the *ciliary ganglion* and paralyze the *ocular muscles*. This is achieved by a diffuse infiltration of the posterior portions of the muscle cone, with care taken to avoid danger zones, especially the orbital apex, where the optic nerve, veins, and other structures are in such close proximity that they will not yield to an advancing needle and are therefore highly vulnerable to puncture (Fig. 136). An important factor in the avoidance of undesired lesions is the quality of the cannula with regard to tip shape, rigidity and length (Fig. 137).

In **transcutaneous injection,** the cannula reaches the muscle cone by piercing the lid, orbital septum, fascia and orbital fat

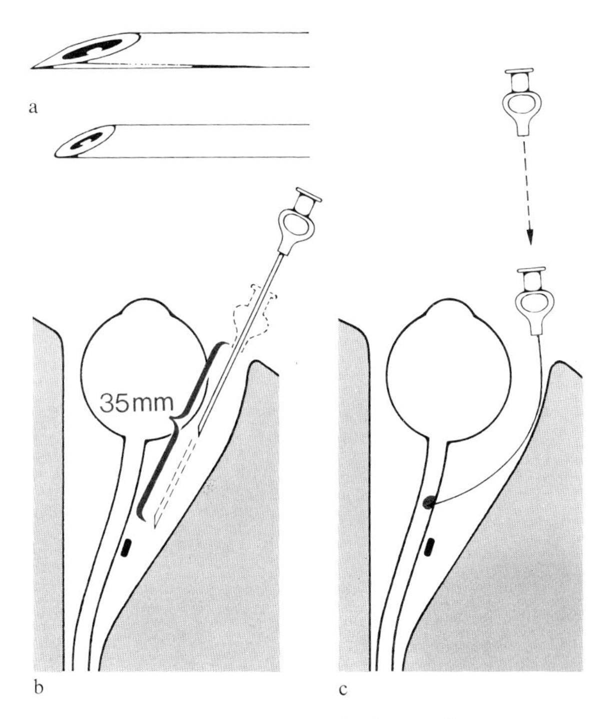

Fig. 137. **Requirements of the injection needle**

a *Tip:* Should have blunt shape to reduce cutting ability (*below*).

b *Length:* Should not exceed 3.5 cm (from orbital margin) so that it cannot reach the apex.

c *Rigidity of cannula:* Rigid needles do not deviate from the guidance direction (see also **b**). Flexible needles, on the other hand, follow the path of least resistance and often deviate in unpredictable ways. If then a correction is attempted by guiding the cannula more forcibly in the desired direction, the opposite effect is achieved

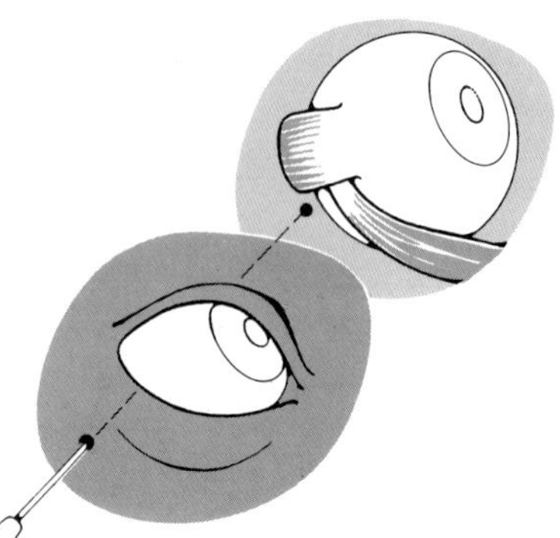

Fig. 138. **Transcutaneous injection.** Puncture is made in the lower temporal quadrant about 6 mm from the lid margin (below the tarsus, which would hinder puncture; sufficiently above the bony orbital margin, which would hinder corrective movements of the cannula). If the patient looks upward, the inferior oblique muscle is removed from the needle path. At the same time, the peribulbar fascial tissue is stretched and so is more easily pierced by the needle

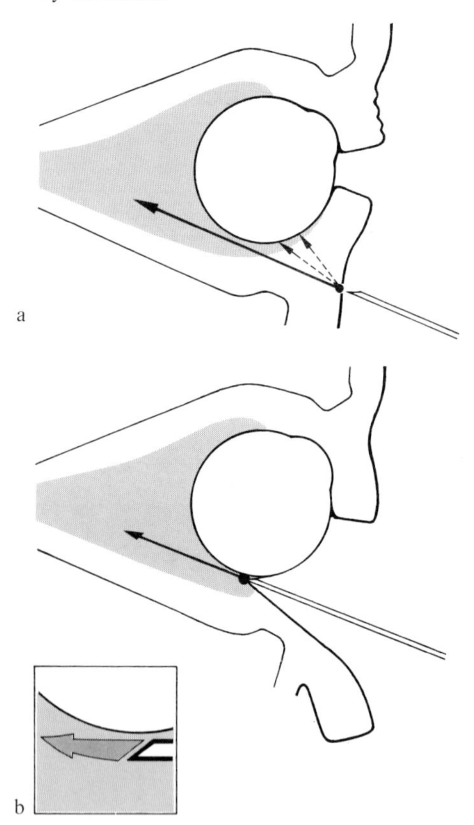

Fig. 139. **Comparison of transcutaneous and transconjunctival injection**

a *Transcutaneous injection:* If inserted at a steep angle, the needle may enter nearly perpendicular to the globe surface (especially in the elongated myopic eye), with a danger of perforation.

b *Transconjunctival injection:* Inserted behind the equator, the cannula will always bypass the globe at a tangent. Inset: If the blunt side of the needle tip is against the globe, the tip will glide harmlessly along the sclera and optic nerve sheath

(Figs. 138 and 139a). In this case the relatively high superficial cutaneous resistance makes it difficult to judge the resistance offered by deeper structures.

In **transconjunctival injection,** the cannula is inserted at the fornix and passed through the peribulbar fascia directly into the muscle cone (Fig. 139b). The main difference between transcutaneous and transconjunctival injection is that in the latter, the cannula tip is inserted *beyond* the largest globe diameter and so is unlikely to perforate the eyeball.

3.5 Infiltration Anesthesia of the Superior Rectus Muscle

Upward eye movement combined with closure of the lids (Bell's phenomenon) is one of the characteristic defensive movements of the eye. To prevent this movement, which removes the upper operative field from the palpebral aperture, the superior rectus muscle is anesthetized by direct infiltration.

The muscle is reached by inserting the needle through the superior fornix (Fig. 140) and advancing it toward the orbital apex.

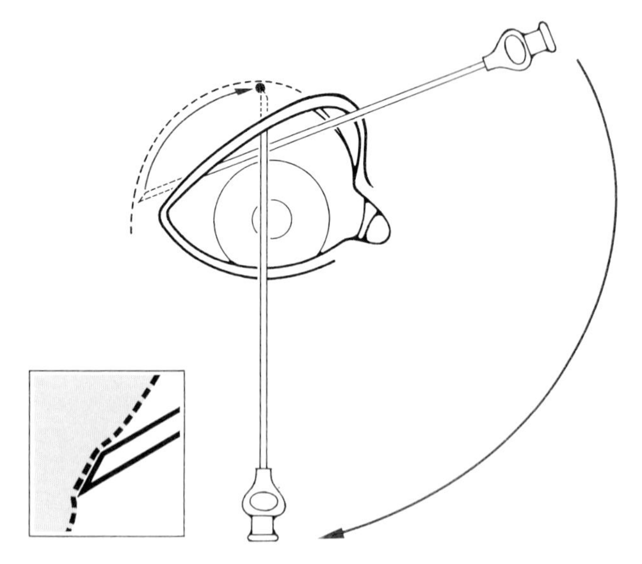

Fig. 140. **Infiltration of the superior rectus.** The poorly-accessible superior fornix is reached by applying the needle tip at the easily-accessible lateral fornix and (with the blunt side leading!) allowing it to sweep upward beneath the upper lid in a swiveling motion. The needle is then inserted and advanced toward the orbital apex

4 Maintaining Separation of the Lids

Simple spreading of the lids (Fig. 141) is an imitation of the *natural opening movement,* and all movements are consistent with the normal function of anatomical structures. However, this form of separation provides only a small exposure and does not eliminate lid pressure on the eye.

In **retraction of the lids** (Fig. 142), the lids are pulled away from the globe, and an *unphysiologic deformation* of the lid region results. Specifically, the margins of the lids are stretched and tend toward a circular shape, forming what we shall call the "palpebral circle" (Fig. 143). The upper and lower margins are pulled outward and orbitally, the lateral margin inward and frontally.[6] The final position of the palpebral circle, when the lid margins are on maximal stretch, depends on the resistance of adjacent tissue structures. Theoretically (i.e., in the absence of anatomical obstructions) it lies on the plane between the lateral palpebral ligament insertions at the orbital margin.

The movements associated with lid retraction cause a widespread shifting of tissue which may influence the passive mobility of the globe: If the palpebral circle is raised away from the globe when formed (Fig. 144a), pressure on the orbit is relieved and ocular mobility is increased. If on the other hand the circle is lowered toward the globe (Fig. 144b), resistance from the orbital cushion increases, and ocular mobility is reduced. If the globe comes in direct contact with the lid margins or lid retractors, there is an imminent danger of deformation, i.e., of a decrease in the margin of deformation.

[6] In theory, both the inner and outer canthus should move inward. Due to the strong fixation of the nasal canthus, however, only the lateral canthus is mobile.

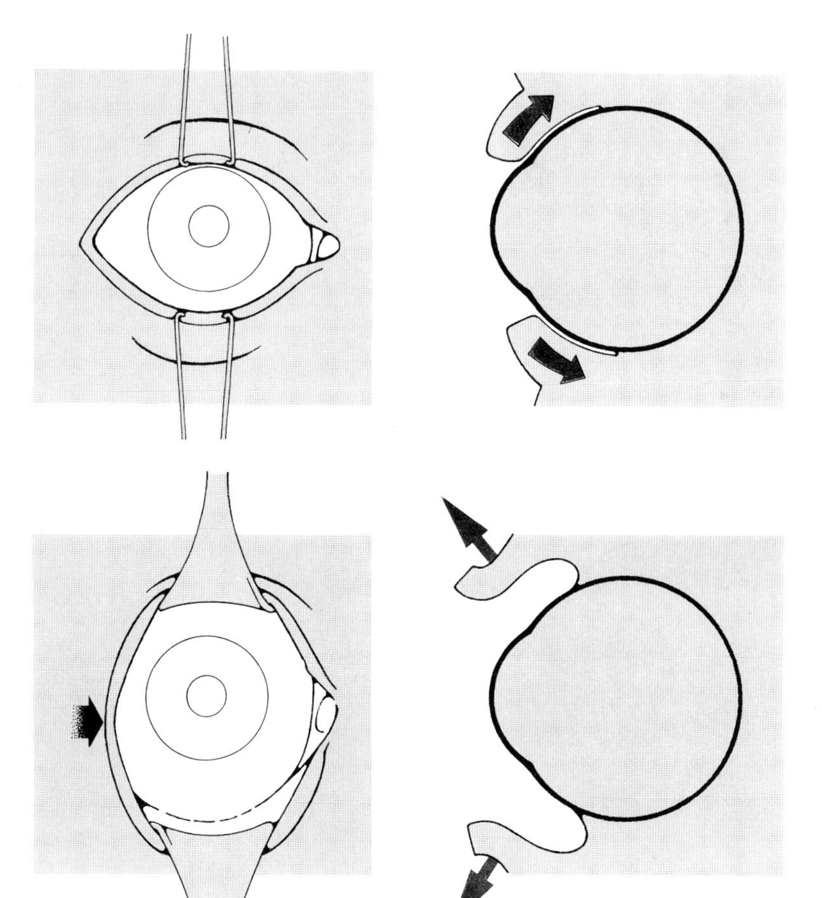

Fig. 141. **Simple spreading of the lids.** Normal palpebral aperture with normal direction of traction

Fig. 142. **Retraction of the lids.** The palpebral aperture is enlarged by lifting the lids away from the globe

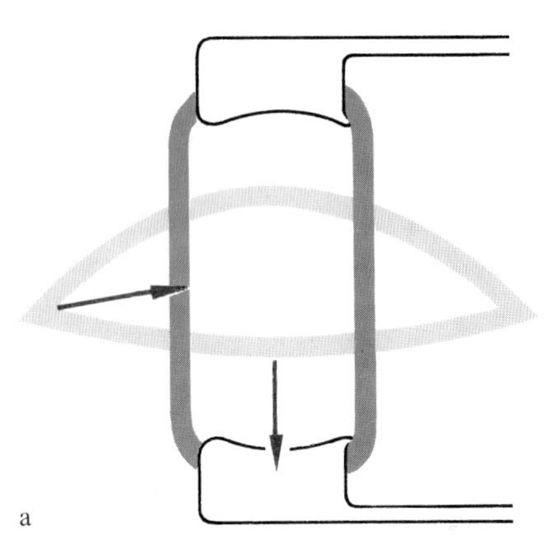

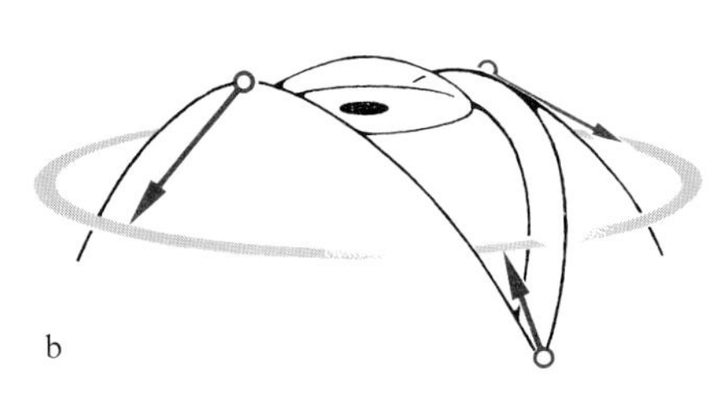

Fig. 143. **Formation of palpebral circle by stretching of the lid margins.** When stretched, the lid margins tend toward circularity.

a When the palpebral aperture is increased in a vertical direction, its horizontal diameter is reduced and the lateral lid margin is pulled inward. If tension is uniform, a circle results. Maximum tension with lid retractors produces an upright ellipse.

b In an attempt to lie in a single plane, the upper and lower lid margins move outward and downward, while the lateral margin moves inward and upward

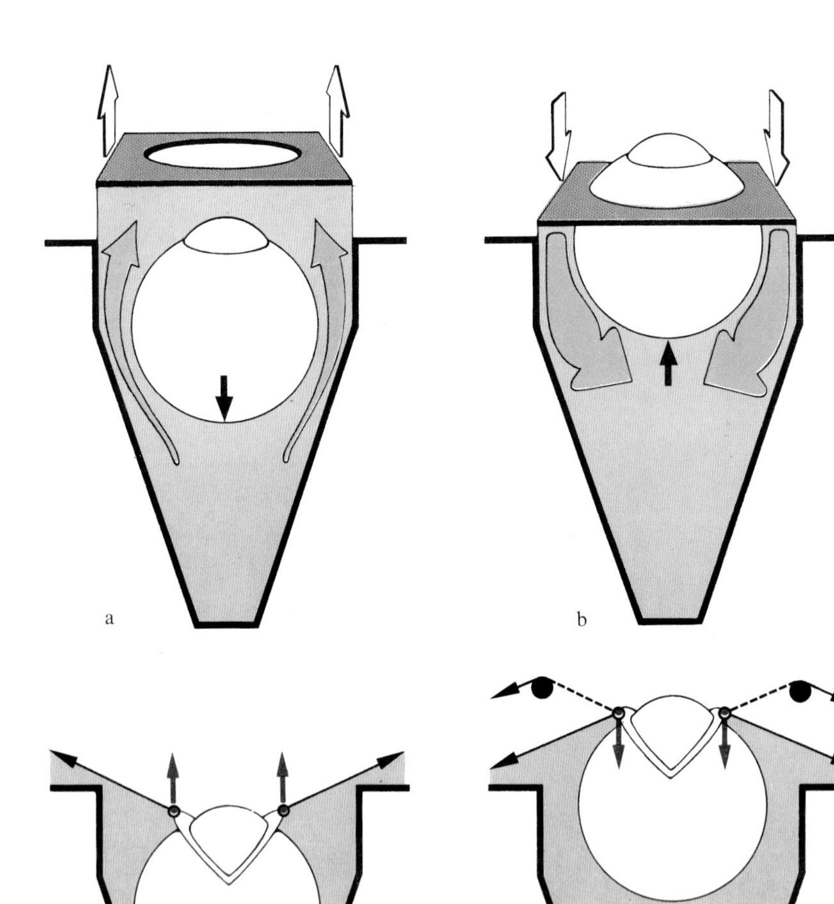

Fig. 144. **Movement of the palpebral circle in relation to the globe**

a If the circle is raised, tissue from the orbital cavity is pulled along with it; the globe recedes, the eye muscles relax, and passive mobility of the globe is increased.

b If the circle is lowered, orbital tissue is compressed; the globe is pressed forward, and passive mobility is decreased

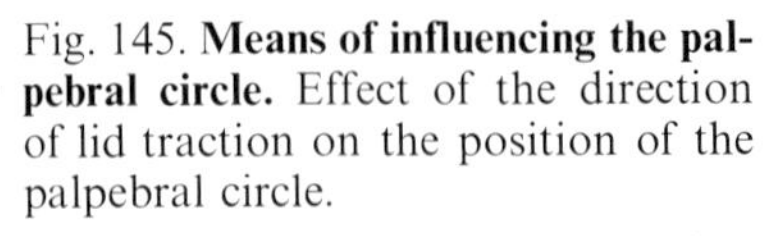

Fig. 145. **Means of influencing the palpebral circle.** Effect of the direction of lid traction on the position of the palpebral circle.

a If the globe is deeply set, lid traction toward the orbital margin creates outward-directed vectors, and the palpebral circle is raised.

b If the globe is protuberant, lid traction toward the orbital margin (*A*) has an inward-directed component, and the palpebral circle is lowered. To raise the circle, the direction of traction must be altered by struts or supports (*B*) to create conditions as in **a** (*broken line*)

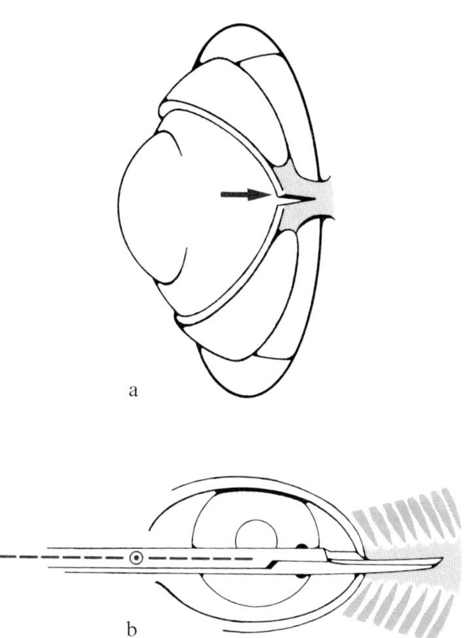

Fig. 146. **Canthotomy**

a The incision to increase the palpebral circumference causes little trauma if made along the lateral muscle raphe.

b This raphe lies on the line connecting the inner and outer lid margins and is engaged by applying a straight scissors to the temporal canthus such that its handle is directly over the nasal canthus. To keep the contiguous tissue layers (skin, fatty tissue, muscle and lateral palpebral ligament) from shifting during cutting, they are divided with a single snip of the scissors; the tissue layers can be thinned beforehand by compression with a clamp to facilitate cutting

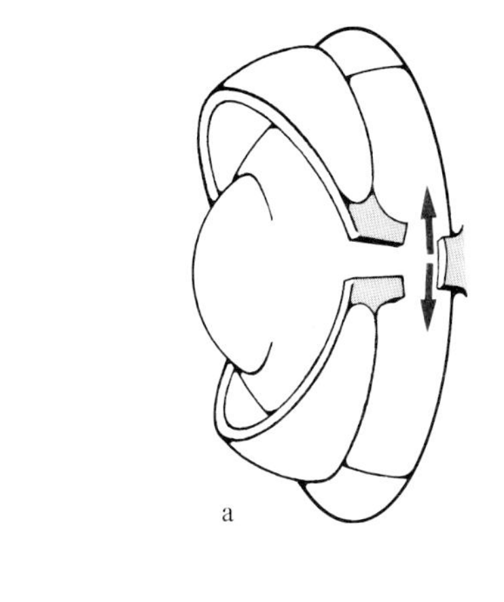

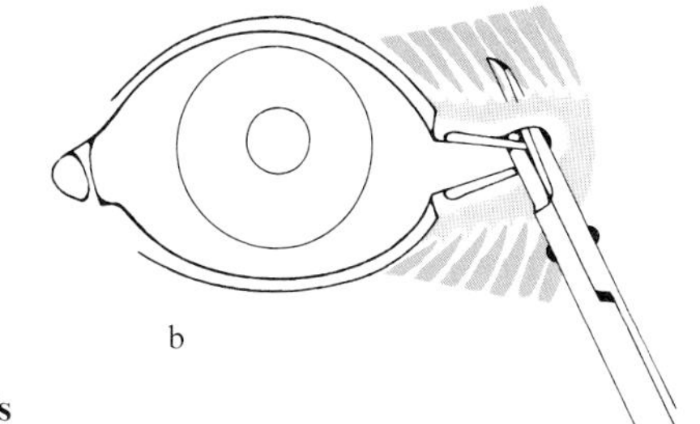

Fig. 147. **Cantholysis**

a If the tight lateral ligament prevents raising of the palpebral circle, its limbs are separated from their periosteal attachment.

b The ligamentous attachments are located from the canthotomy incision by probing upward and downward along the inner margin of the orbit. Cutting directly over the periosteum will help prevent hemorrhage. Traction on the tarsus makes it easier to identify the ligaments and judge the effect of the procedure

For these reasons, an attempt is made to *raise* the palpebral circle away from the globe. If this does not happen spontaneously by virtue of the anatomical configuration of the orbital region (Fig. 145a), active *outward traction* must be applied during lid separation (Fig. 145b). This is especially necessary in the protuberant eye, because here the palpebral circle is always drawn against the orbita. This requires special apparatus[7] to redirect the traction in an outward direction. Anatomically, the possibilities of raising the level of the palpebral circle are limited by the extensibility of the lateral palpebral ligament.

The configuration of the palpebral circle can be surgically altered by *canthotomy* (Fig. 146), which increases the palpebral circumference and thus relieves pressure from the lateral lid margin. *Cantholysis* (Fig. 147), or section of the palpebral ligaments, is employed if these bands prevent the palpebral circle from being adequately raised.

Instruments for maintaining lid separation: Traction sutures (Fig. 148) are suitable for *simple spreading of the lids*. If used for lid retraction, difficulties may arise: They have a tendency to evert the tarsal margins if the globe is recessed, and lower the palpebral circle if the globe is protuberant (Fig. 145b) unless passed over special supports on the cheek and forehead.

Lid hooks are inserted beneath the lid margin to effect *retraction* of the lids. The diameter and level of the palpebral circle can be adjusted as needed with **simple lid hooks** (Fig. 149), but they must be handled by an

[7] Example: Traction sutures passed over a support on the forehead; lid retractors fitted with special struts.

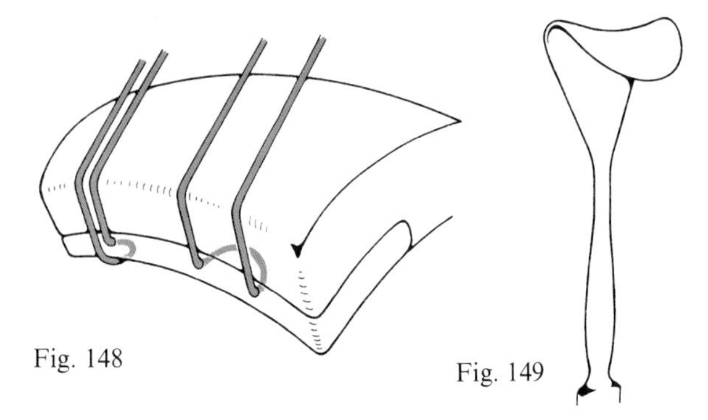

Fig. 148. **Traction sutures.** If passed through the tarsus, traction sutures are firmly anchored owing to the strength of the tissue and there is no danger of hemorrhage from the muscle and marginal artery

Fig. 149. **Simple lid hooks.** The back of the hook is curved to conform to the shape of the globe

experienced assistant who can recognize special situations as they arise. In the **self-retaining lid retractor (lid speculum),** the hooks for the upper and lower lids are interconnected. If the speculum is of the spring-tension type, the palpebral aperture depends entirely on the interaction between lid tension and the spring tension and cannot be adjusted (Fig. 150a). If retraction is maintained by a *screw thread* or *screw clamp,* a specific aperture can be set and adjusted as needed (Fig. 150b). The net weight of the instrument determines whether it can ride upward (i.e., outward) with the palpebral circle. Heavy retractors depress the circle and must be supported on the bony orbital margin by mechanical means.

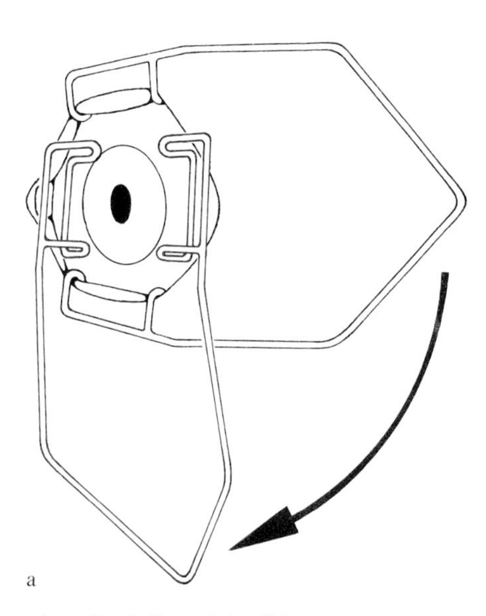

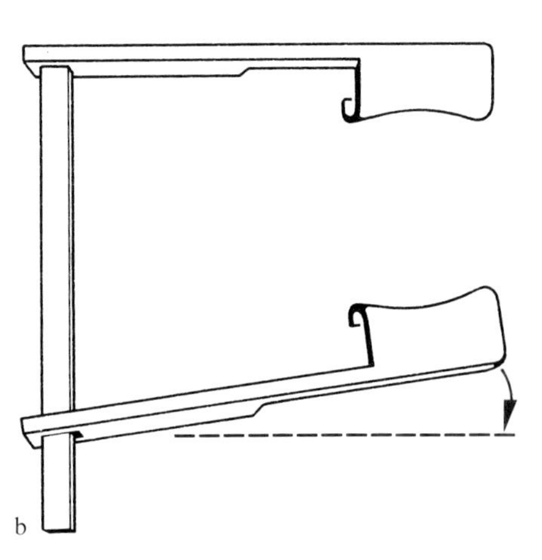

Fig. 150. **Self-retaining lid retractors**

a Light wire speculum with spring tension. The retractor is removed by rotating it out of the palpebral fissure.

b Lid speculum based on the screw-clamp principle. To remove, the branches are grasped near the connecting post and are first spread apart slightly (*arrow*) to loosen, then are slid together

5 Fixation of the Globe

Fixation serves to limit the passive mobility of the globe so that the force vectors of the operative instruments can be optimally applied. However, if forces act on a fixated globe which are independent of the operator (muscular traction, for example), there is a danger of deformation which can be averted only by *immediately releasing the fixation* to restore ocular mobility.

In **point fixation** (Fig. 151), passive movements of the globe are prevented only if the force vector passes through the center of rotation of the eye and the point of instrument fixation. All vectors from other directions will cause the globe to rotate sideward. Thus unplanned forces tend to displace, rather than deform, the globe.

Zonal fixation (Fig. 152) immobilizes the eye against vectors from various directions. However, one result of this stronger fixation is that unplanned forces [8] now have a tendency to deform the globe rather than displace it.

The quality of the fixation depends on the firmness of the tissue between the fixation instrument and sclera. Of course it is best when the globe is grasped directly by the sclera.

[8] Example: Resistance to a blunt cutting instrument.

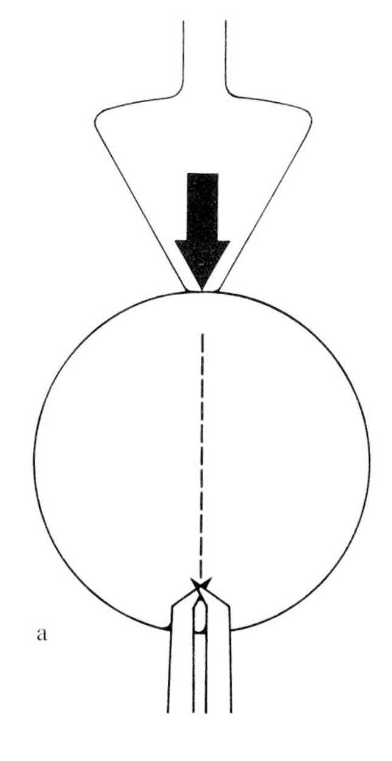

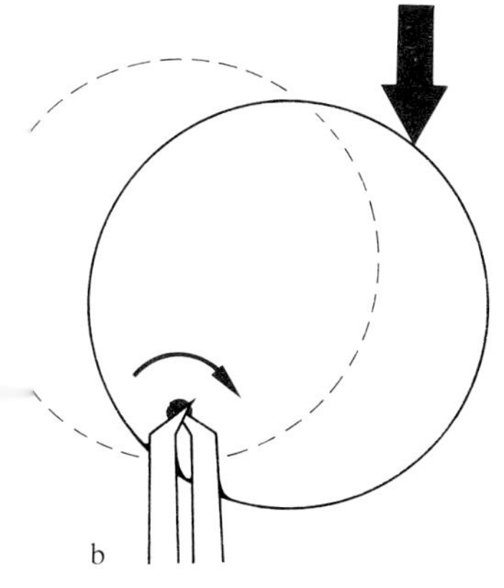

Fig. 151. **Effect of point fixation**

a Point fixation resists only that force vector which passes through the ocular center of rotation and the fixation site.

b If vectors from other directions are applied, passive eye movements acquire a new center of rotation, namely the point at which the fixation instrument is applied

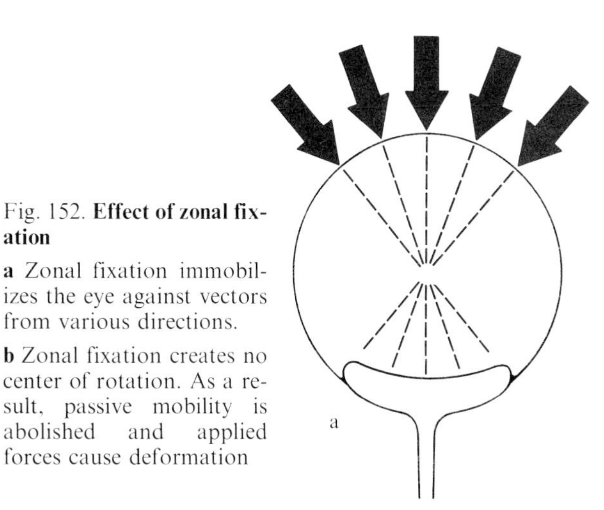

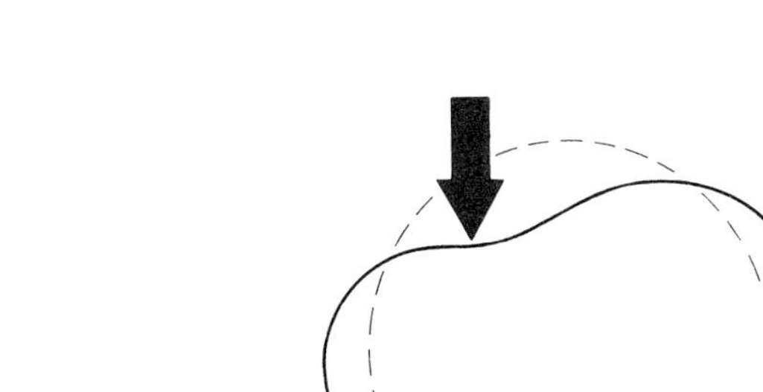

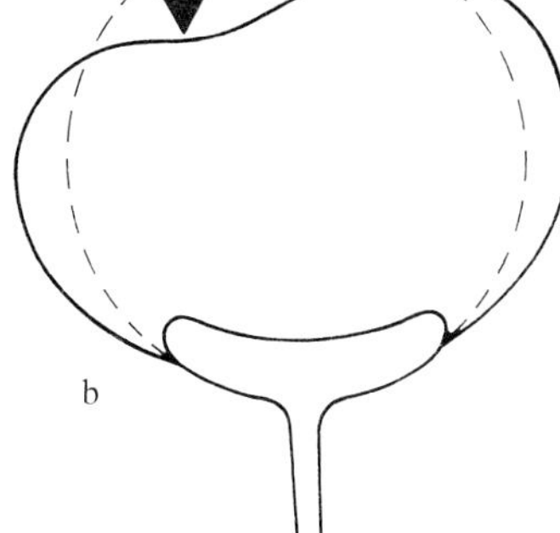

Fig. 152. **Effect of zonal fixation**

a Zonal fixation immobilizes the eye against vectors from various directions.

b Zonal fixation creates no center of rotation. As a result, passive mobility is abolished and applied forces cause deformation

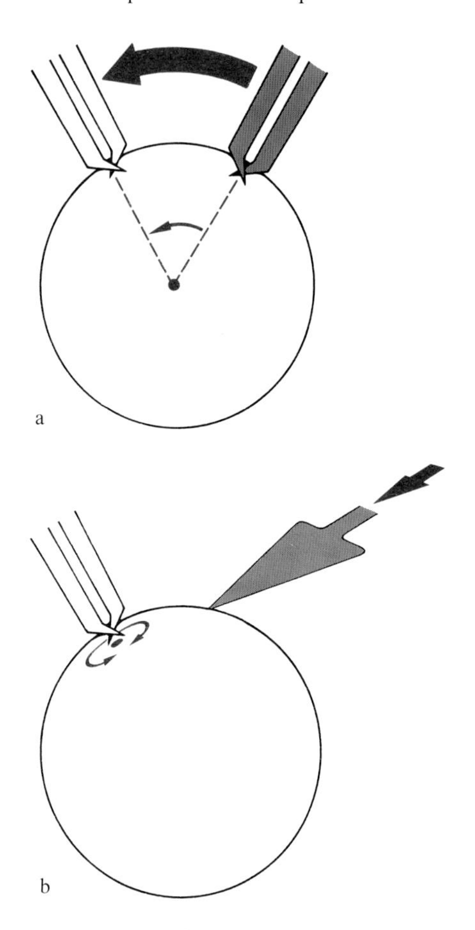

Fig. 153. **Centers of rotation during passive ocular movements**

a Intentional rotation of the eye with fixation instruments takes place about the center of rotation at the center of the globe.

b In contrast, the center of rotation for compensatory movements during operative manipulations on the fixated eye lies at the application point of the fixation instrument

Fixation at ocular adnexa is most effective if applied close to their attachment (e.g., the insertion for muscles, the limbus for the conjunctiva).

Note: Eye movements take place about the center of rotation at the globe center during manipulations with fixation instruments, and about the fixation point during manipulations with operative instruments.[9] As a result, the right and left hand rotate the globe about different points! (Fig. 153).

6 Traction Sutures for Orienting the Globe

Traction sutures are used to rotate a particular part of the globe into the operative field. The rotation achieved depends on the site of suture placement relative to its fulcrum (Fig. 154).

The sutures can be attached directly to the sclera or the adnexa. If the tissue between the suture and sclera is firm,[10] the control of ocular rotation is improved, but the fixation effect is correspondingly increased.[11] If the tissue is more yielding, only part of the traction will be transmitted to the globe.[12] The eye then remains somewhat mobile, and this may be advantageous from a safety standpoint, especially if the free ends of the traction sutures are not controlled by an assistant but are immovably clamped in place.

[9] In some cases, i.e., if resistances dictate, the operative instrument may produce a fixation effect of its own.

[10] Example: Attachment to the sclera or a muscular insertion.

[11] Immobilization is not the true purpose of traction sutures! Should a fixation effect occur, the suture must be released at once if the eye is moved by unplanned forces, e.g. active muscular contraction.

[12] Example: Attachment to a tendon or muscle belly.

7 Sutured-On Corset Rings

Local rings (Fig. 131 d) stabilize the wound edges during excisions from the globe wall and thus facilitate the accurate fitting of grafts.

Rings for *protecting the vitreous chamber* (Fig. 132) are applied to prevent complications in case of diaphragm rupture, i.e., if the diaphragm is already damaged prior to operation or if its intraoperative destruction is anticipated.

Applied too tightly, rings are themselves a source of deformation (Fig. 155). Therefore the sutures should be left somewhat *loose*. This will not impair the corset function, since the rings become part of a scleral system which in itself is not absolutely rigid.

a

b $\alpha > 0$ c $\alpha = 0$

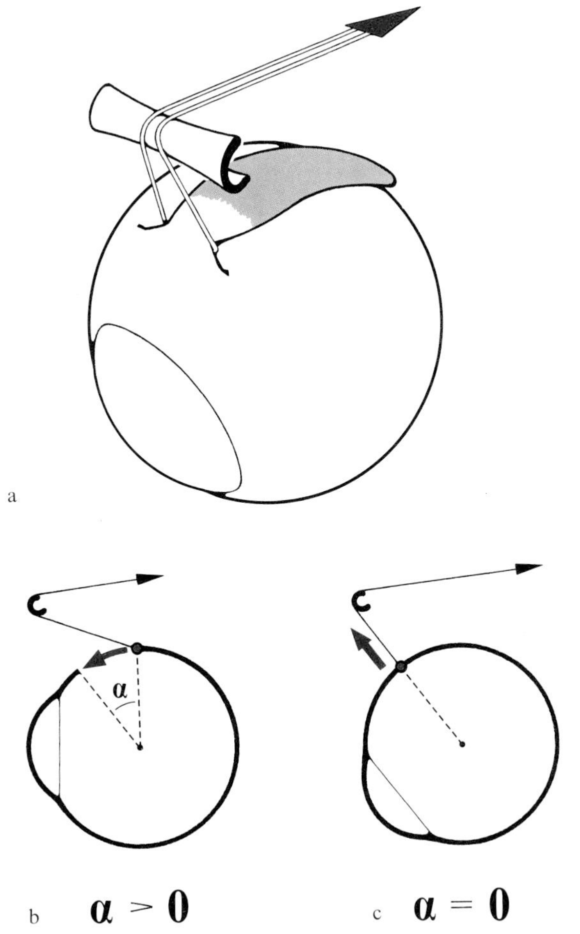

Fig. 154. **The action of traction sutures**

a The suture is passed back over the fulcrum formed by the edge of the lid retractor.

b The resulting rotation is determined by the angle α between the line joining the center of rotation with the fulcrum, and that joining the center of rotation with the point of suture attachment.

c If $\alpha = 0$, rotation ceases. Pulling the suture only raises (and may deform) the globe

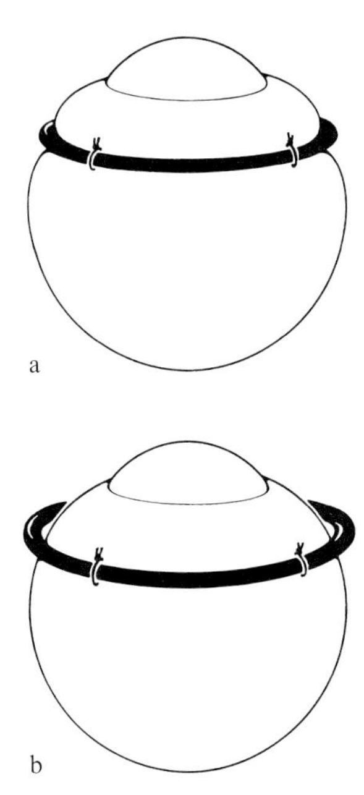

Fig. 155. **Sutured-on corset rings**

a If sutured on too tightly, the rings deform the globe.

b Slightly loose attachment preserves the shape of the zone of diaphragm attachment

8 Placement of Transconjunctival Muscle Stutures

If traction or corset-ring sutures are to be attached to an ocular muscle, the tendon must be grasped and pierced transconjunctivally, and thus under conditions of poor vision (Fig. 156).

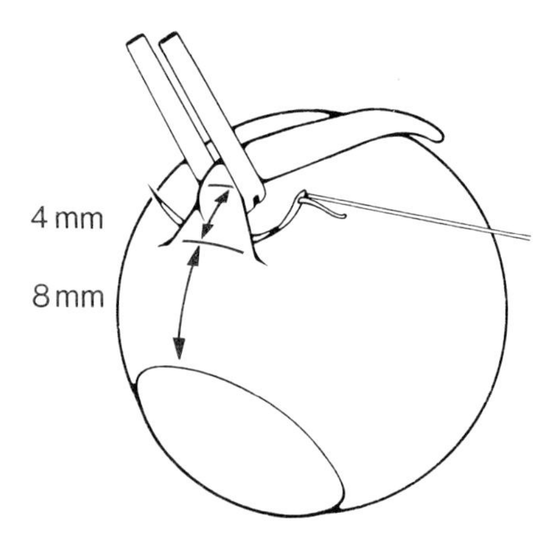

Fig. 156. **Transconjunctival muscle suture.** The tendon is grasped far enough behind its insertion that it can be pressed into a bulge. The needle is passed close to the scleral surface

The muscle is grasped through the conjunctival layer with a *mouse-tooth forceps* whose tooth length is commensurate with the thickness of the tissue layer to be traversed (Fig. 157). Since the teeth can grasp the muscle tendon only when perpendicular to the globe surface, the intended grasping site must be rotated into view either with a second instrument[13] or with the grasping forceps itself (Fig. 159).

To avoid perforations, the needle tip is guided *parallel* to the globe surface when inserted, so that no vectors directed toward the sclera are produced (Fig. 158).

[13] Examples: Forceps applied at the lower limbus; squint hook thrust into the lower fornix.

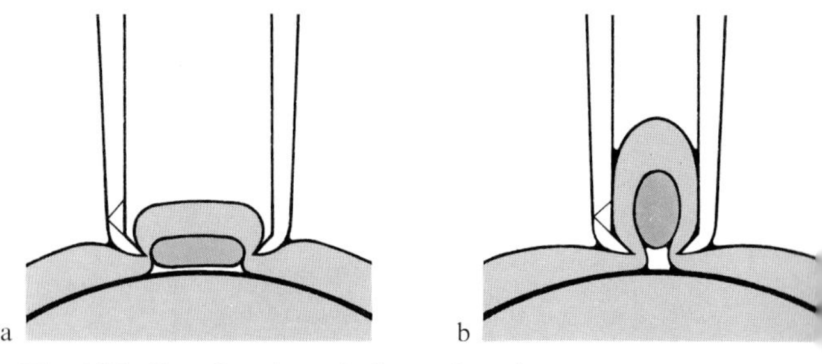

Fig. 157. **Grasping through the conjunctiva**

a To grasp the muscle, the forceps blade spacing must be greater than the width of the muscle so that the teeth can slip below the tendon.

b By bringing the blades together, the tendon is made to bulge away from the globe surface

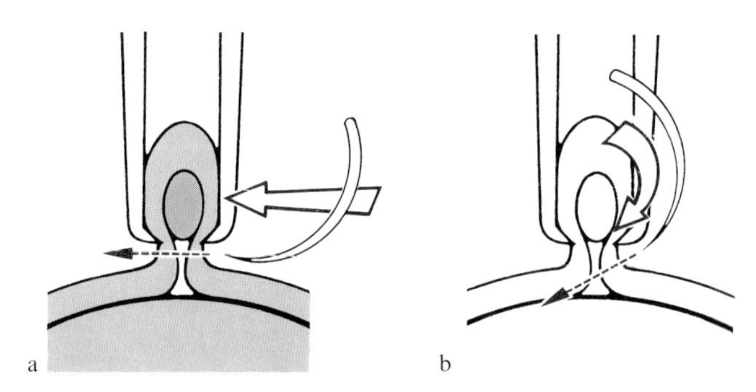

Fig. 158. **Passing the muscle suture**

a The needle tip is pushed through the tendinous bulge strictly parallel to the scleral surface.

b If the needle is passed in a rotary movement, vector components directed toward the sclera are created, with a danger of perforation

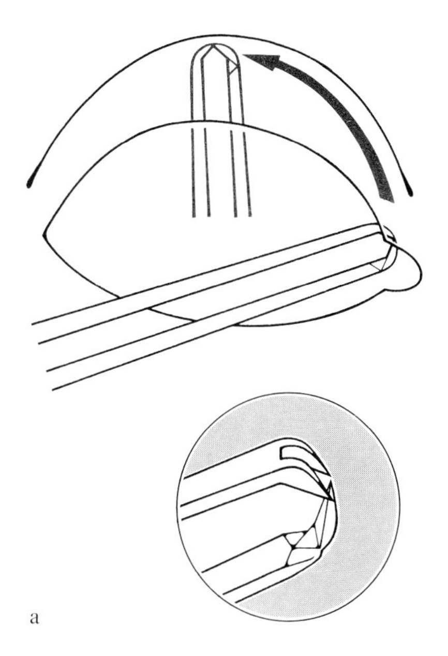

a

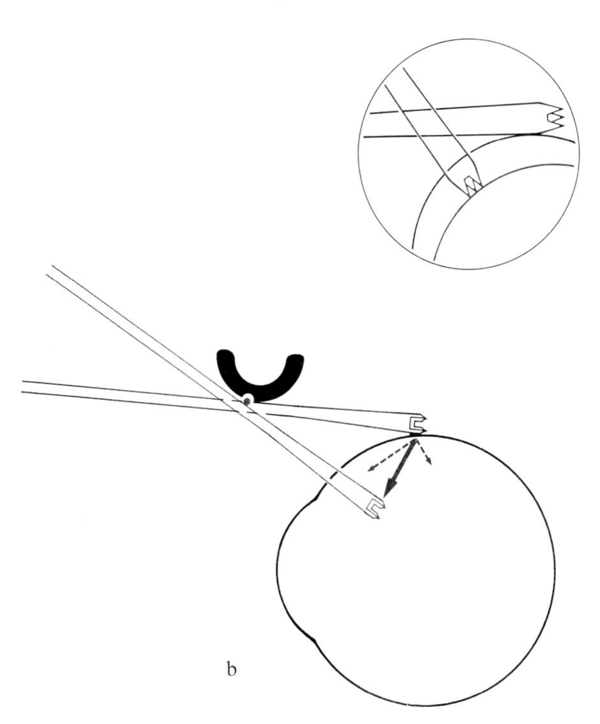

b

Fig. 159. **The presentation of tendons covered by the tarsus**

a *Use of the forceps for rotating the eye:* The forceps is applied laterally at an accessible part of the fornix and from there is swept upward beneath the lid. *Inset:* To allow the forceps to glide smoothly into place, the blades are closed until the tips just touch (closure is not complete). The two-toothed blade leads, protecting the tissue from the tip of the single-toothed blade (*inset*).

b Lest the teeth slip off the muscle, they are pressed against the surface of the globe (once in place) by bracing the forceps against the fulcrum of the lid retractor. The teeth are not closed until they are perpendicular to the globe surface (inset), because only then is their grip effective

IV Operations on the Conjunctiva

1 General

From a surgical standpoint, the conjunctiva can be subdivided into three layers: The *epithelial lamella,* comprised of the epithelium and an underlying layer of connective tissue; a *subepithelial fibrous layer;* and the *episcleral space* (Fig. 160). The **epithelial lamella** is closely interlaced with the underlying fibrous layer and presents as a layer only when surgically dissected. It is then found to be compliant but of *low elasticity,* and thus tends to maintain any position assumed. It also exhibits an extensive surface area (Fig. 161), which is not ordinarily apparent due to the constricting effect of the adherent **subepithelial fibers.** [1] Directly adjacent to the globe is the **episcleral space**, which contains a small number of loose connective fibers (Fig. 162). This space does not extend all the way to the corneal margin, for in a zone from 1 to 2 mm wide about the limbus the subepithelial

[1] This surface area is necessary to permit broad excursions of the eyeball. The elasticity of the subepithelial layer ensures that the epithelial lamella does not wrinkle during eye movements.

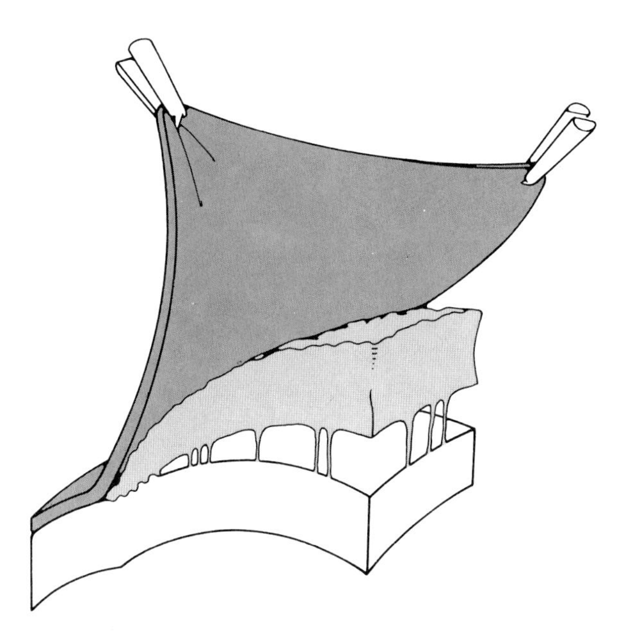

Fig. 161. **Separating the epithelial lamella from the subepithelial fibrous layer (formation of large sliding flaps).** If the epithelial lamella is separated from the contractile fibrous layer, it can be expanded to its full size

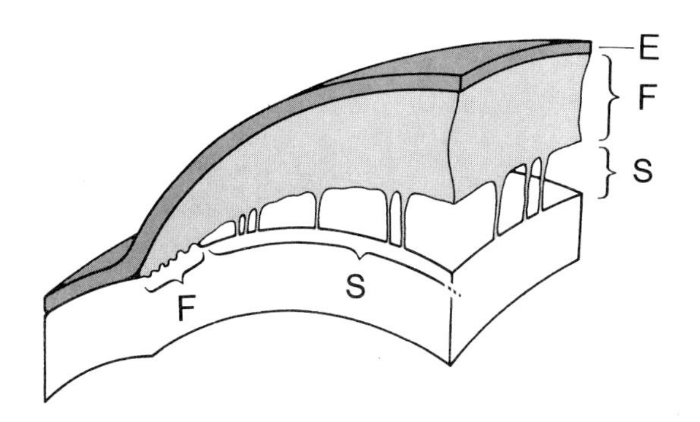

Fig. 160. **Structure of the conjunctiva.** *E* The superficial epithelial lamella is continuous with the corneal epithelium. *F* The subepithelial fibrous layer extends to the limbus. *S* The episcleral space terminates a small distance from the limbus

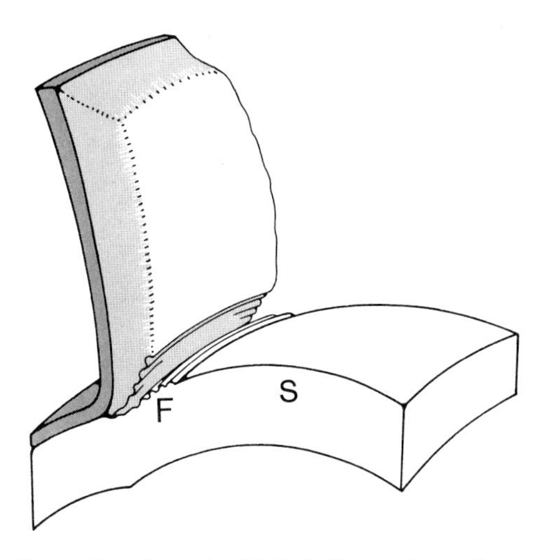

Fig. 162. **Separating the subepithelial fibrous layer from the sclera (exposure of the globe surface).** After the loose connective fibers in the episcleral space (*S*) are detached and the perilimbic fibrous zone (*F*) is sectioned, the conjunctiva can be raised to expose the sclera. The conjunctival flap will contract somewhat if the subepithelial fibers are sufficiently elastic

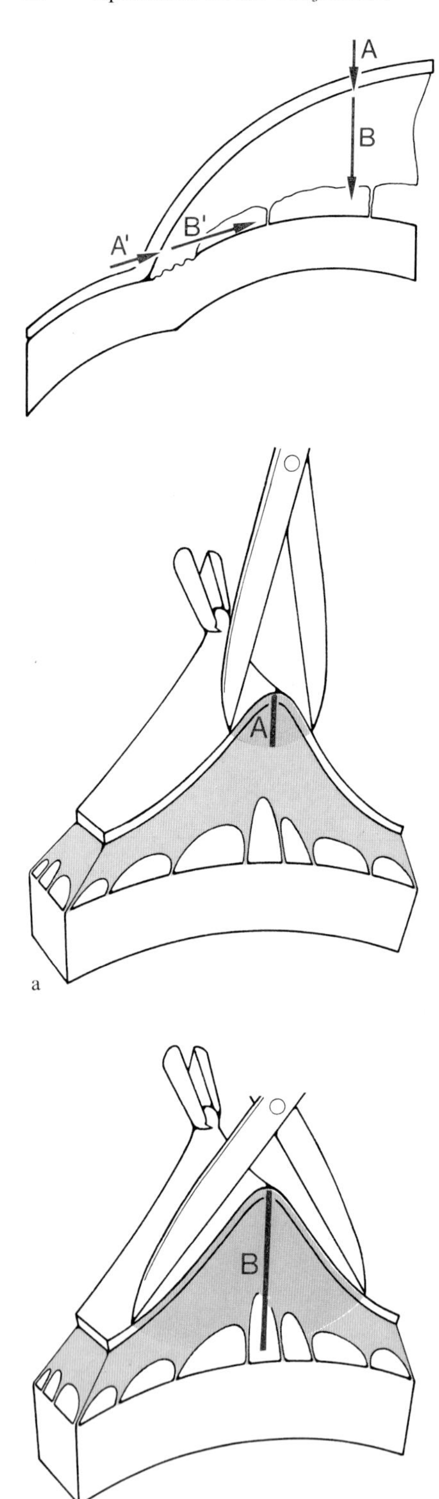

Fig. 163. **Means of approaching the deeper tissue layers.** Over the sclera, the conjunctival layers are incised in a perpendicular direction to the globe. (*A*, *B*). Starting from the limbus, the desired depth is reached in a parallel direction (*A′*, *B′*)

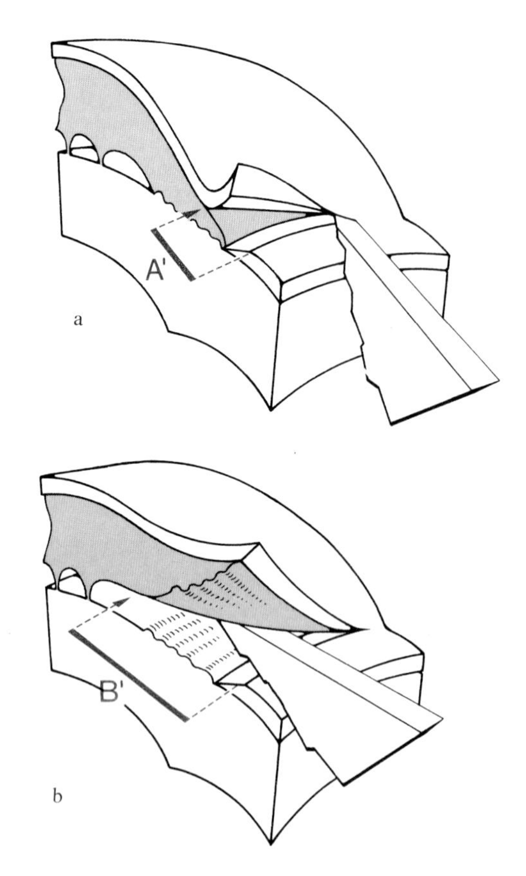

Fig. 164. **Incising the conjunctiva in a perpendicular direction.** The position of the blade tips determines the depth of incision.

a If only the most superficial layer is to be sectioned, the blades are held farther away from the sclera.

b To reach the episcleral space, the blade tips are held as close as possible to the scleral surface (*A*, *B* see Fig. 163)

Fig. 165. **Incising the conjunctiva at the limbus.** The distance of the blade tip from the limbus determines the depth of incision.

a If the blade tip is guided close to the limbus, only subepithelial fibers are incised.

b If the tip is more than 2–3 mm from the limbus, the episcleral space is opened (*A′*, *B′* see Fig. 163)

fibers are firmly adherent to the sclera (the "perilimbic fibrous zone").

Approach to the deep conjunctival layers is parallel to the globe surface starting from the limbus, and perpendicular in all other regions (Figs. 163–165).

The delicate conjunctival tissue is in itself highly susceptible to injury. The fact that it is seldom injured in practice is due to its high **displaceability** and consequent *poor sectility*.

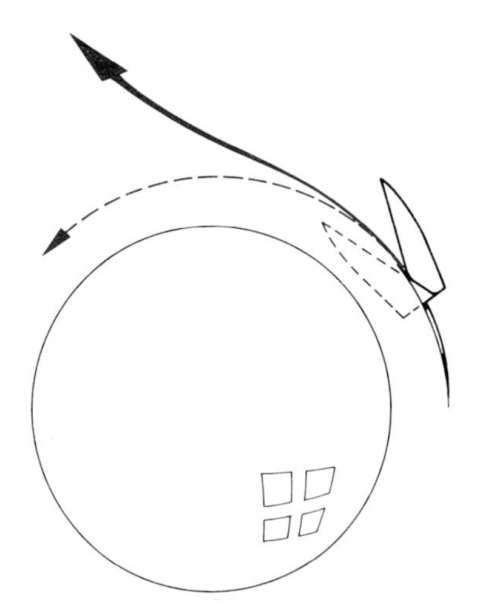

Fig. 166. **Cutting the loose conjunctival tissue.** Due to the shifting tendency of the conjunctival tissue, cuts parallel to the limbus gradually deviate in the direction of the fornix (see Fig. 40); this tendency varies with the distance from the limbus

However, this protection is lacking in places where the conjunctiva is firmly adherent, specifically, at the *limbus* and at *scars* (and at *points where forceps are applied*). The closer to such fixation zones the conjunctiva is grasped or cut, the greater the *danger of inadvertant perforation.*

The displaceability of the conjunctiva also causes *cuts to deviate* from the intended path (see Figs. 39, 40). The smaller the distance of the cutting edge from the fixation zones mentioned above, the greater the likelihood of deviations (Fig. 166).

Displaceability can also be a problem during *grasping*, because the tissue is then strongly deformed and displaced. Incisions will assume a different shape and position from that intended as soon as the tissue is released (see Fig. 41). If only moderate precision is required, the resulting inaccuracies are of little consequence. Of more practical importance, however, are those deformations on grasping which become *sources of perforations,* i.e., the folds which come to lie in the interblade area and are thus sectioned on closure (Fig. 167a). The formation of such folds can be avoided either by keeping the interblade area small (cutting with a small blade aperture) or by the proper regulation of traction (Fig. 167b).

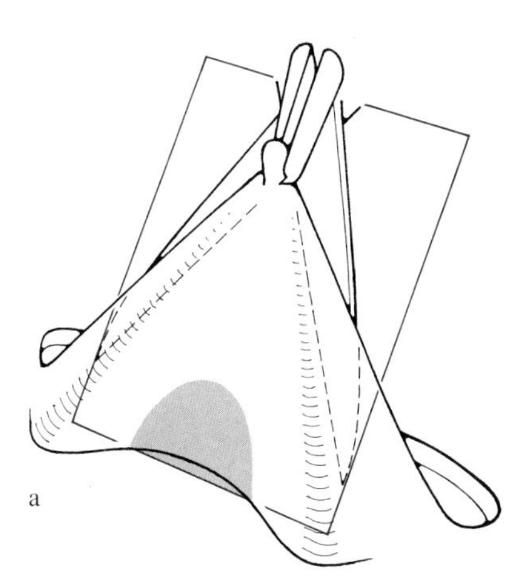

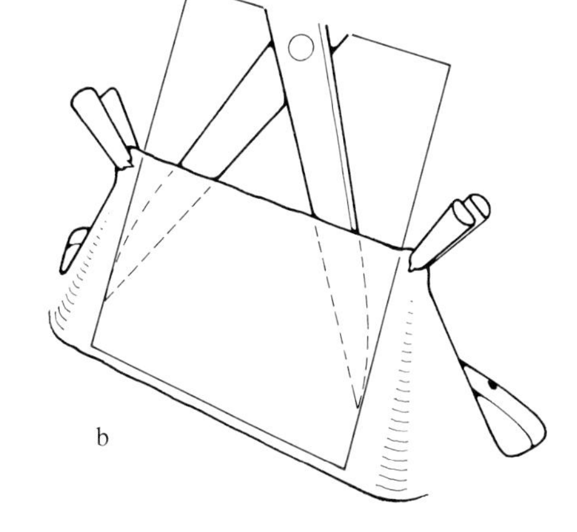

Fig. 167. **Deformation of the conjunctiva on grasping**

a If infolds are formed when the conjunctiva is lifted, there is a danger of perforation if the scissors is held such that its guidance path intersects the folds.

b If the conjunctiva is stretched out flat so that it parallels the guidance path, however, the scissors can cut close along the surface without perforating it.

The guidance path of the scissors (i.e., the surface on which the cutting edges move during closure) is outlined in red

2 Episcleral Dissection ("Deep" Dissection)

"Deep" dissection exposes the episcleral space and affords *access to the extraocular muscles, sclera* and *interior of the eye* (Fig. 162). Where difficult to discern, the episcleral space can be visualized by infiltration with a fluid which enlarges the space and makes the interstitial fibers tense (Fig. 174b). To reach the episcleral space, it is necessary to transect the epithelial lamella and subepithelial fibrous layer (Figs. 164b, 165b). When the space is exposed, the use of *rounded blade tips* will spare the scleral surface and muscular attachments. The blunt dissection can be best controlled by keeping the scissors pressed firmly against the surface of the globe where the episcleral fibers are anchored and are thus the most sectile (Fig. 168).

On the other hand, the firm fibers at **fixation sites** (perilimbic zone, scars) require *sharp instruments* such as blades (Fig. 169) or scissors (Fig. 170) with sharp or semi-rounded points. There is, of course, a *danger of perforation* of the conjunctival flap when sharp instruments are used, but it can be reduced by reg-

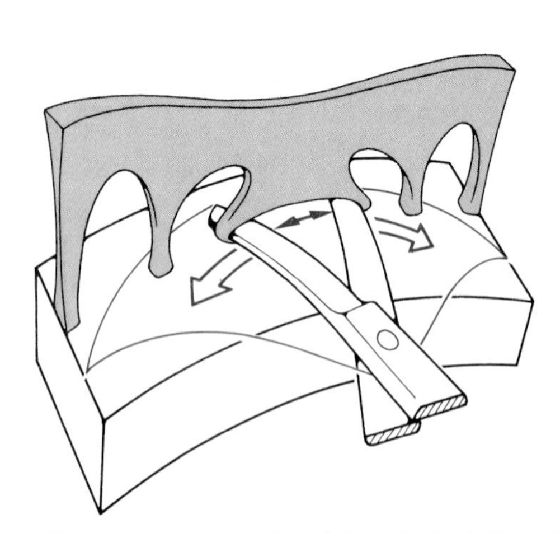

Fig. 168. **Blunt dissection of the episcleral tissue.** The ends of the blades are pressed against the sclera so that they contact the fibers near their point of attachment. If the guidance path of the blades follows the surface of the globe, the surrounding structures are spared

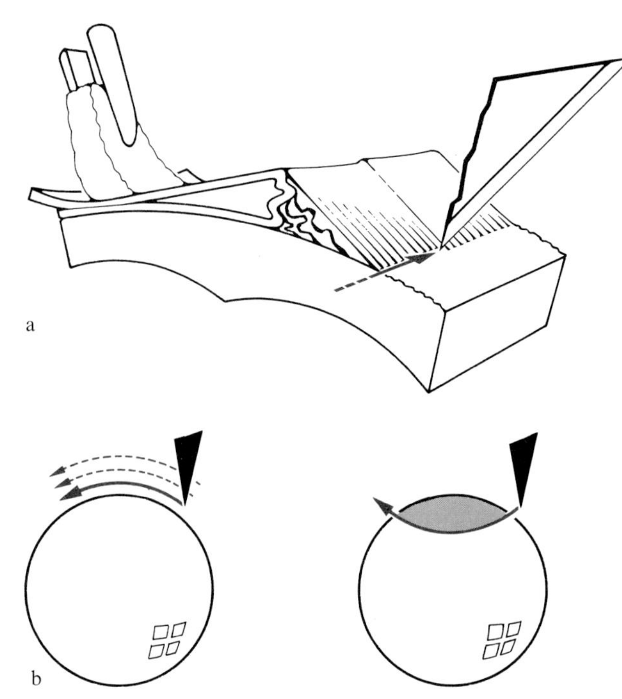

Fig. 169. **Prevention of perforations**

a Selective fiber tension at the margin of fixation zones. If the dissected conjunctival flap is reflected onto the globe, selective tension is exerted on the peripheral fibers exposed directly to the cutting edge. Meanwhile, the more central fibers and vulnerable epithelial layer are relaxed and are therefore less sectile (see also Fig. 32).

b Guidance direction during dissection of the limbus. To avoid injury to the conjunctival flap, no vectors should be directed toward the cornea.

Left: During "hatching" (see Fig. 44) the cutting point is directed parallel to the limbus to avoid vectors in the corneal direction.

Right: "Slewing movements" produce vectors in the corneal direction and thus endanger the conjunctival flap

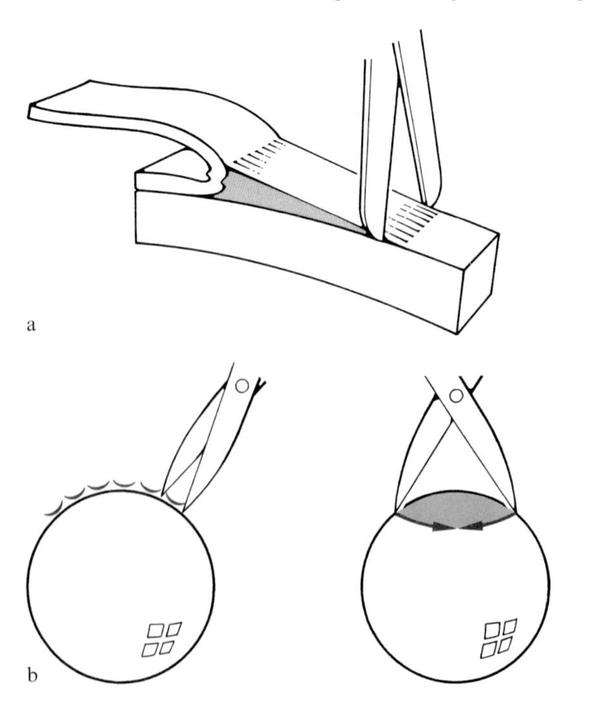

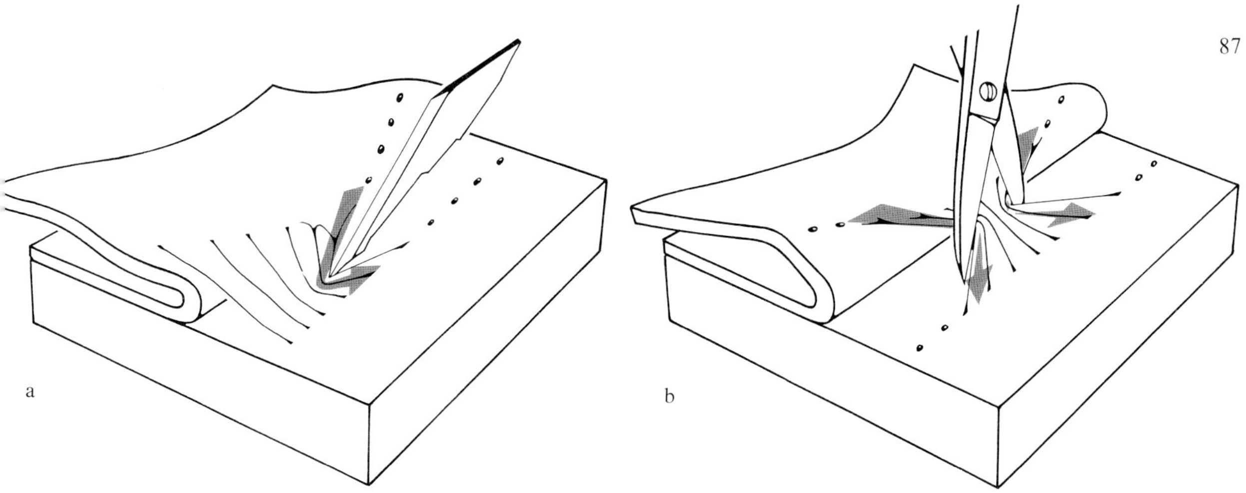

Fig. 171. **Effect of lateral shifting tendency during dissection at the limbus.** If a blade moves parallel to the limbus, the fibers before it are shifted from the reflected flap toward their scleral attachment. The greater the distance travelled by the blade, the more tissue is shifted scleralward. Ultimately, the conjunctival surface may enter the cutting path and become sectioned.

a Lateral shifting tendency when cutting with a razor blade tip.

b Shifting tendency when cutting with scissors. Tissue is pulled between the blades during closure. Since the danger of perforation depends on the distance travelled by the cutting point, it varies with the aperture angle and can be reduced by dissecting with a small aperture (i.e., in many small steps, see Fig. 170b)

ulating sectility by means of selective fiber tension (Fig. 169), and by avoiding potentially harmful vectors when guiding the instrument (Figs. 169b, 170b).

When a blade is directed *parallel to the limbus,* the tissue demonstrates a lateral shifting tendency which gradually brings the surface of the conjunctival flap into the cutting path (Figs. 171, 172). The danger of conjunctival perforation is reduced by exerting a countertension on the flap to offset this tendency.

If all the subepithelial fibers up to the limbus (or scar) have been sectioned, the fold at the reflected epithelial lamella appears as a sharp *step* – the sign that the episcleral dissection is complete and that any further cuts would merely perforate the flap itself (Fig. 173).

Fig. 170. **Dissection of the perilimbic fibrous zone with scissors**

a When the conjunctival flap is reflected (as in Fig. 169), the subepithelial fibers are stretched parallel to the globe surface, and the scissors must be positioned accordingly (see Fig. 63).

b Cuts are made in small steps to avoid injury to the conjunctival flap.

Left: On closure from a small aperture angle, the tips of the scissors are moved nearly parallel to the limbus. *Right:* On closure from a large aperture, the tips are directed toward the reflected conjunctival flap and may perforate it

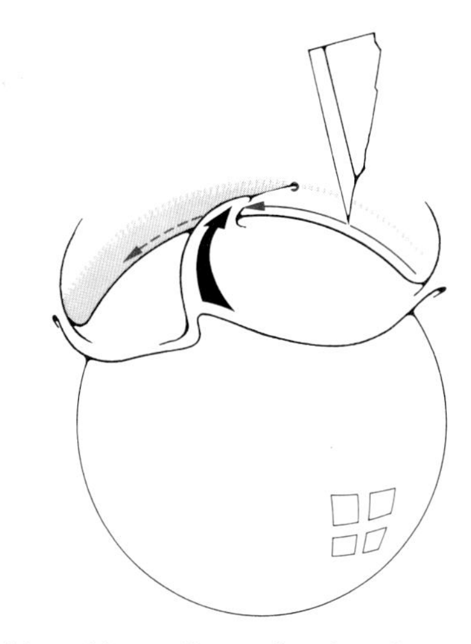

Fig. 172. **Early recognition of impending perforation.** Conjunctival folds appearing during dissection parallel to the limbus indicate lateral shifting and are an important warning sign. *Gray:* still undissected perilimbic fibrous zone

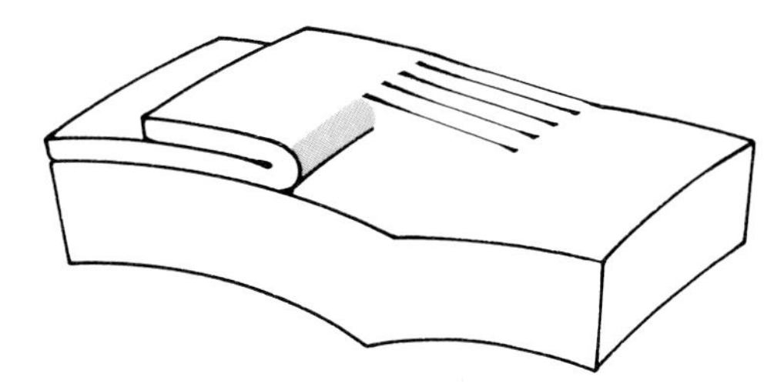

Fig. 173. **The completion of deep episcleral dissection.** If the last subepithelial fiber connections have been separated, a distinct step (*gray*) is formed where the epithelial lamella is reflected. Where fibers are still present, the flap surface appears to be continuous with the sclera

3 Subepithelial Dissection ("Superficial" Dissection)

The epithelial lamella can be separated from the subepithelial fibers (Fig. 161) to produce *sliding flaps* for repairing tissue defects.

The attainable size and mobility of these flaps depend upon how carefully the contractile fibers have been dissected away. The more stringent the requirements in this regard, the closer the cut must be to the epithelial lamella. But as the lamellar thickness decreases, the danger of perforation increases, and so an extremely high degree of precision must be strived for, at least if the flaps to be dissected are very large.[2]

[2] Example: Conjunctival flaps for covering the entire cornea.

This degree of precision is made difficult by the poor sectility of the tissue. However, conditions can be improved by *increasing the sectility* on the one hand, and by *exploiting the shifting tendency* of the tissue to direct the cut more superficially on the other.

Sectility is increased by exerting tension on the subepithelial fibers, whether by infiltration with a fluid (Figs. 174–176) or with instruments such as the scissors tips themselves (as shown in Fig. 177). However, this can be done only as long as the fibers are *firmly anchored* to the sclera and thus create a lateral shifting tendency which directs the cut toward the surface (Fig. 178). If this fixation is absent, as when the episcleral space is opened, the opposite effect is achieved: The cut is driven deeper into the tissue, and a thick surface lamella is obtained. Any attempt to correct the situation by applying stronger tension (as by lifting the scissors) will only bring more fibers toward the surface and thicken the lamella even more. Therefore, it is essential in superficial dissection that the episcleral space be spared and

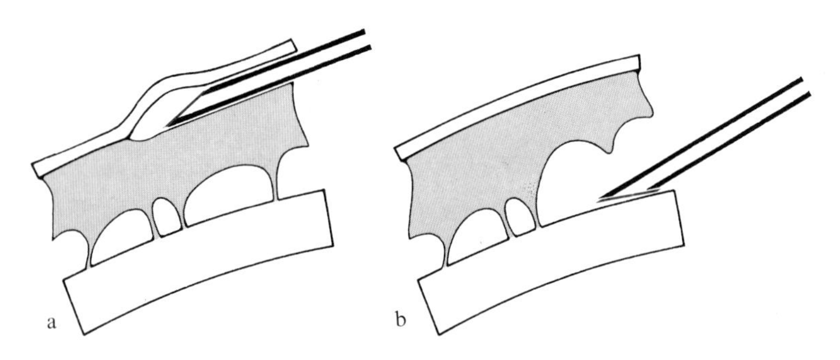

Fig. 174. **Infiltration of the conjunctiva with fluid**

a Superficial infiltration to make the subepithelial fibers tense. The cannula is inserted just below the conjunctival surface, with its blunt side upward to avoid epithelial injury.

b Infiltration to visualize the episcleral space. The cannula glides smoothly over the scleral surface if its blunt side is pointed downward

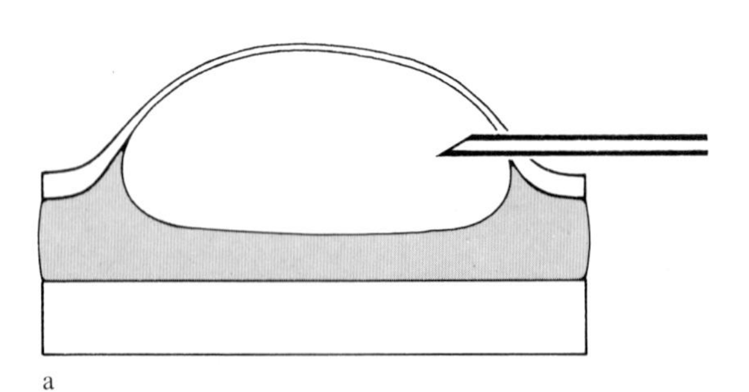

b

Fig. 175. **Technique of subepithelial infiltration**

a If fluid is injected from a cannula held stationary, a large vesicle is formed which ruptures the finer fibers and thus creates a cavity. When incised, the vesicle collapses and cannot maintain tension during dissection.

b If the cannula is advanced during injection, numerous small fluid chambers are formed which ensure tension even during progressive superficial dissection

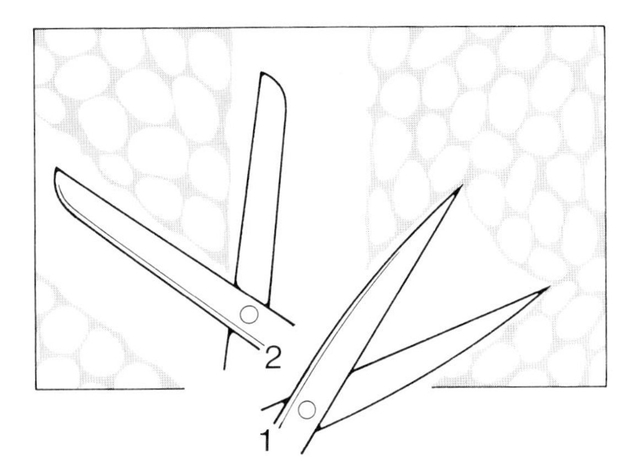

Fig. 176. **Dissection of the infiltrated conjunctiva.** To maintain tension in the infiltrated region as long as possible, isolated tunnels are first cut through the tissue (*1*), leaving infiltrated "pillars" to maintain tension. Then these intermediate pillars are sectioned in a second step (*2*)

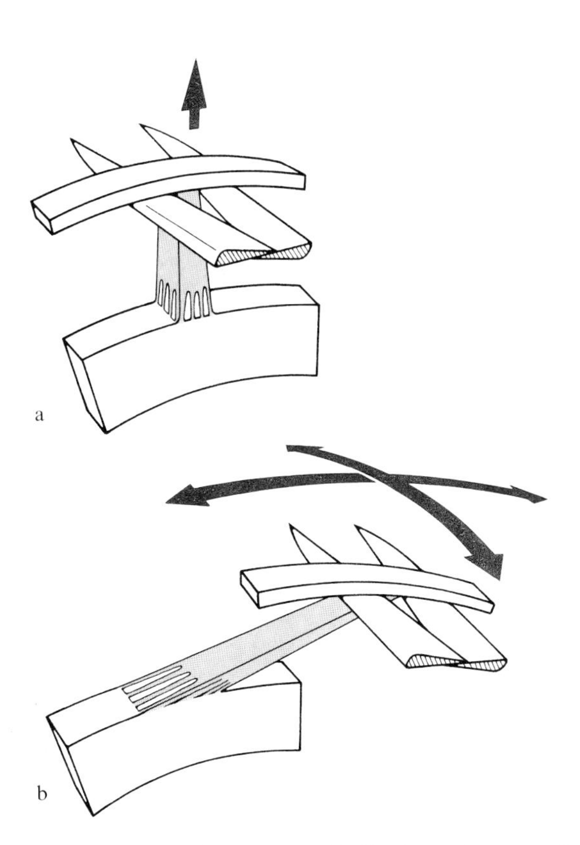

Fig. 177. **Stretching the subepithelial fibers** increases their sectility and exploits their retractile tendency (Fig. 41) to place the cut nearer the surface.

a Stretching the fibers by lifting the scissors vertically from the globe.

b If the fiber tension produced by this measure is insufficient, it can be increased by also moving the scissors parallel to the surface

not opened either by the incision (Figs. 164a, 165a) or during the course of further dissection.

The situation is analogous for *fluid infiltration*. The tensing effect is lost as soon as the episcleral space is filled. Thus, great care must be taken to inject the fluid just below the conjunctival surface (Fig. 174a). It should not be injected into a single large compartment, since this will collapse completely once opened, and the desired tension will be lost. Instead, the fluid is distributed throughout numerous small compartments during injection (Fig. 175), some of which are spared during cutting in order to maintain tension as long as possible (Fig. 176).

For anatomical reasons there is always an absence of deep fixation when operating at an increasing distance from the globe, i.e., when dissecting in the direction of the fornix. Should the effect of fluid infiltration be insufficient in this case, there is often no recourse but to produce a deep fixation artificially with forceps or traction sutures. This leads to yet

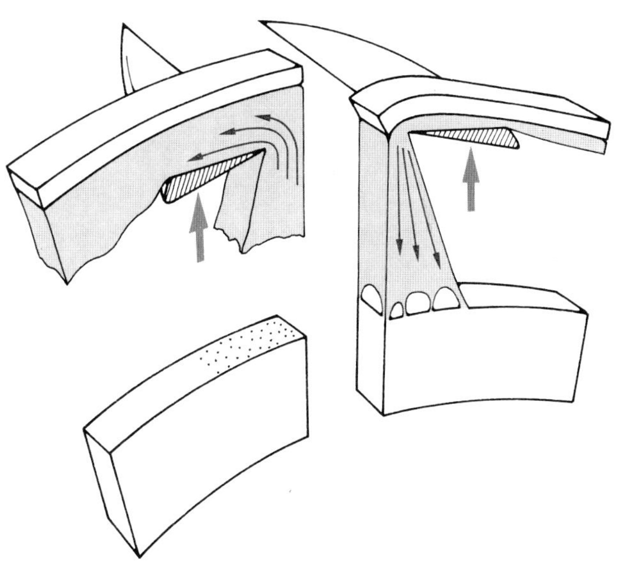

Fig. 178. **Utilization of lateral shifting tendency in conjunctival dissection.** When stretched, the fibers ahead of the advancing blade are shifted in the direction of strongest fixation. *Right:* Fibers securely anchored to the sclera are driven scleralward from the blade. The more tension is exerted, the greater the downward shift of fibers and the thinner the dissected superficial layer. *Left:* In the absence of scleral attachment, the epithelial lamella becomes the strongest fixation point, and the subepithelial fibers are shifted toward it by the blade. The result is a thick dissected layer, which becomes even thicker as more upwards tension is exerted

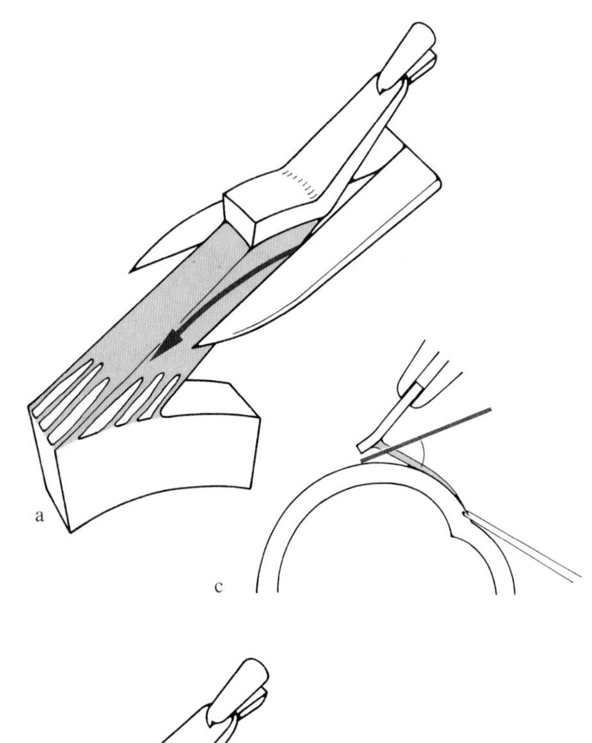

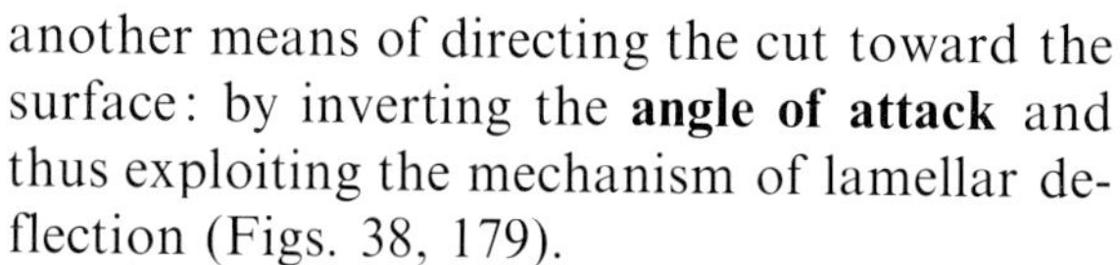

another means of directing the cut toward the surface: by inverting the **angle of attack** and thus exploiting the mechanism of lamellar deflection (Figs. 38, 179).

The tension on the subepithelial fibers which is necessary for superficial dissection again raises the danger of perforation, since it tends to produce infolds between the scissors blades (see Fig. 167). Superficial dissection therefore requires a skillful blending of tension and countertension, a continual adjustment to ever-changing tensions, and a close monitoring of the "danger zone" between the scissors blades.

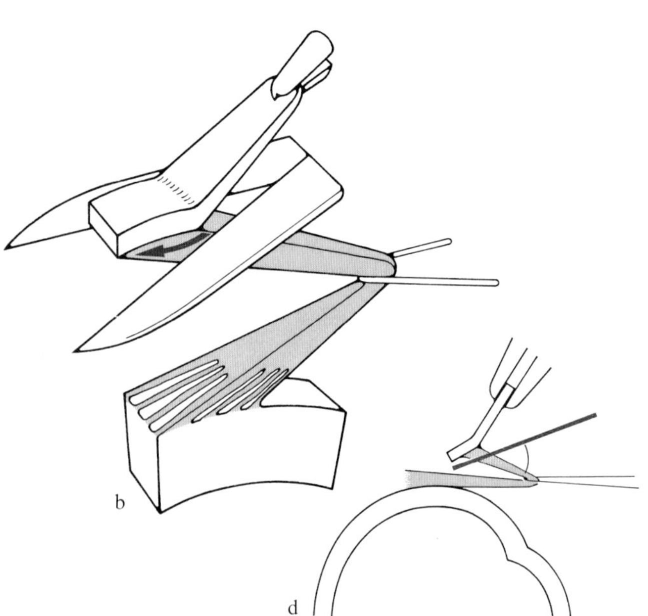

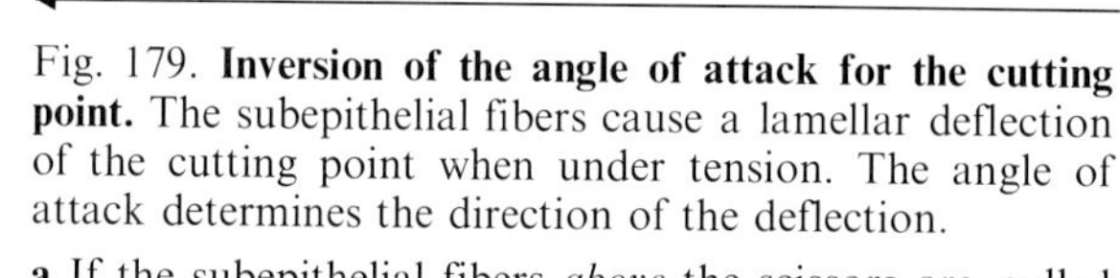

Fig. 179. **Inversion of the angle of attack for the cutting point.** The subepithelial fibers cause a lamellar deflection of the cutting point when under tension. The angle of attack determines the direction of the deflection.

a If the subepithelial fibers *above* the scissors are pulled toward the scissors joint, as by traction on the epithelial lamella, they present to the cutting point in such a way as to deflect it downward (toward the sclera), and the resulting superficial layer increases in thickness.

b If the subepithelial fibers *below* the scissors are pulled in the direction of the scissors joint, the angle of attack is inverted, the cutting point is driven upward and the lamella becomes thinner.

c Inversion of the direction of attack by traction on the globe (traction suture through the *sclera*) during the dissection of fibers fixed at the sclera.

d Inversion of the direction of attack by means of traction sutures through the *subepithelial fibers* in areas lacking adequate deep fixation (e.g., the conjunctiva of the fornix)

4 Suturation of the Conjunctiva

The edges of conjunctival wounds have a tendency to curl due to the elasticity of the subepithelial fibers. To obtain correct apposition of the layers during suturation, this retraction must be reversed by *countertraction on the subepithelial fibers*. They are engaged with the teeth of an open forceps or seized directly with a fine forceps and stretched out. This expands the overlying epithelial lamella, which can then be engaged at its edge (discernible by its distinctive vascular pattern) with a needle.

The inherent flexibility of the conjunctiva allows great freedom in the choice of suture form. Tissue deformations by the suture rarely jeopardize the operative goal. They are even utilized to produce the compression necessary for the uniting of tissues.

The postoperative *adherence* of the conjunctiva is extremely good and rapid on a vascular substrate, but poor on avascular surfaces. **Conjunctival flaps** for covering the cornea should be fixed to the vascularized circumcorneal tissue, therefore (Figs. 180, 181, 184). Flaps for partial covering of the cornea may obtain their necessary tension from a shortening of the wound margin. But this tension cannot withstand large opposing forces and is, for example, insufficient to seal fistulous openings that are under aqueous pressure. Here the compression must come from the suture itself (Figs. 182, 183).

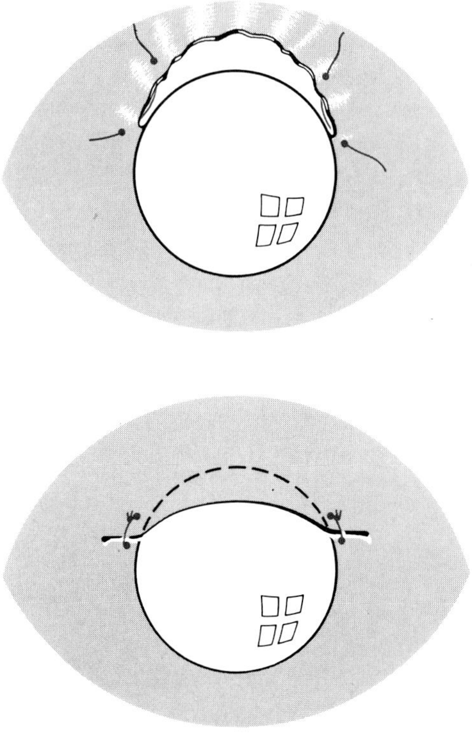

Fig. 180. **Forming a conjunctival flap by shortening the lateral wound margin.** The lateral wound margin is shortened by suture and fixed episclerally. This shortening exerts tension on the flap and presses it onto the cornea. The tension achieved depends on the number of contractile subepithelial fibers still adherent. But this also increases the retractile tendency of the flap, causing it to gradually recede

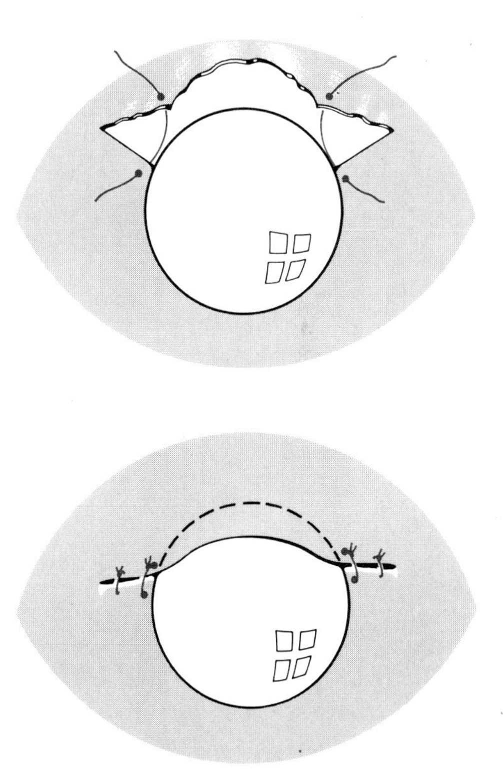

Fig. 181. **Forming a conjunctival flap by lateral triangular excisions.** Shortening by excision of excess conjunctival tissue avoids bulging as in Fig. 180 and promotes rapid adhesion in the area of attachment

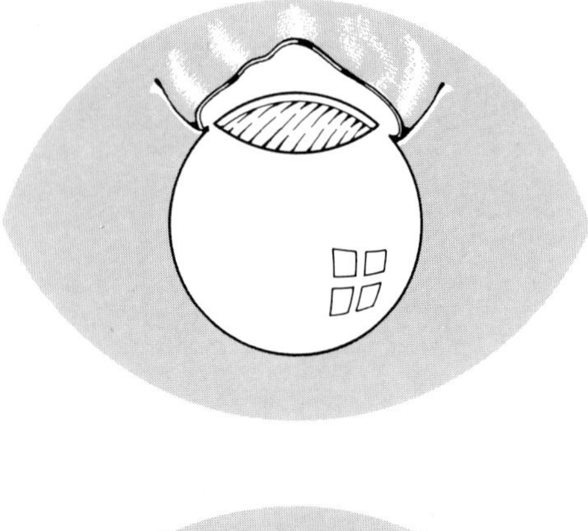

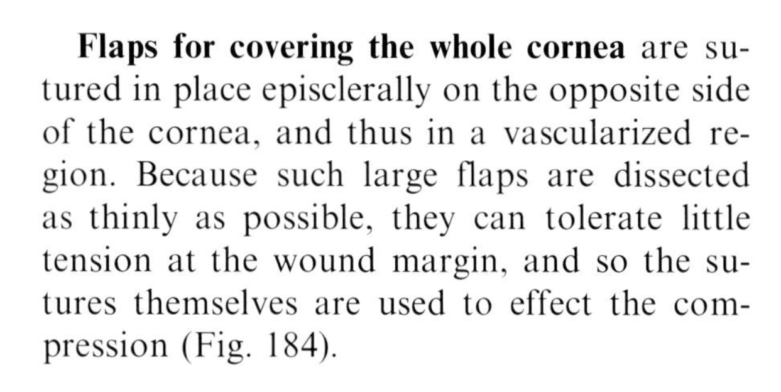

Flaps for covering the whole cornea are sutured in place episclerally on the opposite side of the cornea, and thus in a vascularized region. Because such large flaps are dissected as thinly as possible, they can tolerate little tension at the wound margin, and so the sutures themselves are used to effect the compression (Fig. 184).

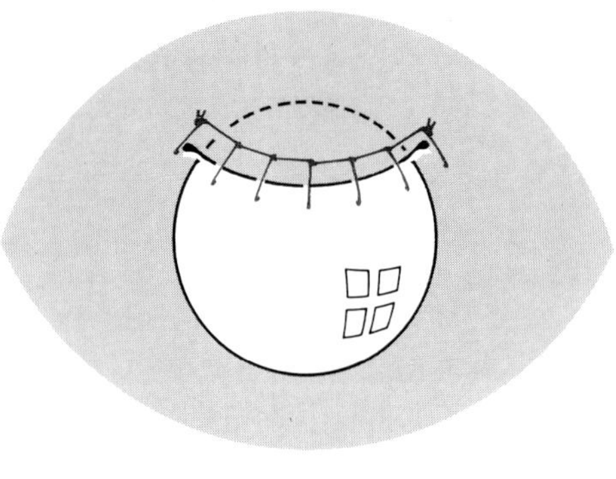

Fig. 182. **Covering aqueous fistulas.** A lamellar keratectomy creates a more adherent substrate. The conjunctival flap is stitched on watertight by continuous chain suture. Note the curvature of the wound line, which regulates the position of the overlying loops in the desired direction (see also Fig. 87)

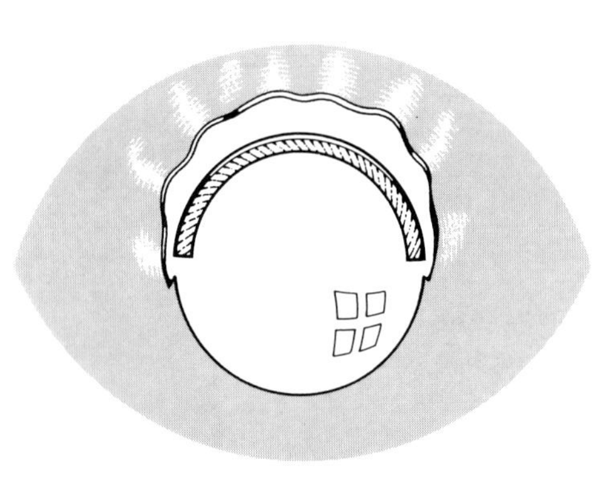

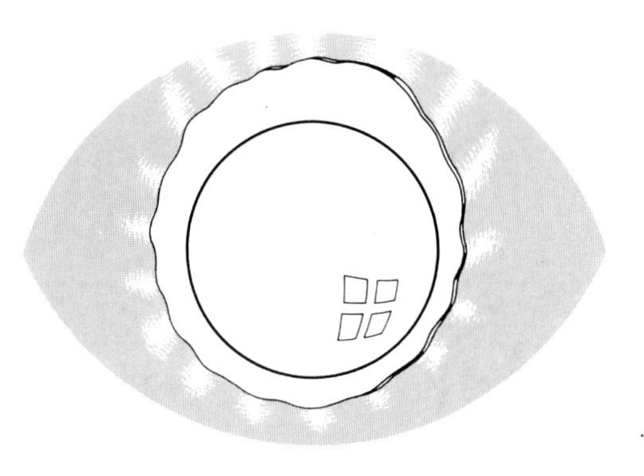

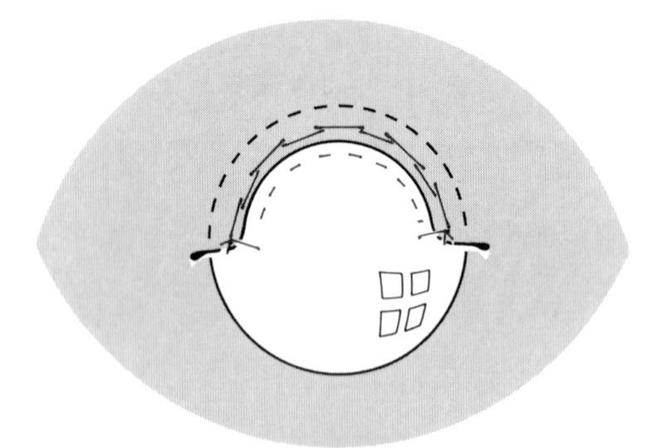

Fig. 183. **Covering a large keratectomy parallel to the limbus** (e.g. in repair of a ruptured cataract wound). The flap is affixed by an inverted meander suture, which will maintain the overlying bridges on the flap and press it watertight onto the cornea. (With a continous chain suture the bridges would slip away from the flap on account of the curvature opposite that in Fig. 182)

Fig. 184. **Whole-cornea conjunctival flap.** The thin, fragile flap is stitched onto the sclera with a continous chain suture. Due to the curvature of the suture (similar to Fig. 182) the overlying loops move to the side of the flap and press it onto the scleral surface

V Operations on the Cornea and Sclera

1 General

The wall of the eyeball has fairly homogenous mechanical properties. The main difference between the cornea and sclera lies in their *thickness* (Fig. 185) and the *regularity of their lamellar arrangement,* which change (along with transparency) in the bluish-gray transition zone at the limbus (Fig. 186).

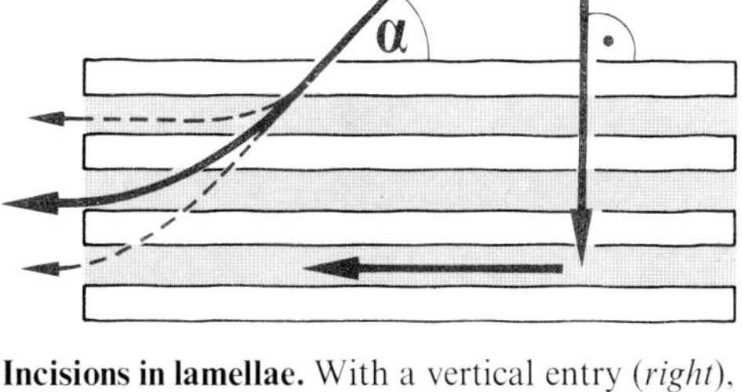

Fig. 187. **Incisions in lamellae.** With a vertical entry (*right*), the depth of the incision and its endpoint can be accurately controlled. With an oblique entry (*left*), the incision is deflected within the lamellae. The endpoint is indeterminate, and due to lamellar deflection it may even be impossible to reach the target layer

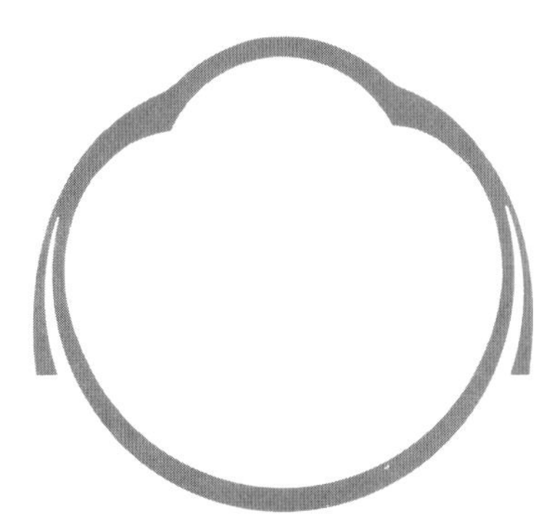

Fig. 185. **Thickness of the globe wall.** The corneoscleral tunic is thickest at the limbus and thinnest at the corneal center and muscular insertions

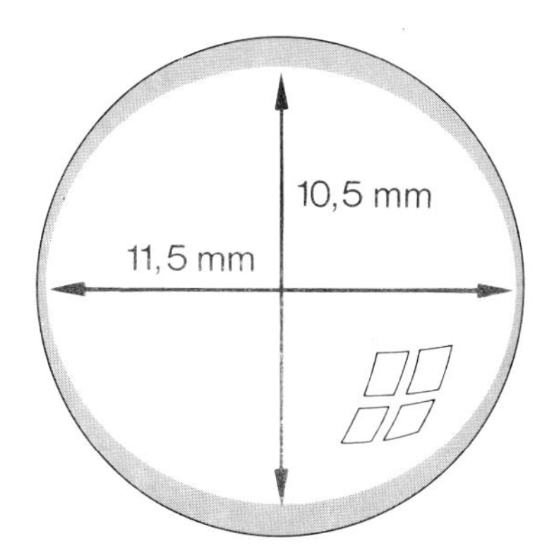

Fig. 186. **Corneoscleral boundary.** Externally, the vertical corneal diameter appears smaller than the horizontal, but internally the diameters are approximately equal in both directions. Thus the overlap zone at the limbus is wider superiorally and inferiorally than laterally and medially

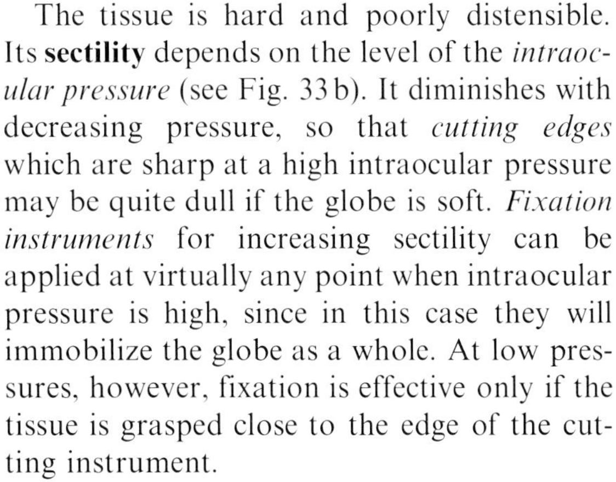

The tissue is hard and poorly distensible. Its **sectility** depends on the level of the *intraocular pressure* (see Fig. 33b). It diminishes with decreasing pressure, so that *cutting edges* which are sharp at a high intraocular pressure may be quite dull if the globe is soft. *Fixation instruments* for increasing sectility can be applied at virtually any point when intraocular pressure is high, since in this case they will immobilize the globe as a whole. At low pressures, however, fixation is effective only if the tissue is grasped close to the edge of the cutting instrument.

The path of incisions in the cornea and sclera is strongly influenced by the phenomenon of **lamellar deflection** (see Fig. 38). The accuracy of the cut is impaired as soon as the blade is applied at an oblique angle to the lamellae. Thus, if high precision is required it is advisable to minimize the unpredictable deflections by making the incisions either *perpendicular* or *parallel* to the lamellae (Fig. 187).

When a *vertical incision* is employed, the depth of the incision is monitored by estimating the length of blade immersed in the tissue (Fig. 188) or by repeatedly pushing the blade aside slightly to reveal the base of the inci-

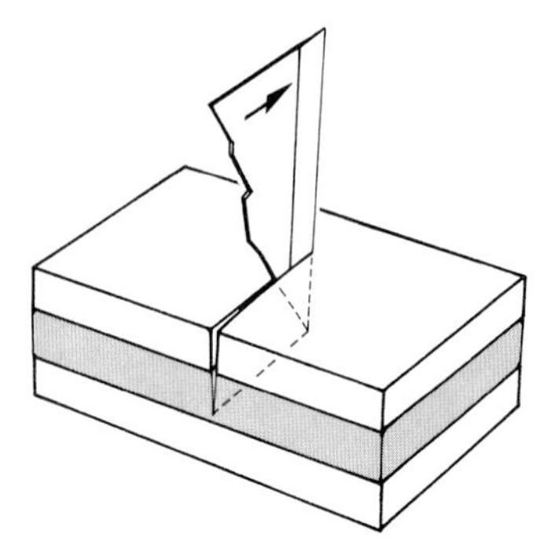

Fig. 188. **Vertical incision.** The depth of a vertical incision can be estimated by the length of blade immersed in the tissue

sion.[1] It is easier to maintain a given depth of incision if the blade is fitted with a *stop* (Fig. 189).

When *cutting parallel to lamellae* ("lamellation"), *blunt dissection* makes it easier to remain in a particular layer but offers limited possibilities for regulating the depth of the cut. To advance to other depths or to maintain the lamellar level in an irregular structure, *sharp dissection* is required (see Fig. 46).

When **lamellae** are dissected **in situ** (Fig. 190), and thus left in their anatomic position, visibility is obstructed by the dissected lamella. If the globe cannot be rotated sufficiently to improve visibility, the blade position can be checked indirectly by lifting the blade slightly to form a visible bulge in the tissue surface.[2]

If the dissected portion of the **lamella is reflected** as the dissection proceeds, a clear view of the cutting edge is afforded. This fold *alters the direction* of the interlamellar fibers, however, requiring a corresponding adjustment of cutting technique (Fig. 191).

[1] See footnote 2; p. 3.

[2] See footnote, p. 2.

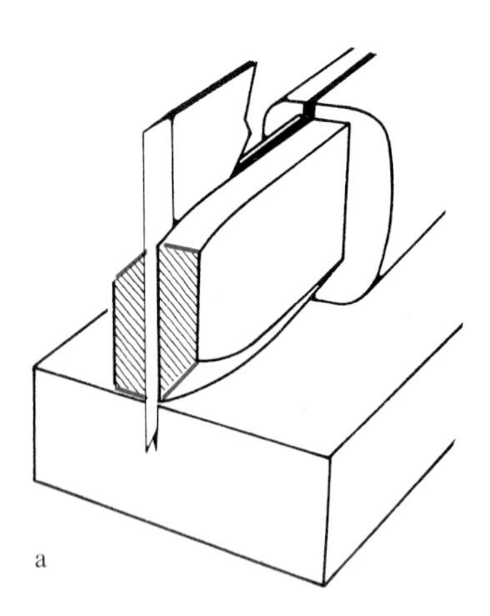

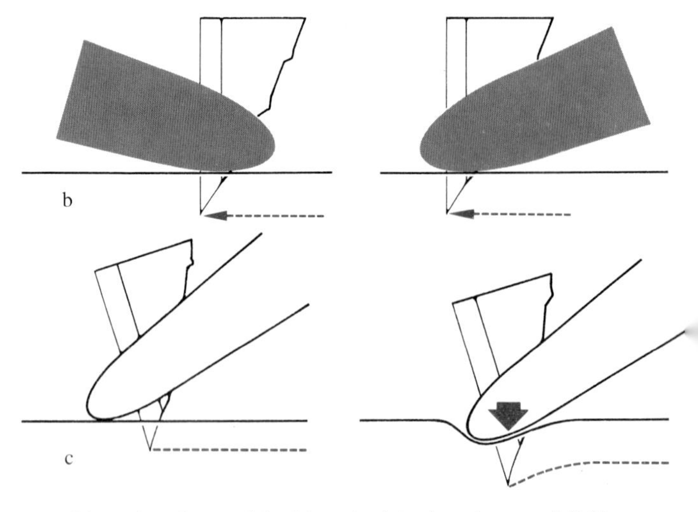

Fig. 189. **Incision with preset depth**

a A sample stop arrangement is shown: one jaw of the razor-blade holder is square-edged and acts as a depth stop; the other jaw, which faces the operator, is cut at an angle to afford a better view.

b The results are determined by the guidance direction of the cutting edge. They are not influenced by whether the blade is "pushed" or "pulled" through the tissue, although a forward incision (*right*) gives better visibility of the tissue to be cut.

c The preset depth is reached only when the blade holder is held in a specific position. In other positions the entire blade tip may not penetrate the tissue (*left*). If the holder is pressed down it adapts the tissue surface (*right*), and the blade will advance until reaching the preset depth

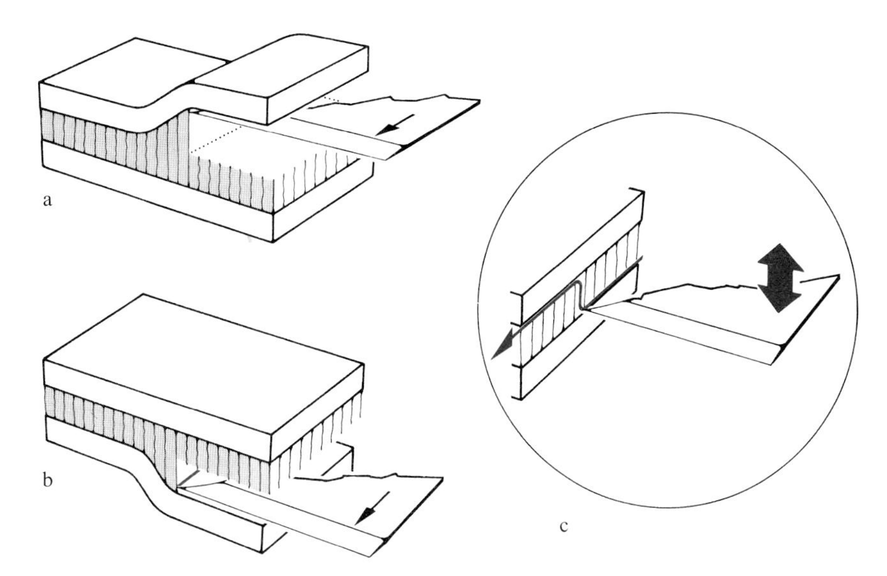

Fig. 190. **Dissection of lamellae in situ (guidance path parallel to the lamellae)**

a If the blade is lifted, the interlamellar fibers are sectioned close to the surface; the upper lamella contains little tissue and is thin.

b If the interlamellar fibers are sectioned deeper, they remain attached to the surface lamella, which is therefore thicker.

c To change the lamellar thickness, the blade is moved *at right angles* to the lamellae (i.e., parallel to the interlamellar fibers)

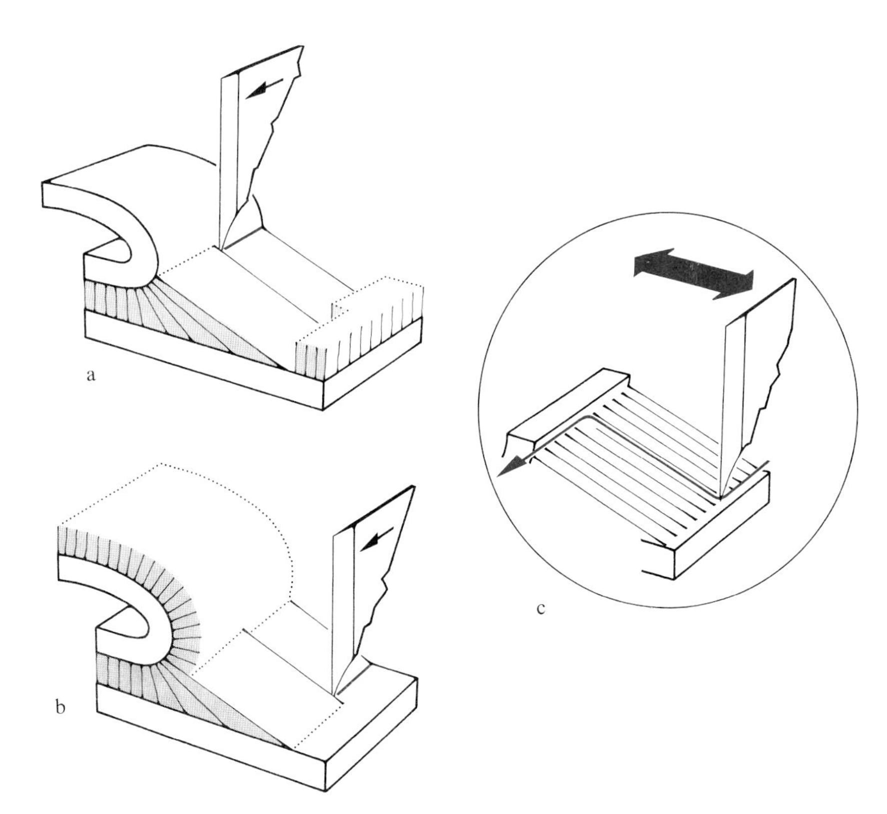

Fig. 191. **Dissection with reflection of the lamella (guidance path perpendicular to lamellar direction).** With the dissected part of the lamella folded back, the interlamellar fibers are stretched almost parallel to the lamellae.

a Section close to the fold produces a thin surface lamella.

b Section at the basal attachment of the interlamellar fibers (i.e., at some distance from the reflected flap) yields a thick surface lamella.

c Here the lamellar thickness is changed by moving the blade *parallel* to the lamellae

2 Planning the Approach to the Eye Interior

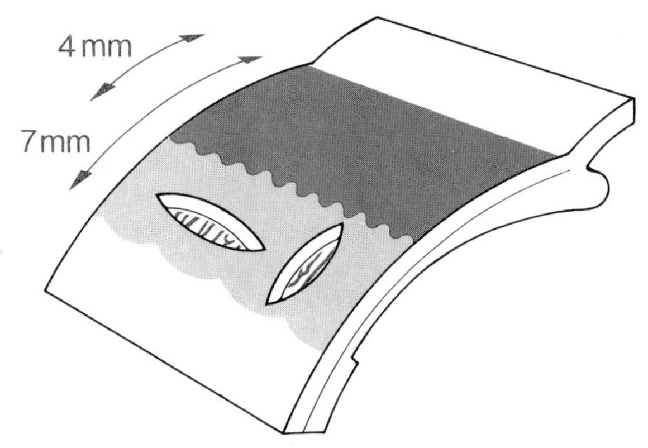

Fig. 193. **Approaches to the vitreous chamber.** The danger of hemorrhage on perforation of the vascular uvea depends on the direction of the incision relative to the vessels. Incisions which cross the vessels (*left*) expose several vascular branches, and an adequate point of access can be found between them. Incisions parallel to the vessels (*right*) can be made longer without vascular lesions, but make it more difficult to find a vessel-free interval. The dark-shaded area represents the ciliary zone which absorbs more light under diaphanoscopic illumination. *Note:* The limbic distance of the ora serrata is smaller nasally (6 mm) than temporally (7 mm)

The planning of a bulbar incision is based not only on the attainable *size of the opening*, but also on the method of closure. The size of an opening is actually limited only by anatomical barriers. The main problem is closure, since good apposition implies not only the restoration of wound geometry, but also *absolute watertightness*.

While *anatomical factors* determine the long-term (=biological) healing tendency of wounds, immediate surgical closure is largely determined by *geometric factors*.

2.1 Anatomical Factors in Opening the Globe

The *vitreous chamber* is best approached from the part of the sclera over the pars plana of the ciliary body, the *anterior chamber* from the limbic region (Fig. 192).

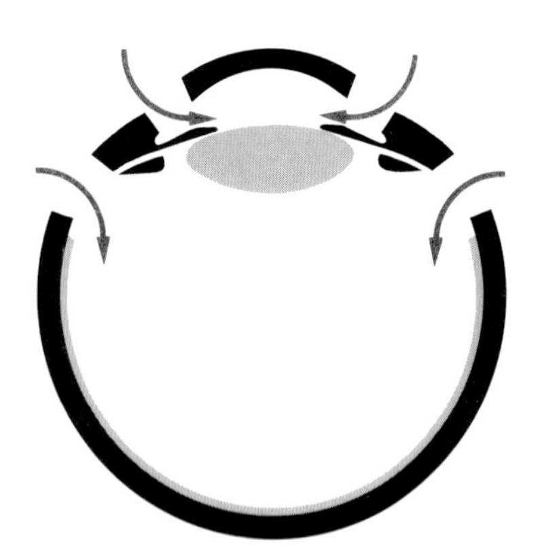

Fig. 192. **Approaches to the eye interior.** The *vitreous chamber* is reached with fewest complications through the pars plana. A more anterior approach is made difficult by the mechanical barrier of the ciliary muscle, and also raises the danger of severe hemorrhage from the vessels of the ciliary processes. Approach behind the pars plana would perforate the retina. The *anterior chamber* is best approached from the limbic region, so that any scars that result will cause no visual disturbance

In opening the **vitreous chamber**, the position of the pars plana can be localized either on the basis of statistical data on the limbic distance, or individually by means of diaphanoscopic transillumination (Fig. 193). Whether a radial incision or one parallel to the limbus is preferred depends on its relation to the direction of the larger *uveal vessels*. The exposed uveal vessels themselves are often difficult to distinguish from their pigmented surroundings by simple visual inspection. They are revealed by either diaphanoscopic transillumination or by their behavior during diathermy, there being less tissue shrinkage over the large vessels. [2]

There are various ways of approaching the **anterior chamber** from the limbic region. One must therefore weigh the advantages and disadvantages attendant upon surgical lesion of the various anatomic structures.

On the *outer surface* (Fig. 194a) the avenues of approach differ in their *vascularity*, a major factor determining the quality and rate of wound healing, as well as the risk of hemorrhage. They also differ in the possibility of

[2] Owing to greater convective heat transfer than in the avascular neighboring tissue (see Fig. 105d).

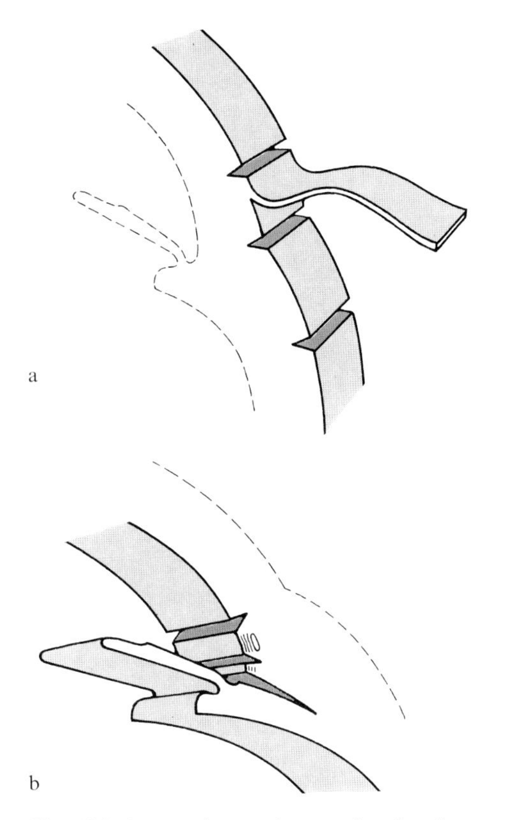

Fig. 194. **Approaches to the anterior chamber**

a *Outer surface*

Scleral incision: vascularized } covered with a
Limbic incision: nearly avascular } conjunctival flap

Corneal incision: avascular

b *Inner surface*

Subciliary approach: implies cyclodialysis

Angular approach: traverses the structures of the chamber angle

Corneal approach: perforates Descemet's membrane and the endothelium

covering with *conjunctival flaps*, which are helpful in effecting rapid closure and wound repair but may obstruct view of the operative field in the anterior chamber.

On the *inner surface* (Fig. 194b) the relations to the structures of the chamber angle must be taken into account. A *corneal approach* facilitates the removal of tissue adhesions during surgery and lessens the danger of synechiae in the postoperative phase owing to the distance from the iris root and ciliary body.

The direct *angular approach* may injure the trabecular meshwork and drainage channels of the canal of Schlemm. Its peripheral location favors the development of synechiae.

A *subciliary approach* requires section of the ciliary attachment at the scleral spur and, if no cyclodialysis is planned, is suited only for narrow openings. It provides excellent access for the separation of angular synechiae, as well as for the injection of air or liquid under high pressure,[3] since the opening is quickly tamponaded by the ciliary body after the cannula is withdrawn.

2.2 Geometric Factors in Opening the Globe

In cases where the incision is made in one stroke (i.e., with no subsequent correction),[4] the **relationship between the surface of the cut and the utilizable opening** must be determined before the section is begun. Both factors, the width of the cut surface and the length of the opening, are dependent upon the *angle of the incision* relative to the globe surface (Figs. 195, 196). If the direction of the incision is referred to the *plane of the iris*, note that the relationship of cut surface and utilizable opening depends on the level at which the incision is made (Fig. 197).

Wounds can be opened by either tangential or perpendicular forces (Fig. 198). When the edges of an incision diverge in a *tangential direction* ("wound gape"), the tangential traction results from an increase in wall tension (i.e., a rise of intraocular pressure). Force vectors acting in a *perpendicular direction* (raising or depressing the wound edge) occur when external forces are applied.[5]

A wound **"gapes"** if the inner edge of the wound on one side can no longer touch the outer edge on the other side, thus forming a communication between the interior of the eye and the outside air (Fig. 199). In the case

[3] To produce a counterpressure in cases of high vitreous pressure.

[4] Example: Keratome or cataract knife incision, trephine incision.

[5] By instruments from without, by ocular structures from within (lens, vitreous).

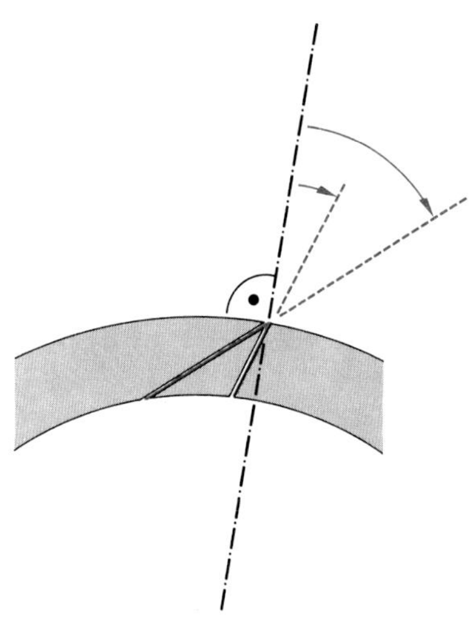

Fig. 195. **Width of the cut surface.** The width of the cut surface depends on the angle of the incision to the perpendicular on the globe surface

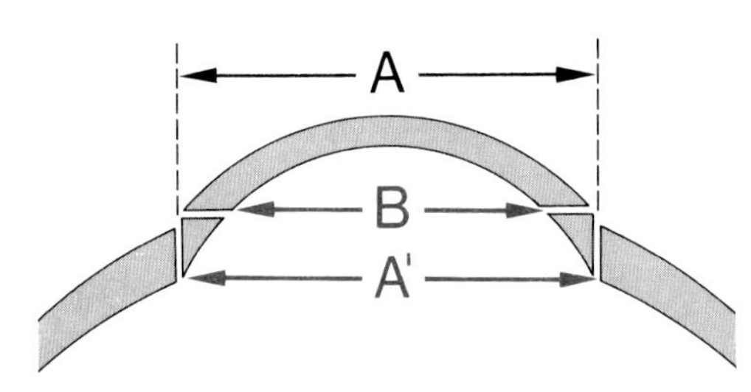

Fig. 196. **Useful opening.** For a given external approach *A*, the useful opening is equal to *A* in the trephine incision (*A'*) but is considerably smaller in a flap incision parallel to the iris (*B*)

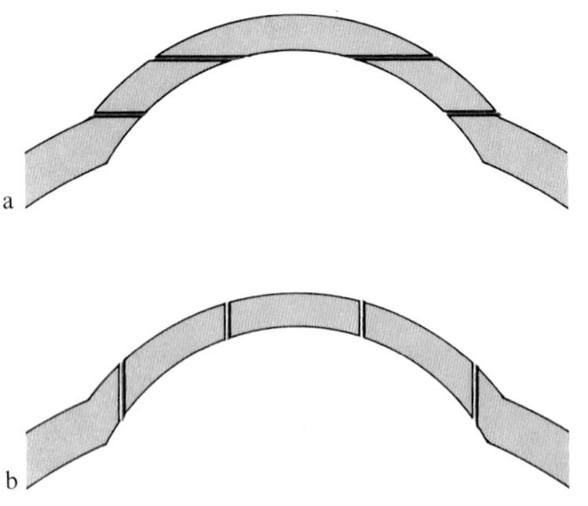

Fig. 197. **Change in the cut surface on parallel shift of the incision.**

Parallel incisions on a thick-walled spherical mantle (the cornea, for example) have surfaces of varying sizes.

a In incisions parallel to the iris, the area of the cut surface (*red*) increases toward the vertex.

b In incisions perpendicular to the iris plane, the cut surfaces become smaller toward the vertex

of a *perpendicular incision,* even the slightest shifting of its edges will produce wound gape (Fig. 199a).

Any incision which deviates from the perpendicular produces a *valvular opening* which will ensure wound closure even if the edges of the incision are shifted somewhat (Fig. 199b, c). The permissible extent of this shift, called the *margin of watertightness,* is expressed in the **valve rule:** *Incisions through the wall of the globe produce valves whose margin of watertightness is equal to the projection of the surface of the incision onto the surface of the globe* (Fig. 200).[6]

Thus, when the intraocular pressure increases, a perpendicular incision will always gape,[7] while a valvular incision will close even more tightly (within the limits of its margin of watertightness).[8] In other words, a valvular incision cannot be opened by a general rise of intraocular pressure. This can occur only when the lip of the incision is raised or depressed, i.e., when forces are applied in a perpendicular direction (Fig. 197b).

This is an entirely different mechanism of wound opening that applies to all wounds which do not follow the path of a great circle (Fig. 201). The movable portion of the ocular wall, called the flap, is rotated about an imaginary **"hinge"** connecting the ends of the wound.

If the tissue is sufficiently rigid, this rotation produces a fold[9] at the hinge (Fig. 202)

[6] The valve rule is valid only if the wound has a "valve capability," or is able to form a functional valve. Incongruent wound surfaces (incongruent grafts, trauma) and the incarceration of foreign material (tissue fragments, foreign bodies, viscous aqueous substituents) interfere with the valve mechanism.

[7] Due to its tendency to gape, the perpendicular incision is suited for producing antiglaucomatous fistulas. It is difficult to make, however, due to the difficulty of maintaining a precisely perpendicular incision through all tissue layers.

[8] It is due to their valvular properties that the keratome and cataract knife incisions could be left unsutured in times when no suitable threads and needles were available.

[9] A fold is produced only if the tissue has a "hinge-fold capability", i.e., if the forces applied to the flap are transmitted to the extremities of the incision. The rigidity necessary for this is either supplied by the tissue or is produced secondarily by applying tension (whether in the open globe with forceps or in the sutured globe by repressurization of the chamber).

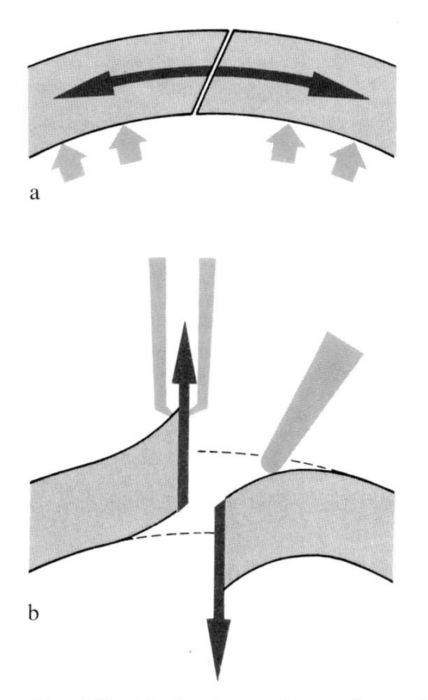

Fig. 198. **Mechanisms of wound opening**

a Gaping: A wound gapes if its surfaces are separated in a tangential direction by tangentially applied forces.

b Raising or depressing the wound edge: A wound can be opened in a perpendicular direction by perpendicularly applied forces (fixation forceps for raising the wound edge, a spatula for depressing it). This mechanism involves the rotation of a tissue flap

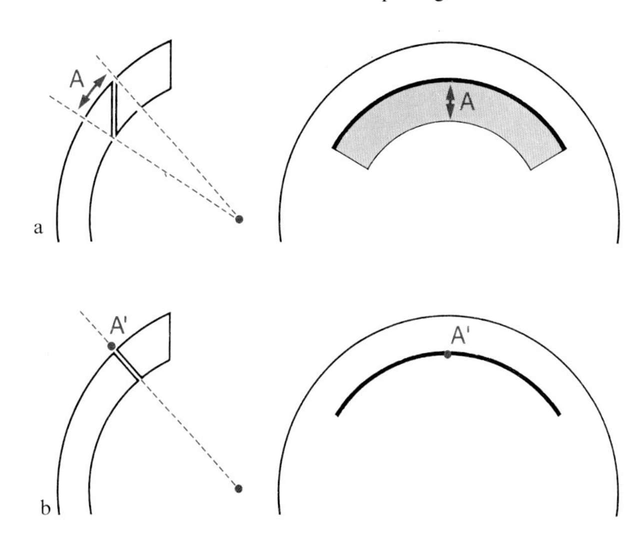

Fig. 200. **Margin of watertightness**

a The larger the projected area of the wound surface onto the ocular surface (*A*), the better the quality of the valve.

b In perpendicular incisions the external and internal edges of the incision (as projected onto the surface) coincide, i.e., the projection of the wound surface is a line. The margin of watertightness of a perpendicular incision is equal to zero

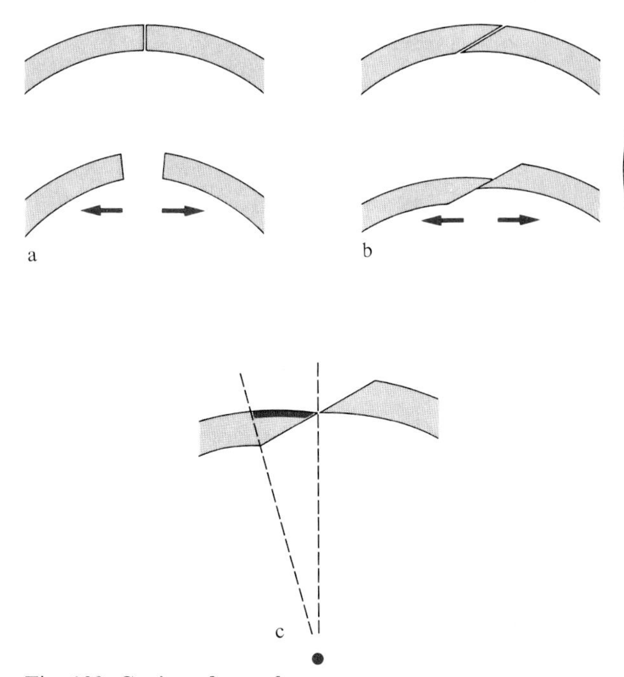

Fig. 199. **Gaping of wounds**

a In a perpendicular incision, the wound gapes at the slightest dehiscence.

b Oblique incisions form valvular openings which remain watertight even when their edges are shifted.

c When the distance of the shift equals the projection of the wound surface onto the surface of the globe (*red*), the incision begins to gape

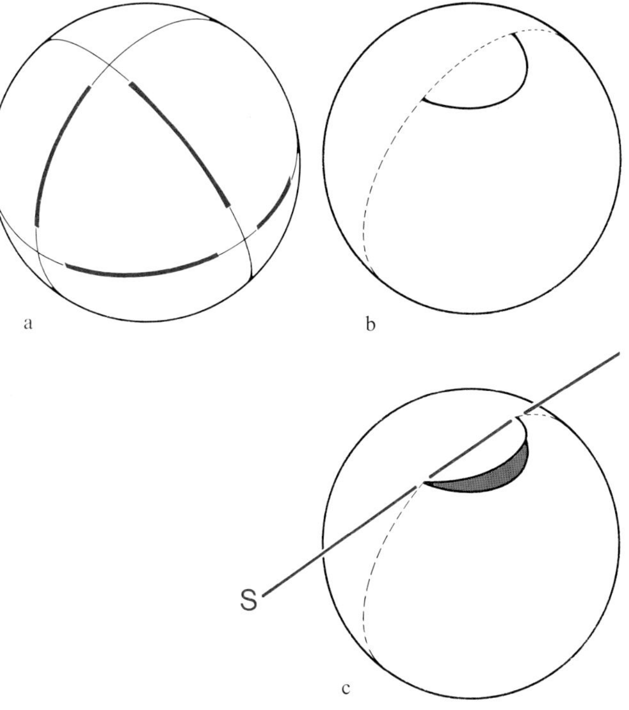

Fig. 201. **Conditions necessary for the rotation of tissue flaps**

a Incisions which lie on a great circle.

b Flap-shaped incision which does not lie on a great circle.

c Flap-shaped incisions can be rotated about an imaginary hinge axis *S* connecting the ends of the incision

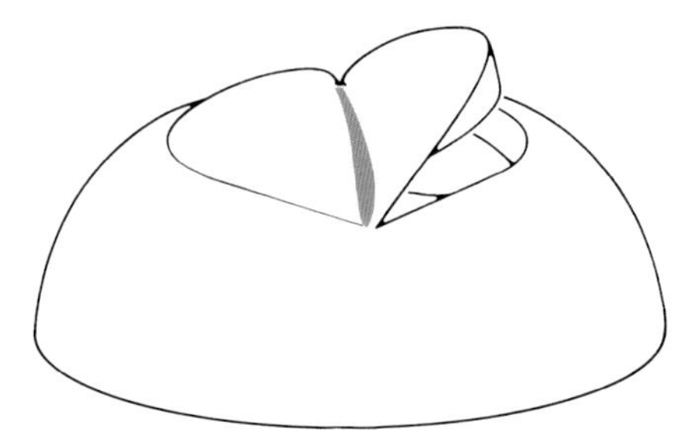

Fig. 202. **Formation of a hinge fold.** Rotating a flap causes an infolding of the domed ocular wall

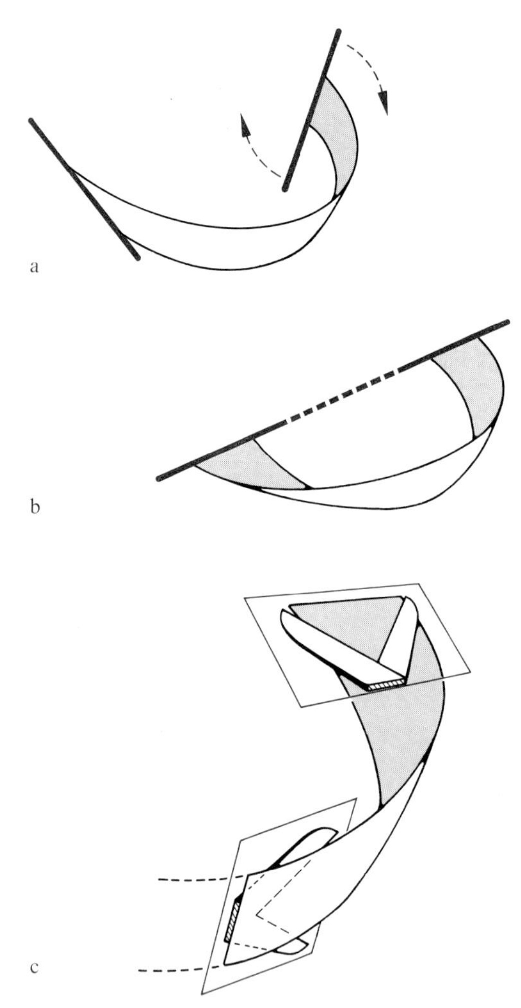

Fig. 203. **Formation of a hinge fold intramurally**

a The ends of the incision are twisted as the hinge is formed.

b The surfaces of the incision are twisted until they lie on the plane of the hinge line; the greater the angle between the real cut surface and the imaginary hinge axis, the more twisting occurs, and the greater is the generalized deformation of the surroundings.

c No deformation occurs if the ends of the cut surfaces lie on one plane from the outset. This condition is met in the keratome and cataract-knife incisions. Scissors must be rotated in the final phase of the cut to produce this effect

as all the tissue parts lying between the ends of the wound are shifted toward the imaginary hinge axis.[10] This shift of tissue encompasses the surfaces of the ends of the incision (the *intramural* part of the hinge fold), which are twisted until they lie in the same plane (Fig. 203), as well as the external portions of the ocular wall between the ends of the wound (the *extramural* parts of the hinge fold), which are flattened until they lie on a straight line (Fig. 204). In the process, the lateral ends of the wound diverge, and if this divergence is opposed by a resistance,[11] the dome is bowed inward.

Thus, rotating a flap is always accompanied by an *overall deformation of the globe,* and so requires an adequate margin of deformation[12] (Fig. 205). The extent of the deformation depends on the height of the dome or (since the curvature of the globe is a given) on the distance between the ends of the wound. Owing to this, the deformation can be minimized by shaping the flap so as to reduce this distance (Figs. 206, 207).

Whether the flap can be rotated outward or inward (i.e., can be raised or depressed) depends on whether the outer or inner wound margin is overriding. Whether a communication will then be formed between the interior of the globe and the outside depends on the location of the hinge axis and is defined in the **"hinge rule":** *A wound acted upon by perpendicular forces will remain watertight if its hinge lies entirely within the wound surface.*

For **flaps which rotate outward,** the hinge rule says that the wound will remain watertight if the imaginary hinge axis does not intersect the inner edge of the wound when both are projected onto the ocular surface (Fig. 208). We can thus make a distinction between wounds which are watertight by

---

[10] The appearance of a transverse fold is a sign of incipient wound opening. If it appears spontaneously, it is an important *warning sign* of impending prolapse through internal forces (muscular activity, expulsive hermorrhage).

[11] Examples: High rigidity of the tissue; corset ring sutured on close to the ends of the wound.

[12] If the anterior chamber is flat, for example, the lens is pushed inward and the vitreous is pressed outward: "...The anterior chamber was scarcely opened when vitreous appeared!"

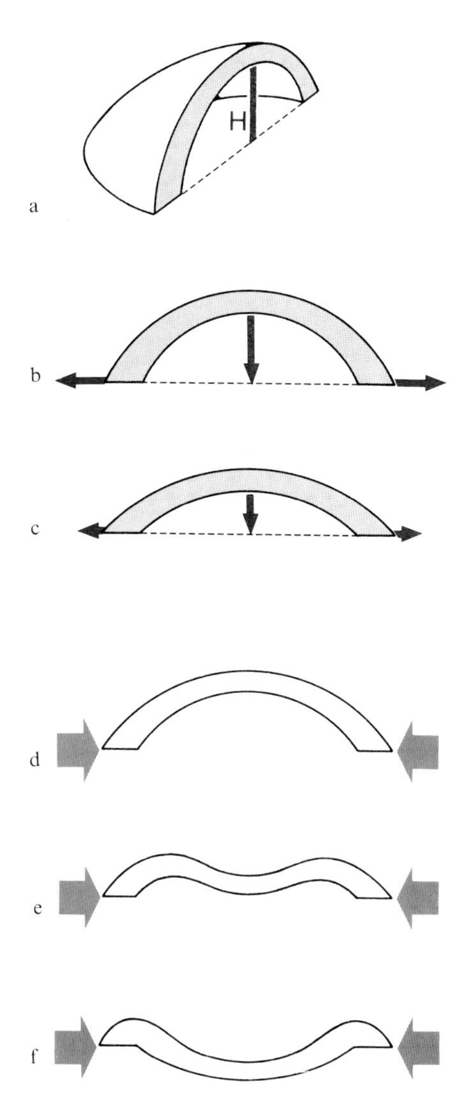

Fig. 204. **Formation of a hinge fold extramurally**

a When the hinge fold is formed, all parts of the dome lying between the ends of the incision are forced onto a straight line. The resulting deformation depends on the difference in length between the spherical segment and chord, or the height of the dome (*H*).

b, c The ends of the incision are forced apart as the dome flattens; the higher the dome, the greater this divergence.

d–f If the ends of the incision cannot move laterally, the tissue is compressed and the dome is finally bowed inward

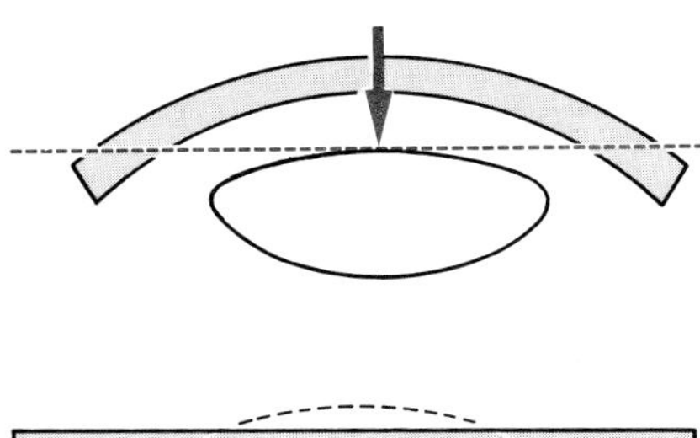

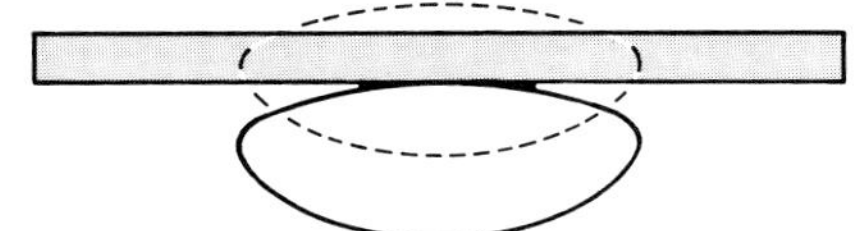

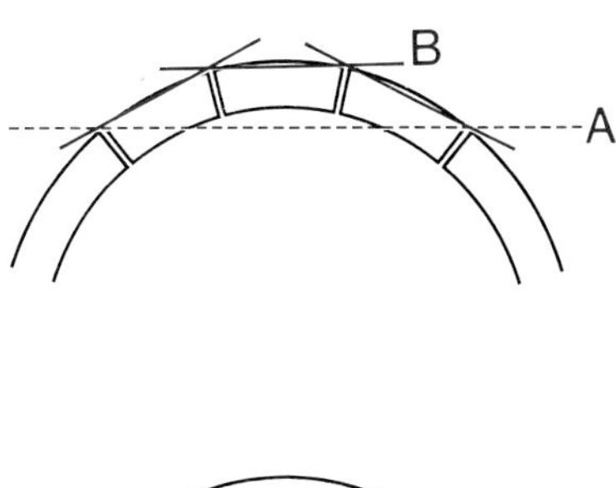

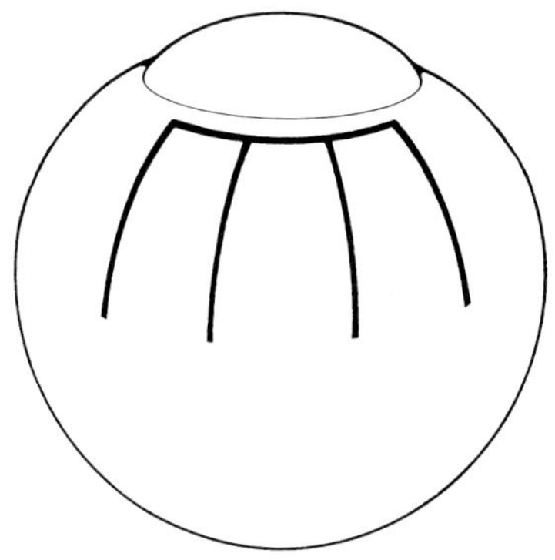

Fig. 206. **Means of reducing deformation by the hinge:** Decreasing the height of the dome. By dividing the flaps into segments, the distance between the ends of the wound is reduced. The dome heights over the segments are smaller than the height above the complete hinge. A – complete hinge. B – segmental hinge

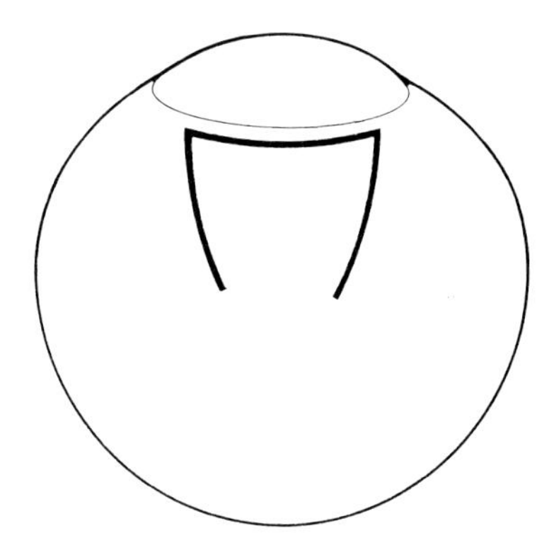

Fig. 207. **Means of reducing deformation by the hinge:** Shortening the hinge. If the sides of the flap are cut so that the ends of the incision are convergent, with increasing flap size the hinge line is shortened and the dome height is correspondingly reduced

Fig. 205. **Reduction of intraocular volume by the hinge fold.** The volume of the space below the dome decreases when the fold is formed. Firm tissue (e.g. the lens) lying above the imaginary hinge axis is pressed inward, and the pressure in the vitreous chamber increases

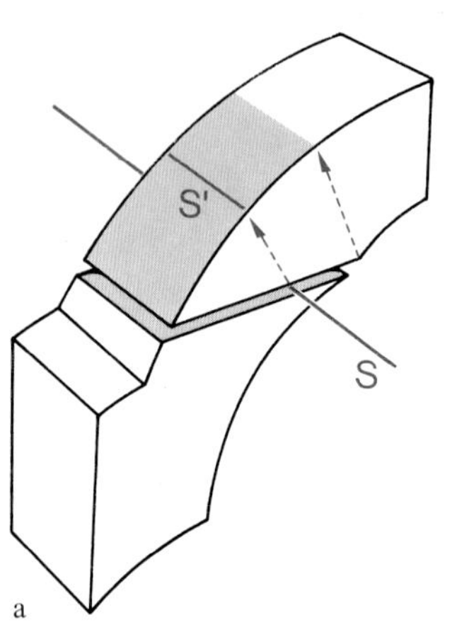

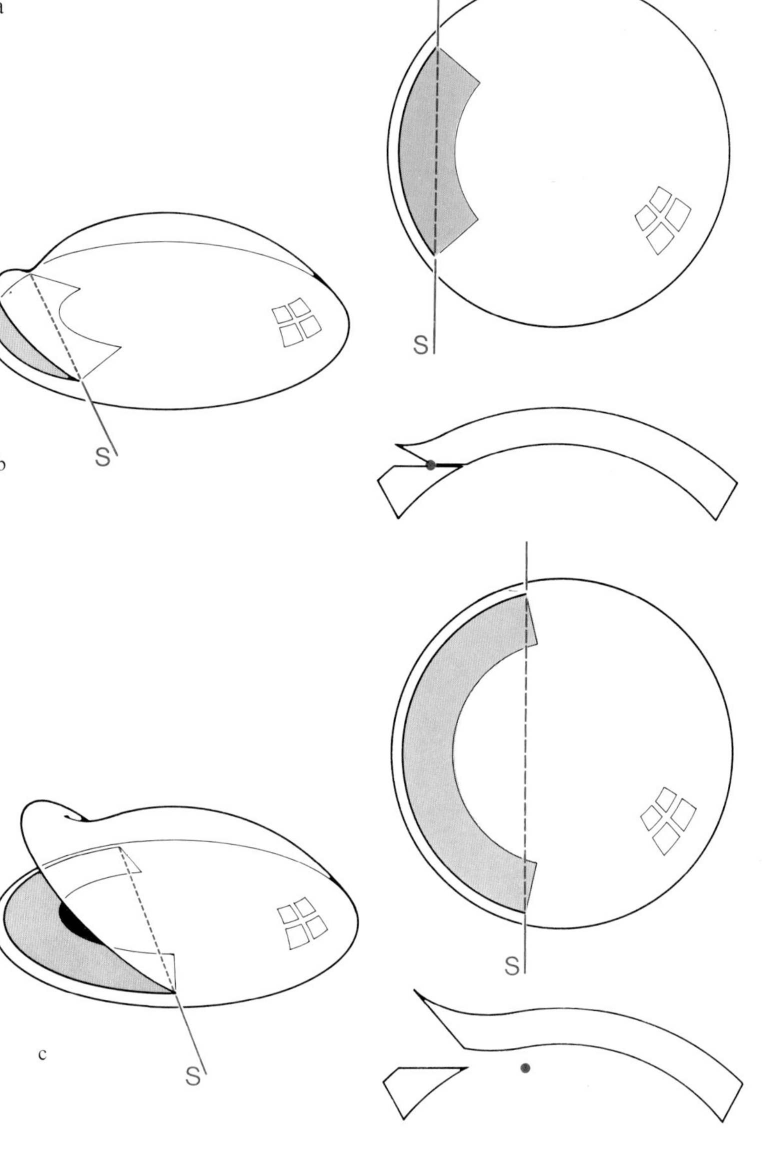

Fig. 208. **Hinge rule for outward-rotating flaps**

a Projection of hinge and wound surface onto the globe surface, as employed in the following illustrations. *S* imaginary hinge axis; *S'* its projection; *pink area:* projection of wound surface.

b Geometrically watertight wound. A line through the outer corners of the wound forms the hinge axis, which lies entirely within the wound surface. When projected onto the globe surface, it does not intersect the inner wound margin; hence the wound is watertight.

c Non-watertight wound. The inner wound margin is intersected by the hinge axis

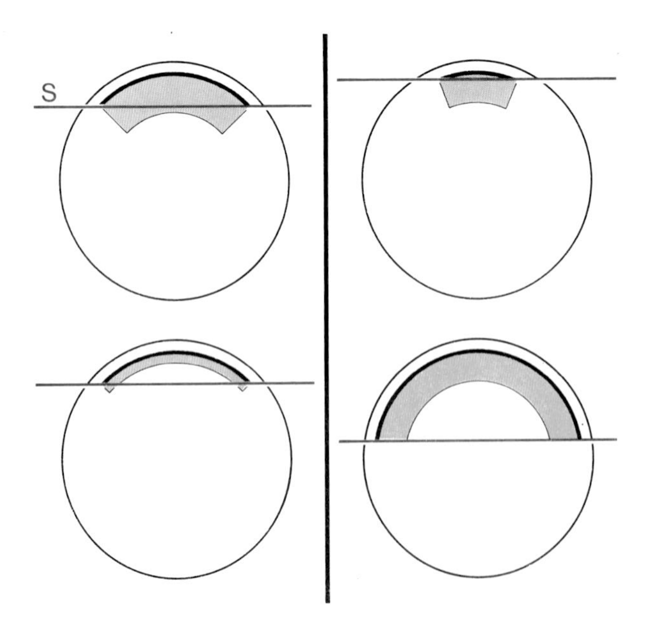

Fig. 209. **Sample applications of the hinge rule.** *Left:* Wounds of equal length: The projection of the wound surface determines whether the wound is geometrically watertight. *Right:* Wounds with surfaces of equal width (as projected onto the globe surface). Here the length of the wound determines whether it is watertight. The incisions in the top row are watertight, while those in the bottom row are non-watertight and thus require suturation for closure

virtue of their geometry, and those which are not. The decisive factor is the length-to-width ratio of the wound surface: Long incisions made at a steep angle are easily opened, whereas short incisions made at a shallow angle tend to remain watertight (Fig. 209). Valvular incisions which follow a great circle path are watertight by the hinge rule, regardless of their length.[13]

Clearly, the distinction between watertight and non-watertight wounds is important from the standpoint of operative tactics. Watertight wounds will remain effectively closed of their own accord,[14] provided there is no obstruction between the wound surfaces.[15] Non-watertight wounds, on the other hand, require sutures for secure closure. These sutures are merely apposition sutures. Their purpose is to divide the wound into segments which, individually, are watertight by the hinge rule. The sutures (or more precisely, the points where the overlying suture segments cross the outer wound margin) function here as the artificial vertices of new hinge axes (Fig. 210). They should be spaced according to the hinge rule such that these new hinge axes do not intersect the inner wound margin[16] (Figs. 211, 212). The *maximum allowable suture spacing* thus depends on the width of the wound surface.[16]

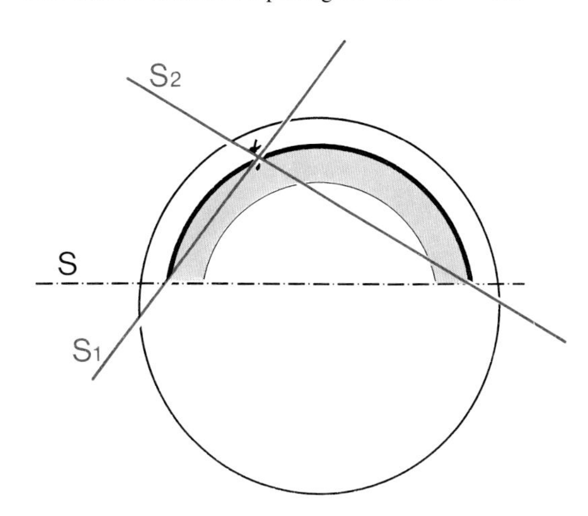

Fig. 210. **Function of sutures in maintaining watertightness.** The suture divides the wound into segments whose watertightness is determined by new hinge axes (S_1 and S_2). The segment with S_1 is watertight, while that with S_2 must be subdivided further

[13] Such wounds are apt to *gape* if the incision is perpendicular, however.
[14] Note: the wound must have a hinge-fold capability if spontaneous closure is to occur. This is ensured by restoring the globe tension if necessary.
[15] Example: Instruments which are introduced into the eye for manipulations (spatula, cannula, viscous aqueous substituents) or tissue parts (iris in iridencleisis, lens, vitreous prolapse).
[16] As projected onto the globe surface.

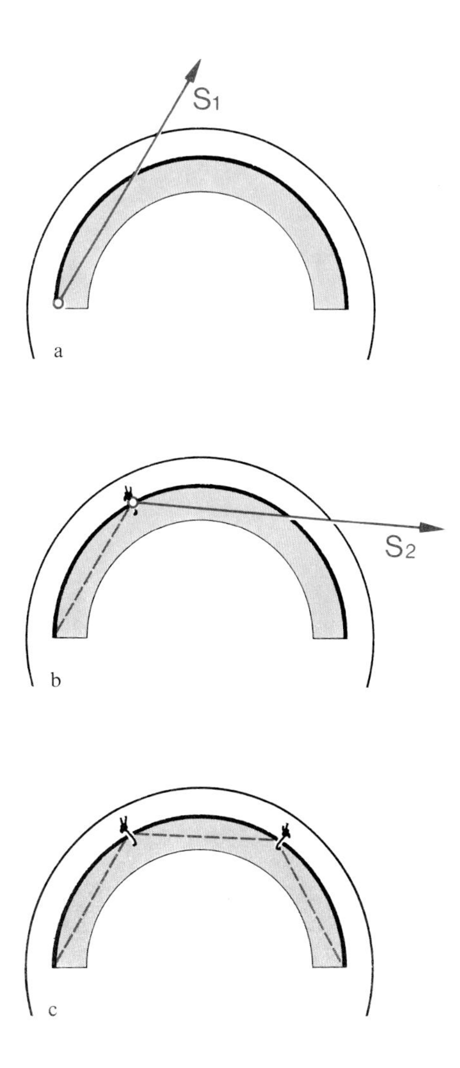

Fig. 211. **Finding the maximum suture spacing**

a To find the location of the first suture, a line is drawn from one end of the incision which just misses the inner margin. The suture is placed at the point where this line crosses the outer margin of the incision.

b Another line (S_2) is drawn in the same way from the first suture, and the next suture is placed at its point of intersection with the outer wound margin.

c A line from the second suture reaches the other end of the incision without intersecting the inner margin (in this example); hence no further sutures are necessary to achieve watertightness

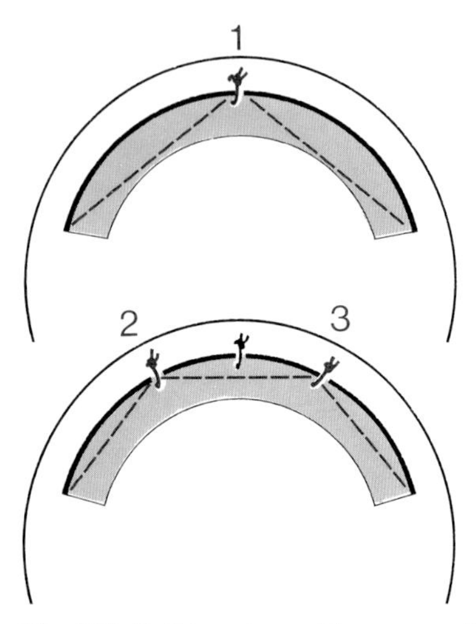

Fig. 212. **Safety sutures.** To ensure effective closure even if a suture placed according to the method in Fig. 211 comes loose, safety sutures are employed. In the drawing above, suture *1* alone is capable of dividing the wound into watertight segments. Sutures *2* and *3* are safety sutures, placed such that their hinge axes do not intersect the inner wound margin. Note that the sutures are not spaced evenly along the wound line, but lie closer to its midpoint

Incisions with narrow surfaces require more sutures to effect closure than those with wide surfaces (Fig. 213). Closure is most difficult in the case of perpendicular incisions, because there is no position in which the inner wound margin is not intersected by a hinge axis.[16] In theory, an infinite number of sutures would be required; in practice, this problem is circumvented by the use of compression sutures.[17]

Incisions whose outer margin follows a *great circle path* (see Fig. 201) represent a special case. Flap-shaped wounds which consist of two such incisions (Fig. 214) can be effectively closed by a single suture, since they are always divided into two watertight segments, regardless of their length and the angle at the apex of the gothic arch.

---

[17] The spacing of compression sutures is determined by the size of the compression zones (see Fig. 75).

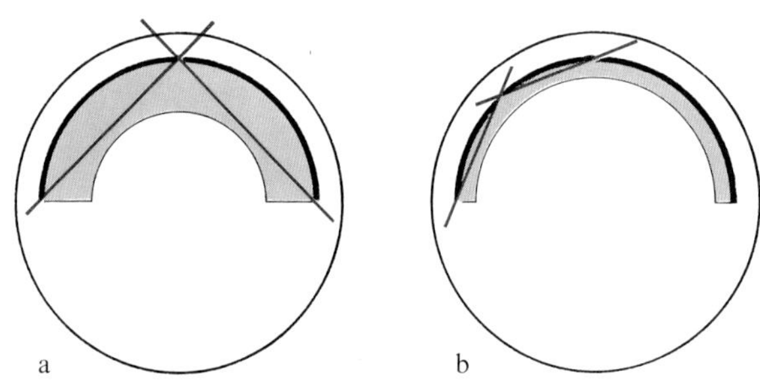

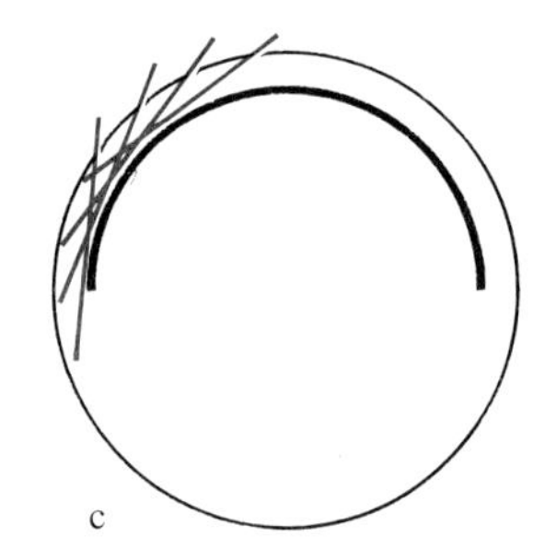

Fig. 213. **Minimum number of sutures needed for outward-rotating flaps**

a If the wound surface is broad enough, a single suture may suffice.

b Narrower wound surfaces require more sutures.

c If the wound surfaces are perpendicular, each hinge axis forms a chord which intersects the wound margin (in projection). Theoretically, an infinite number of sutures are required

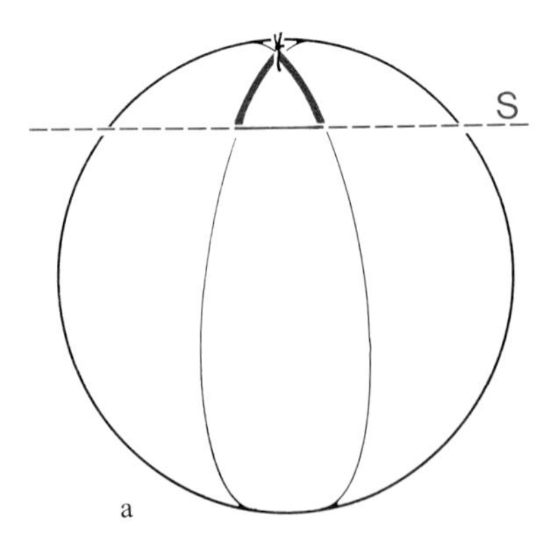

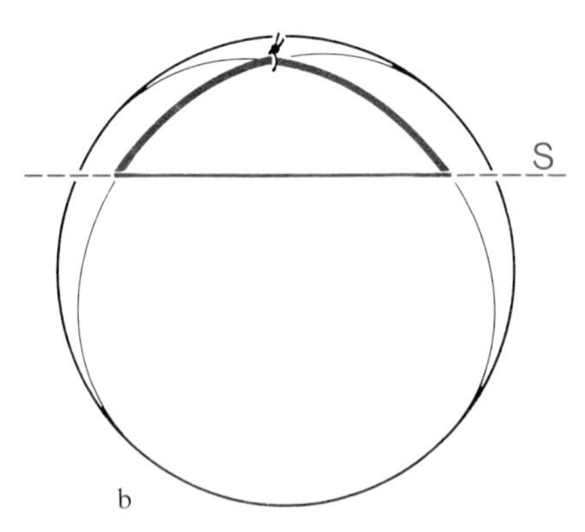

Fig. 214. **Suturation of "gothic arch" incisions.** Flap wounds made by two incisions which follow a great circle path are divided into two watertight segments by a single suture placed at the apex of the arch, regardless of the size of the flap. Only the outer wound edges are shown in the drawings; the projection of the wound surface is omitted (for a practical example of the gothic arch incision, see Fig. 246)

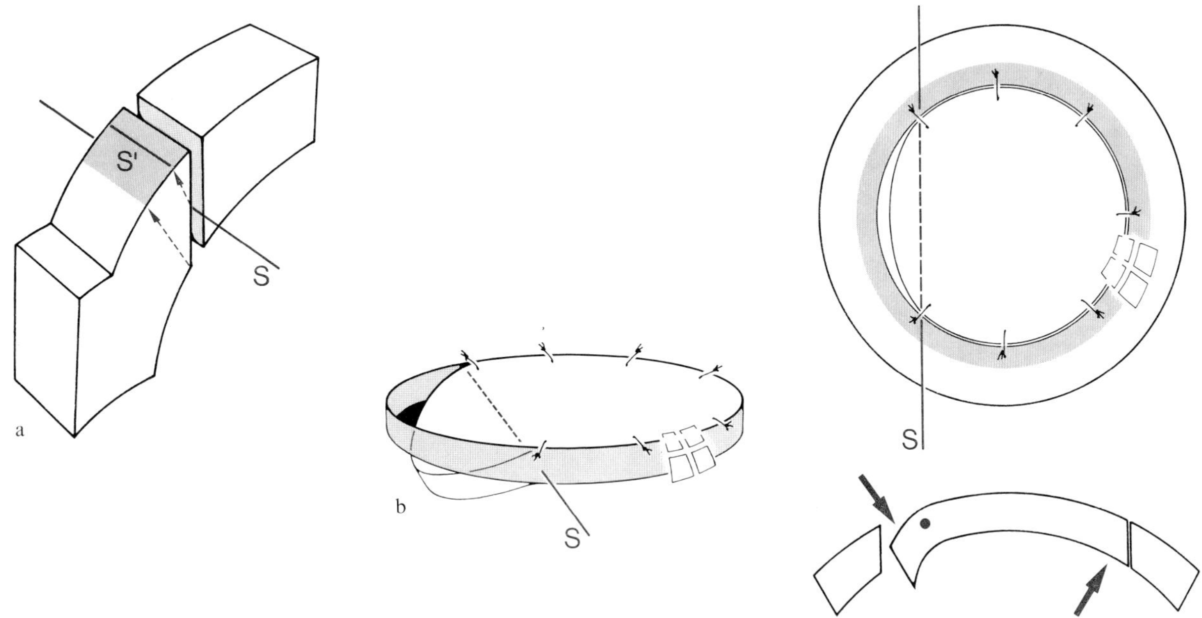

Fig. 215. **Hinge rule for inward-rotating flaps** (suturation of a trephine disk)

a Projection onto the globe surface. *S* hinge axis; *pink area:* projection of wound surface.

b If the projection of the imaginary hinge axis intersects the outer wound margin, the wound is opened when the flap is rotated inward

For **inward-rotating flaps,** wound closure is determined by the relation of the hinge axis to the *outer,* rather than inner, wound margin; and it is the *points of deep suture passage* that form the vertices of the new hinge axis (Fig. 215). According to the *hinge rule,* rotating the flap inward will not cause the wound to open if the imaginary hinge axis does not intersect the *outer* wound margin. [16]

It follows from this rule that the greater the distance of the point of deep suture passage from the surface (Fig. 216), i.e., the broader the wound surface and deeper the suture, the fewer sutures are required (Fig. 217).

The *trephine* produces flaps of the inward-rotating type. As soon as the trephine disk is fixed by two sutures, the first hinge axis is formed. Further sutures serve to shorten the length of the non-watertight segments, whose closure is then governed by the valve and hinge rules. The former, however, applies only if the tissue possesses a *valve capability,* i.e., if the wound surfaces are smooth and congruent; irregular wound surfaces require compression sutures to ensure a contact area adequate for closure. The hinge rule requires a *hinge-fold capability,* i.e., a tissue rigidity sufficient to produce a hinge fold. Thus, the principal task of the sutures in trephination is to make the disk tense, the number of sutures depending on the inherent elasticity of the tissue. Once a hinge-fold capability is present, the hinge rule states that a small trephine disk requires more sutures than a large disk (in relation to the length of the incision), and that more sutures are needed for superficial suturation than for loops passed more deeply.

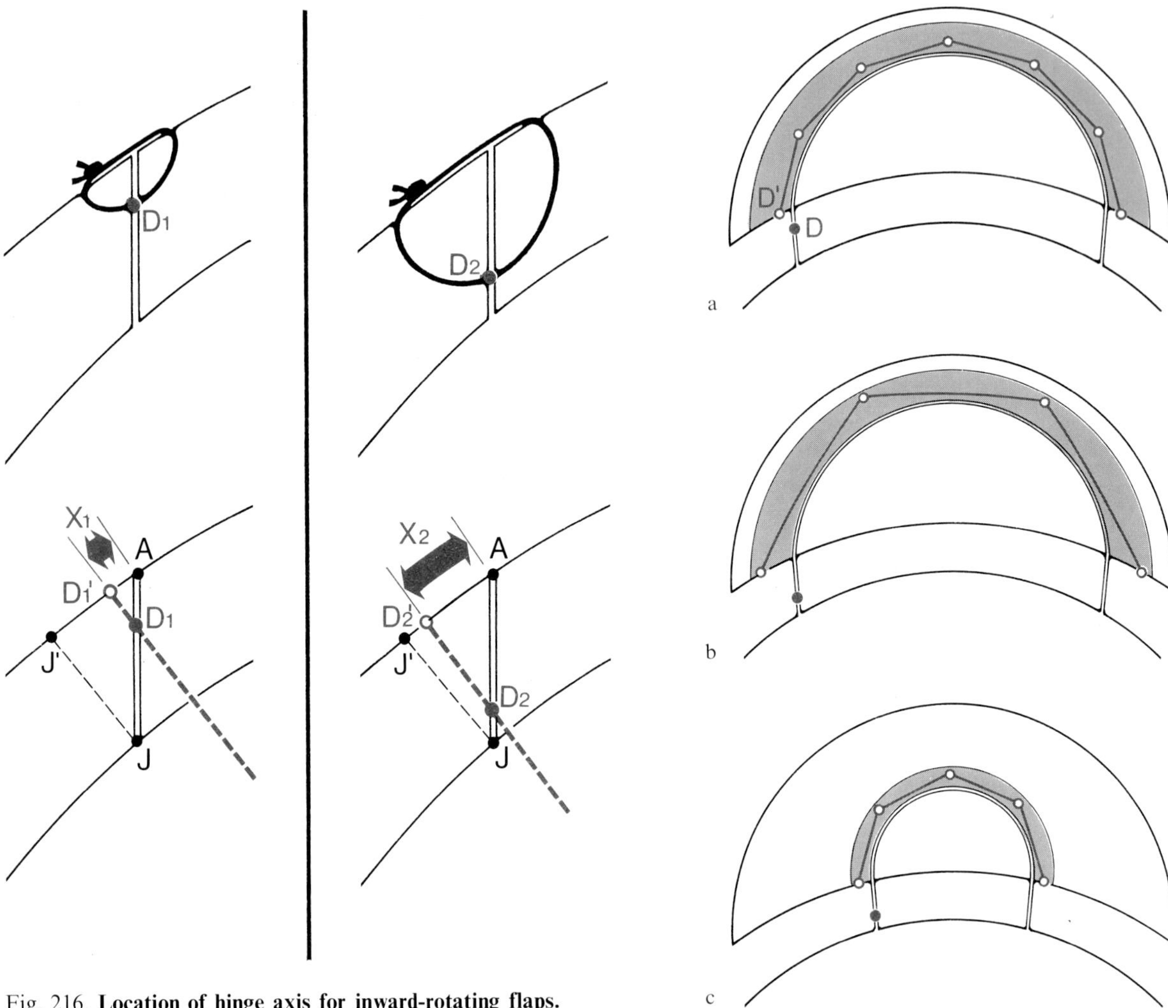

Fig. 216. **Location of hinge axis for inward-rotating flaps.** The points of deep suture passage *D* form the new vertices of the hinge axis. The deeper the suture, the greater the projected distance *X* from the outer wound margin *A*. *J* inner wound margin: *J′* its projection onto the globe surface; *D′* projection of suture passage onto the globe surface.

Left: superficial suture
Right: deep suture

Fig. 217. **Minimum number of sutures needed to divide wound into watertight segments.** Effect of suture depth (*D*) and width of wound surface. *Pink:* projection of the wound surface onto the surface of the globe.

a In the case of superficial sutures, the vertices of the hinge axes project close to the outer wound margin. The number of sutures is correspondingly large.

b In the case of deep sutures, the distance of the vertices from the outer wound margin is increased, and fewer sutures are required.

c If the trephine disk is small, the projection of the wound surface is narrowed, and the distance of the projected vertices from the outer wound margin is reduced (despite the same suture depth as in **b**). Despite the decrease in wound length, there is little decrease in the number of sutures required

2.3 Comparison of Various Incision Profiles

The following criteria must be considered when selecting the profile of the incision:

Freedom of choice of topographic reference points (Fig. 218). When the incision is made in a single plane, the positions of the outer and inner wound margins are correlates of the slope of the incision. In multiple-plane incisions they are mutually independent and can be varied as needed during the course of the incision.

Margin of watertightness (Fig. 219). The tendency of a wound to remain watertight when acted upon by tangential or perpendicular forces is, according to both the *valve* and *hinge rules,* dependent on the width of the wound surface as projected onto the globe surface. This "margin of watertightness" generally characterizes the stress resistance of a wound.

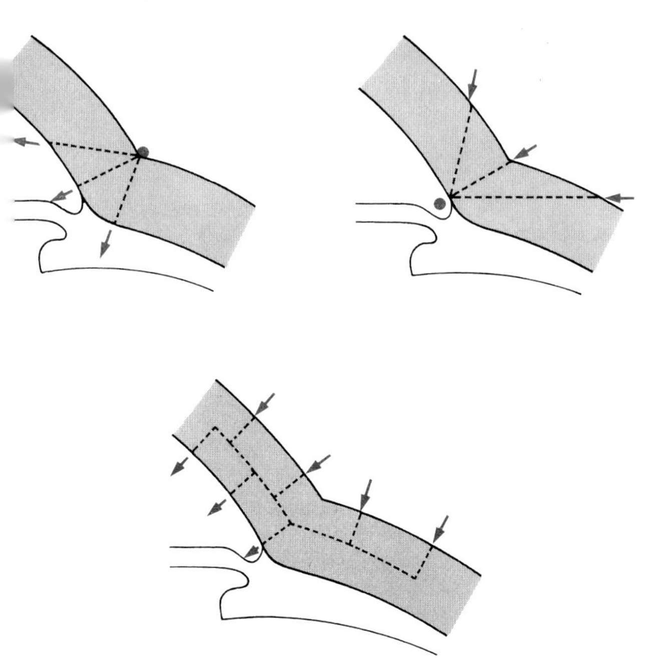

Fig. 218. **Topographic factors in selecting the type of incision**

a Single-plane incisions: if the position of the outer or inner wound margin is established, the choice of the direction of incision (i.e., the width of the wound surface) will also determine the opposite wound margin.

b Multiple-plane incisions: The positions of the outer and inner wound margins are mutually independent and can be varied as needed even during the course of the incision (see also Fig. 194)

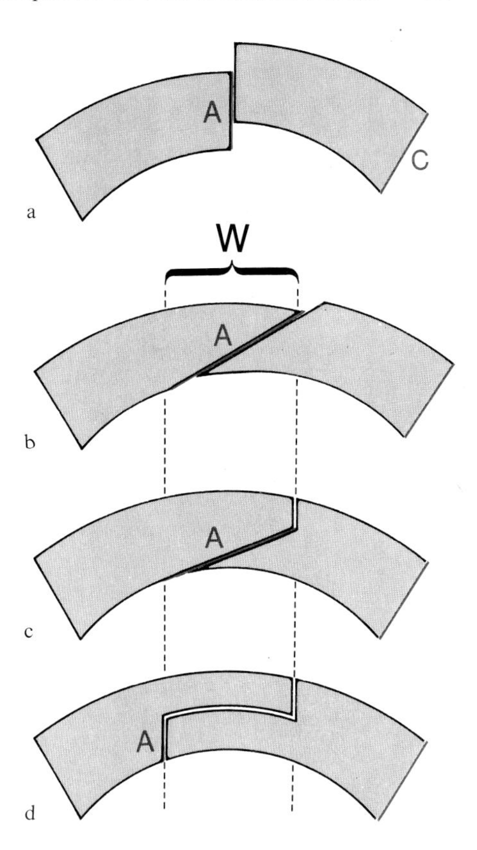

Fig. 219. **The properties of various incisions**

	Margin of watertightness	Apposability	Oblique surfaces	Resistance on opening of chamber	Complexity of incision
a) Perpendicular incision	∅	+	–	$A = C$	+
b) Single-plane oblique incision	W	–	++	$A \gg C$	+
c) 2-plane step incision	W	+	+	$A >=< C$ depending on W	++
d) 3-plane step incision	W	+	–	$A < C$	+++

A = thickness of tissue layer which must be sectioned as a last step prior to entering the chamber.
C = corneal thickness.
W = projection of wound surface onto ocular surface (= margin of watertightness)

Apposability. *Perpendicular* wound surfaces facilitate accurate apposition. The vectors created during suturing cannot shift the wound edges in a tangential direction. Perpendicular shifts create steps which, even if slight, are readily recognized, especially in reflected light. *Oblique* wound surfaces are more difficult to appose, because the edges can easily shift relative to each other (Fig. 219b). Moreover, faulty apposition is more difficult to detect due to the angulation of the wound edges.

Lamellar deflection. Incisions made at an angle to the lamellar direction will be deflected, with a corresponding loss of precision.

Tissue resistance on entering the globe. The lower the tissue resistance in the critical phase of the incision (last step prior to entry into the ocular interior), the less force is required, and the smaller the danger of inadvertant lesions of internal eye structures. This resistance depends on the thickness of the tissue layer that must be sectioned in the last phase of the incision.

Complexity of incision. The complexity of the incision, the technical difficulties involved, and thus the time required to make it increase with the number of direction changes made during the incision.

3 Methods of Opening the Anterior Chamber

3.1 General

If a high degree of accuracy is required, a perpendicular incision is desirable[18] to prevent **deflection of the incision** in the lamellae (Fig. 220).

If it is important to prevent **premature drainage** of the anterior chamber, the instrument itself can often be used to seal the incision. In guidance motions along a straight path, closure is maintained by using a *wedge-shaped* blade (Fig. 222). In swivelling movements, care must be taken that the *center of rotation* always is strictly at the wound entrance (Fig. 232, top).

As soon as part of the instrument has entered the anterior chamber, the polished parts will appear much brighter than the part still in the corneal tissue.

[18] This rule is especially important if intraocular pressure is low, i.e., if tissue sectility is poor.

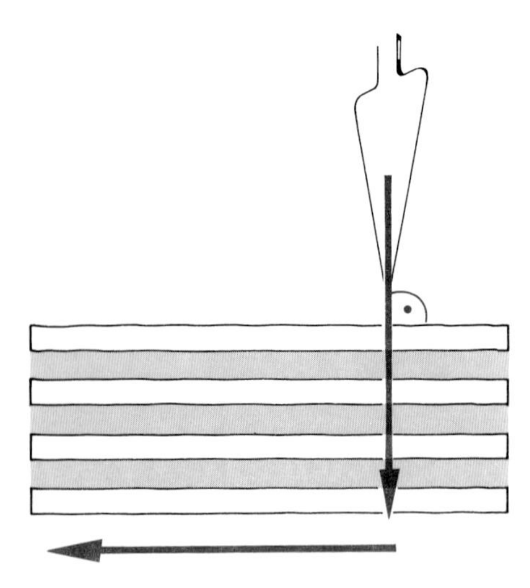

Fig. 220. **Incising the anterior chamber.** Lamellar deflection of the incision is avoided if the blade is first directed vertically toward the planned opening on the posterior corneal surface before it is passed parallel to the iris

Instruments in the anterior chamber also appear to change their **position** due to the high refractive index of the cornea and aqueous fluid (Fig. 221). This presents no difficulties as long as the instrument is used exclusively within the anterior chamber, since all structures are viewed under the same optical conditions. But if the instrument is used to make a *counterincision* from within, its *apparent upward bending* must be allowed for by aiming for a point on the inner corneal surface which is *higher* than the planned point of emergence.

As soon as aqueous escapes, the **wall tension** of the anterior chamber decreases. As a result, the resistance of the orbital cushion becomes a more important factor when the globe is passively moved. To avoid deformations it is always advisable to *lift* the globe somewhat on grasping. The diminished wall tension also reduces tissue sectility. Initially sharp blades become suddenly dull when aqueous drainage occurs. To improve sectility, the tissue fibers must be made tense, either by applying forceps close to the cutting edge or by using scissors to make the cut. If an initial incision is watertight by the hinge rule, sectility for enlarging the section can be increased by restoring the wall tension through the injection of watery fluid or viscous substances.[19]

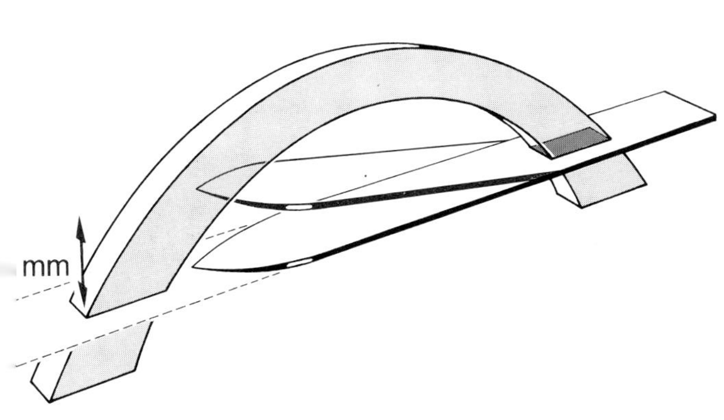

Fig. 221. **Apparent bending of instruments.** Instruments in the anterior chamber appear to be bent upward, the effect varying with the viewing angle. In reality the tip is lower in the chamber (*black*) than it appears from the outside (*red*). If the tip is to emerge at the limbus, for example, the surgeon must aim for a point about 1 mm higher on the outer surface. If he aims directly for the limbus, the tip will emerge too far scleralward

3.2 Keratome Incision

Keratomes are wedge-shaped blades whose preferential paths lie in one plane.[20] The shape of the cutting edge determines the vector components created when the blade is advanced (Figs. 222, 223).

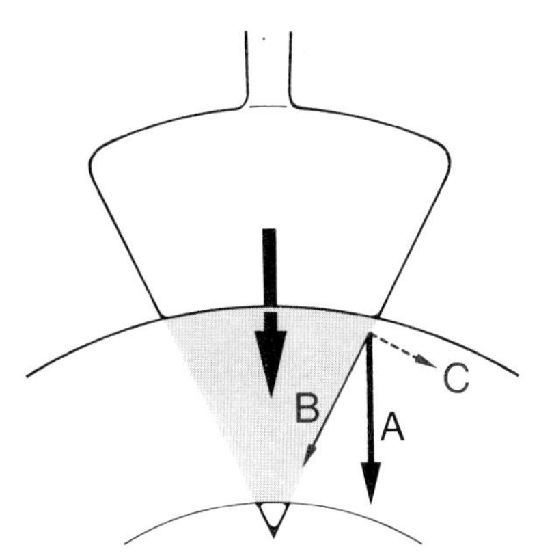

Fig. 222. **Force vectors of keratome.** When the keratome is moved forward (*A*), a thrust component is created (*C*) which expands the incision, as well as a pull-through component (*B*) which improves the cutting properties of the blade

Owing to the wedge shape of the keratome blade, the incision is watertight as long as the blade is advanced. The intraocular pressure remains constant, the tissue remains sectile, and the diaphragm stays in place until the tip reaches the opposite chamber angle. The length of incision attainable under these *optimal conditions* is determined by the width of the keratome blade (Fig. 224). However, this same width will cause the incision to open at the slightest mistake, that is if the blade is raised, lowered or tilted to any degree. This excludes any possibility of *corrections* during the keratome incision (Fig. 226), for the diaphragm surges forward as soon as the chamber drains, and so the incision must be concluded without delay.

When the *keratome is withdrawn*, the tip is first removed from the pupillary region in order to prevent injury to the lens, now in

[19] E.g., to enlarge a corneal incision following the discission of a lens capsule.

[20] If the two cutting edges are asymmetrically ground and thus have preferential paths lying in different planes, the incision will deviate as in Fig. 226.

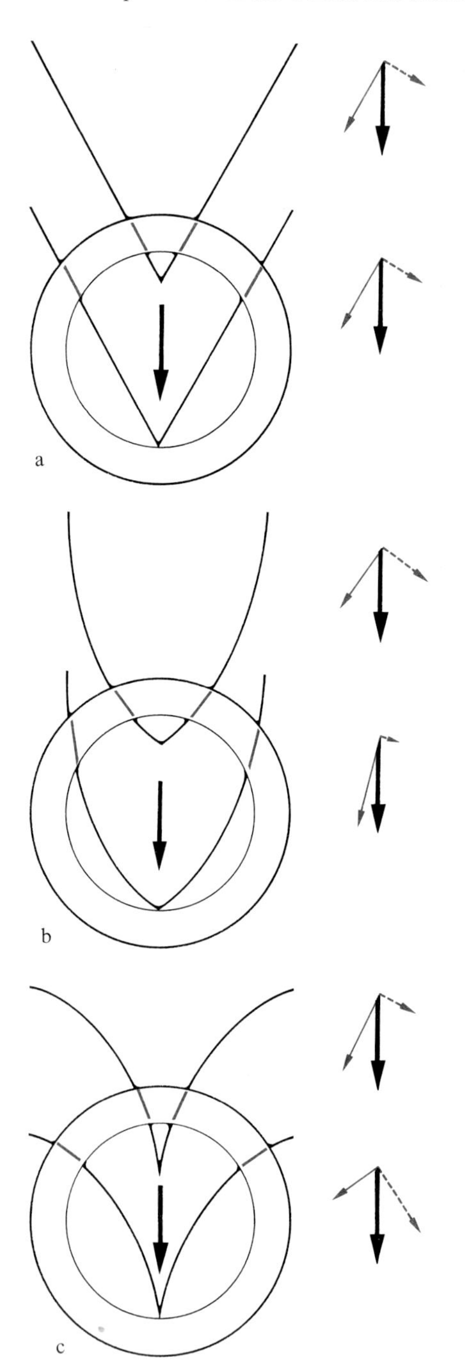

Fig. 223. **Cutting properties of various keratomes**

a In keratomes with straight cutting edges, the relation between the thrust and pull-through vectors remains more or less constant throughout the incision. The length of the tissue segment to be divided increases somewhat and, with it, the resistance.

b In keratomes with convex cutting edges, the ratio is altered in favor of the pull-through vector, so that the cutting ability of the blade constantly increases.

c In keratomes with concave edges, the ratio is altered in favor of the thrust vector. Cutting ability decreases as the incision proceeds. The resulting incision differs from that in **b** by the position of the hinge axis, which in **b** facilitates, whereas here it facilitates opening

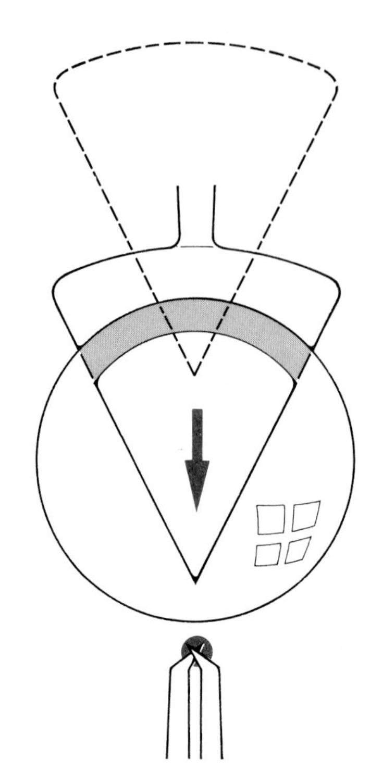

Fig. 224. **Advancing the keratome.** The tip is directed toward the fixation forceps (cf. Fig. 220)

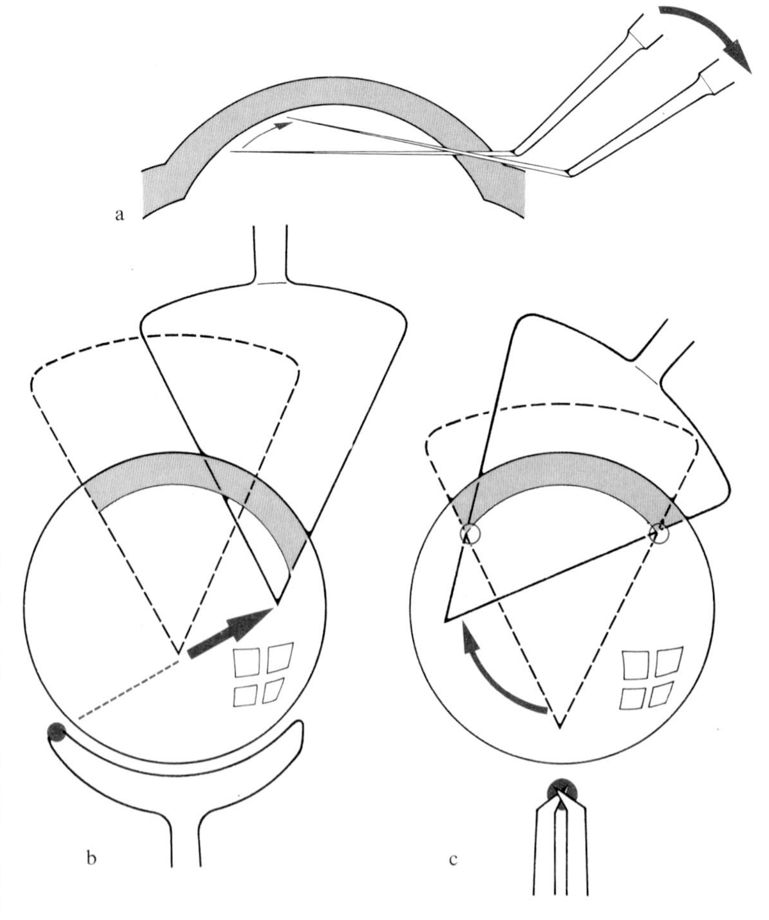

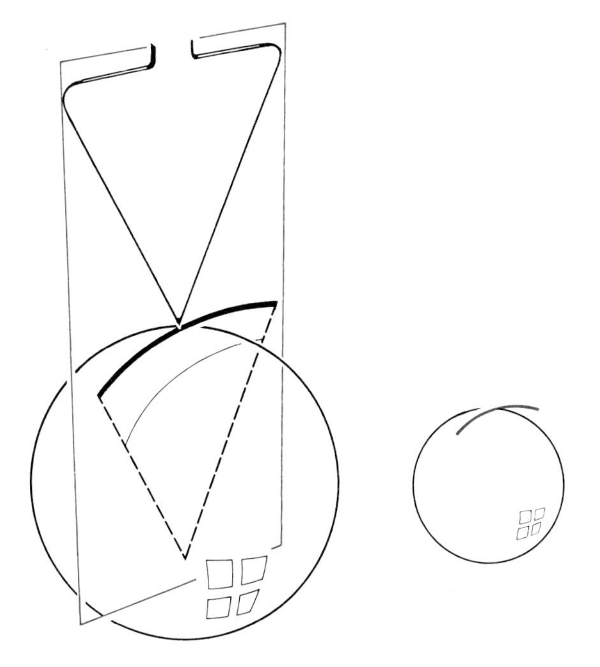

Fig. 226. **If the guidance path of the keratome** is not parallel to the limbus plane, the incision will extend partly too far into the cornea and partly too far into the sclera. No corrections may be made during the incision, or else the aqueous will drain

a more anterior position. This is done by raising the tip and simultaneously moving it to the side (Fig. 225). With the same withdrawal movement the incision can also be extended. If this is done in a *rotary movement,* the wound can be kept watertight, and tissue sectility can be preserved (Fig. 225b). If the keratome is moved *laterally* on withdrawal, however, the anterior chamber will drain in any case. The sectility then decreases, but the pull-through vector component of the cutting edge, which then becomes more effective, will help make it possible to continue the incision despite aqueous drainage (Fig. 225c).

Fig. 225. **Withdrawing the keratome**

a To avoid injury to the protruding diaphragm during drainage of the anterior chamber, the keratome tip is raised (handle is lowered) during withdrawal.

b Lateral blade movement to extend the incision: During withdrawal, the keratome tip is removed from the pupillary region by a lateral movement. Simultaneously, the incision can be extended by a pull-through motion of the blade. A broad fixation forceps facilitates the lateral movement, since it also offers resistance to lateral vectors.

c Rotation of the keratome to extend the incision: The ends of the incision (*red circles*) can be sealed during this movement by keeping the cutting edges in firm contact with them

3.3 Cataract Knife Section

Cataract knives have narrow, sharp-pointed blades which are used first to *puncture* the chamber and then *section* it from within (Fig. 227). The various forms of cataract knife differ chiefly in the shape of the tip, which determines whether the blade will deviate from the guidance direction when thrust into tissue (Fig. 228).

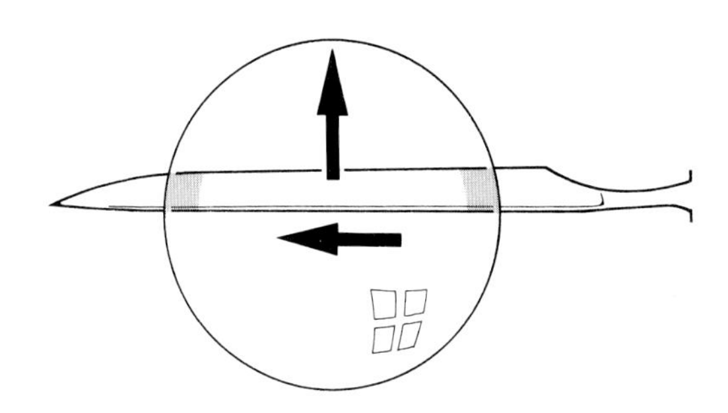

Fig. 227. **Force vectors in the cataract knife section.** The vector for puncturing the chamber and that for making the section are separate from each other and are mutually perpendicular

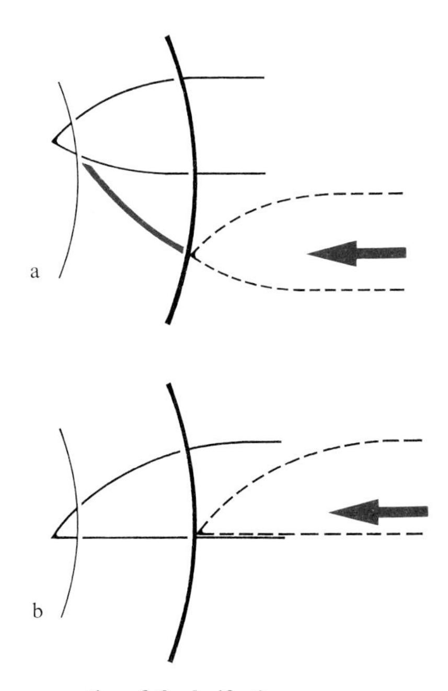

Fig. 228. **Cutting properties of the knife tip**

a Knives with a curved back deviate in the direction of the cutting edge when thrust straight into tissue.

b Knives with a straight back do not deviate from the guidance direction

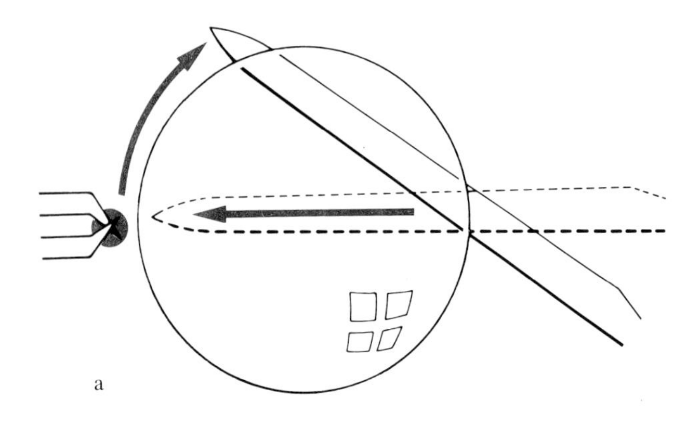

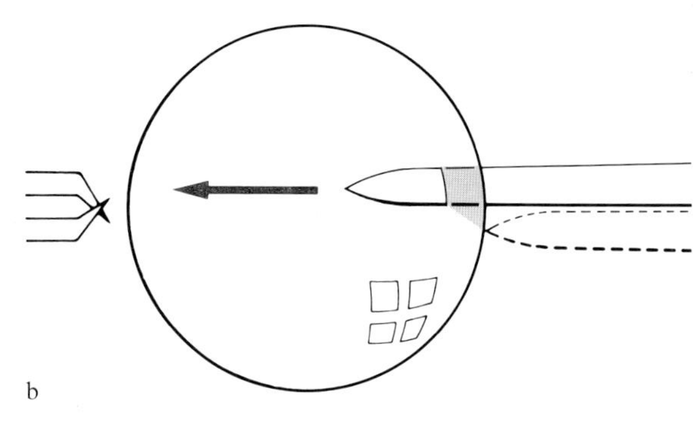

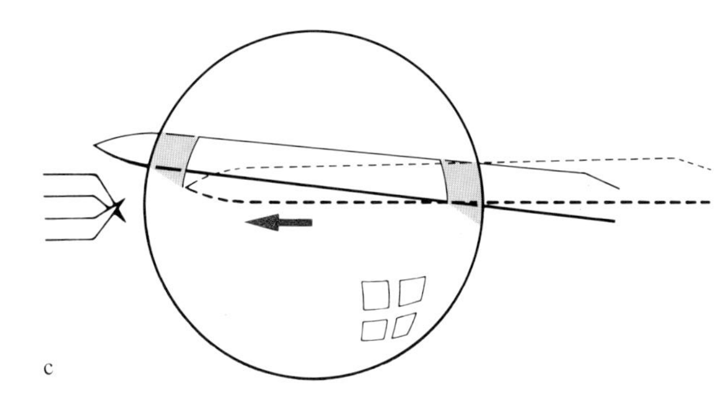

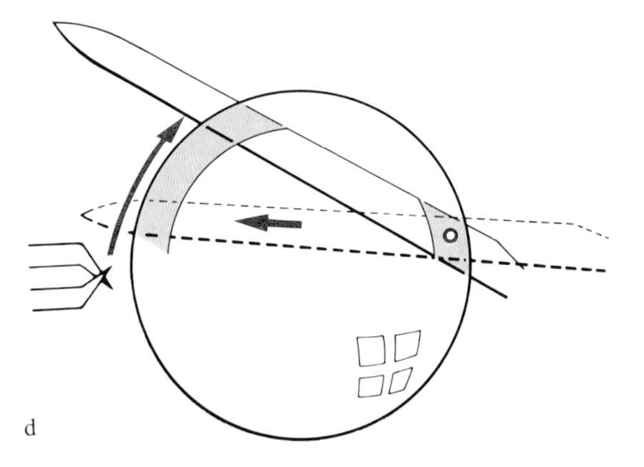

Fig. 229. **Cataract knife section with lateral fixation (favoring the puncturing vector)**

a Principle: The vectors of the puncture and section movements are directed through the application site of the forceps.

b Blade directed toward fixation forceps during puncture (*Note:* forceps should always be raised slightly).

c For the counterpuncture, knives with a rounded back may be directed toward the forceps, since the tip will deviate (see Fig. 228a) and emerge to the side of the forceps. (*Note:* tip is aimed about 1 mm higher for counterpuncture, see Fig. 221).

d Extending the incision by a slewing movement of the knife. The cutting edge is guided in the tissue such that the vectors of maximum tissue resistance are directed toward the point of forceps application. Note: center of rotation is at the entrance opening (*red circle*).

e Terminating the section: The blade is moved away from the fixation forceps.

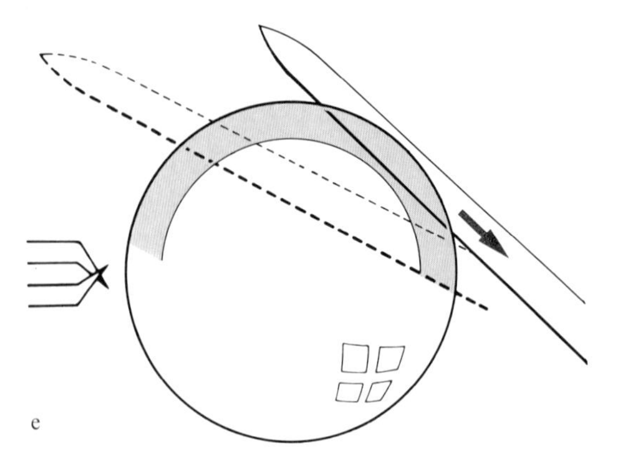

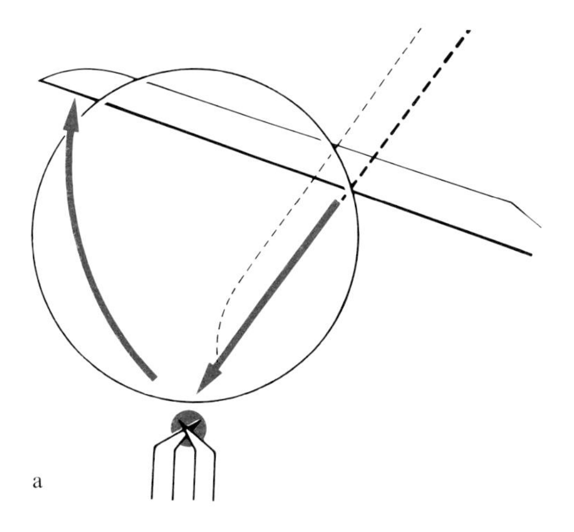

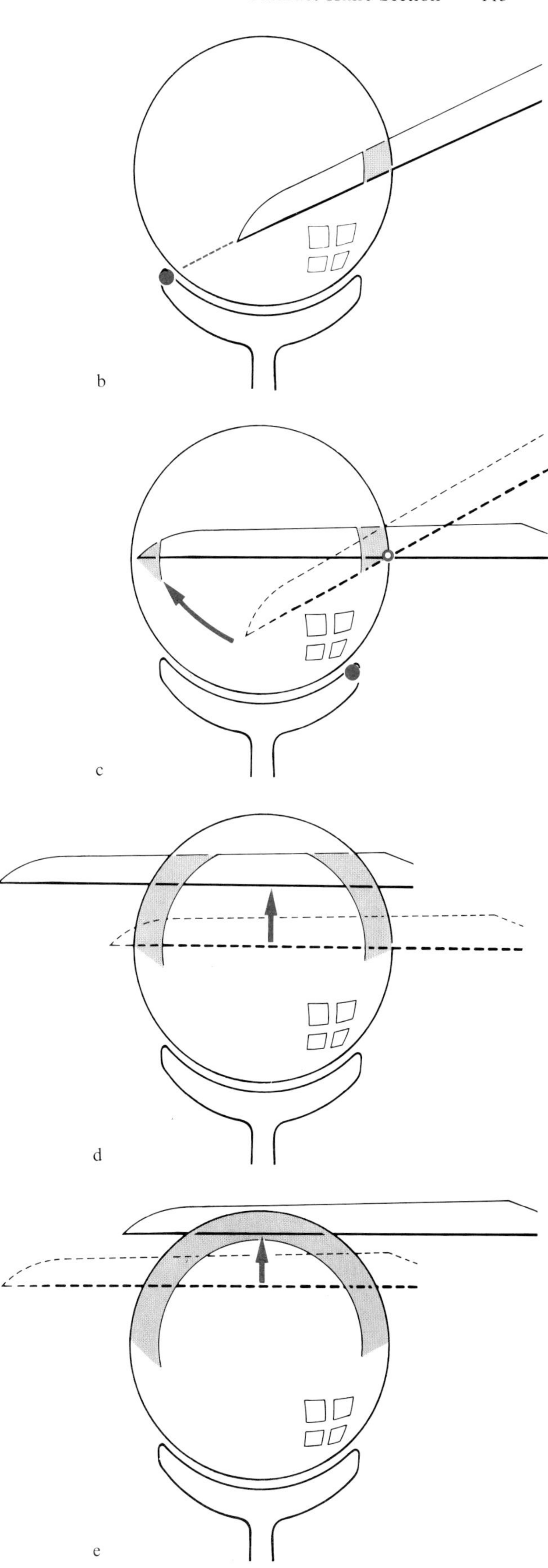

Fig. 230. **Cataract knife section with fixation from below (favoring the sectioning vector).**

a Principle: The vectors of puncture and counterpuncture are directed through the application point of the fixation forceps.

b Inserting the blade in the direction of the fixation instrument. Knives with a straight back make it easier to maintain the initial direction on passage through the tissue. If broad fixation forceps are used, the tip is directed toward the opposite end *(red point)*.

c Emergence with slewing movement, so that the vector of tip motion passes through the point of forceps application. The broader the grasping plate of the forceps, the smaller the angle of the slewing movement, with the result that the guidance of the knife approximates that for lateral fixation.

d, e Completing the section by to-and-fro movement of the knife

Since the puncturing and sectioning movements are separate in the cataract knife incision, both vectors cannot be simultaneously opposed by a *single* fixation. The surgeon must decide, therefore, whether main resistance should be given to the *puncturing vector* or the *sectioning vector*. This will determine whether the fixation instrument is applied opposite the puncture site or opposite the end of the incision (Figs. 229, 230). The disadvantages incurred for the other, "neglected" guidance direction can be eliminated somewhat by compensatory movements whose vectors pass through the forceps fixation point.[21]

Drainage of the chamber can be prevented only during puncture. As soon as the *section* is begun, the incision is made under more difficult conditions, i.e., with lax tissue, diminished sharpness and protruding diaphragm. To keep from wounding the iris during the cataract knife section, the surgeon must pass the knife *beyond the pupillary margin* immediately after the counterpuncture while the chamber still has sufficient depth. He must avoid any corrective maneuvers prior to this, because any tilting, raising, lowering or withdrawal of the blade would cause premature chamber drainage. Only after the pupillary margin is passed may the direction of the incision be corrected. It must be borne in mind, however, that any direction change will also change the width of the opening (Fig. 231).

The cataract knife section requires *great skill,* because the movements of the fixation forceps, the knife, and the relative movements between them have *different centers of rotation* (Fig. 232). A good result is obtained only if these movements are closely coordinated at all times. This is made difficult by the requirement that all movements be performed quickly and smoothly in the initial phase, i.e., before the blade passes the pupillary margin.

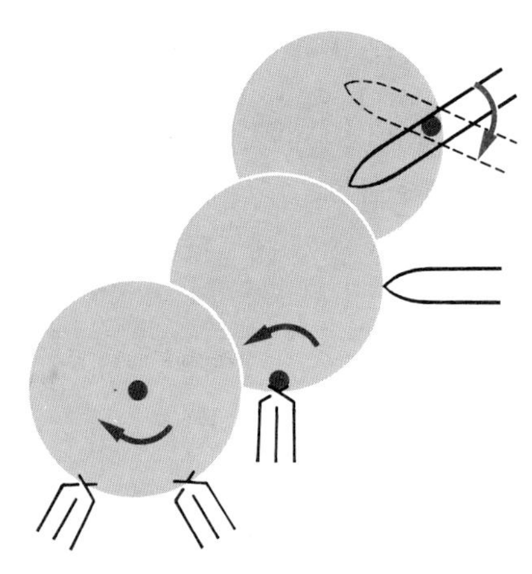

Fig. 232. **Centers of rotation of concurrent movements in the cataract knife section.** The center of rotation for corrective movements of the fixation forceps (see Fig. 153a) lies at the center of the globe (*bottom*). Movements of the knife (see Fig. 153b) cause the globe to rotate about the point of forceps application (*center*). Pivotal movements of the knife (see Figs. 229d, 230b) which are not to drain the chamber are made about the puncture site (*top*)

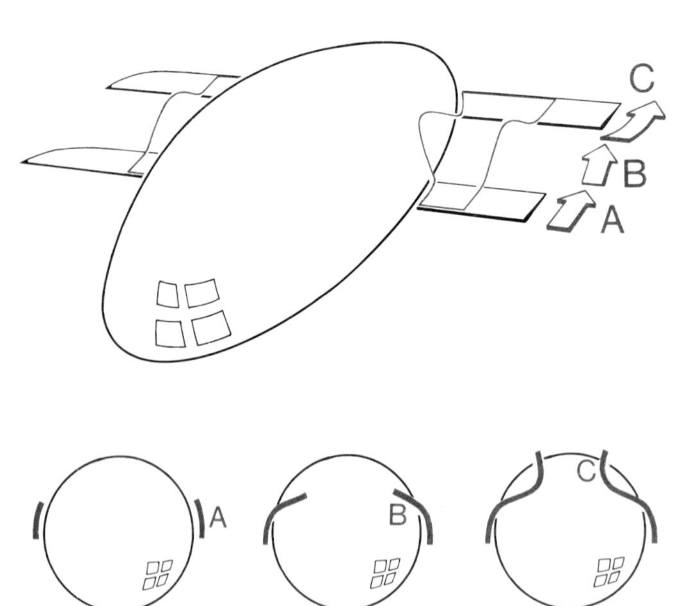

Fig. 231. **Corrective movements with the cataract knife.** The result of the incision depends on the geometric section of the guidance path with the corneal dome. If the blade is not directed parallel to the iris (*A*), the incision will turn inward if it is raised (*B*) or outward if it is lowered (*C*)

[21] The "sharper" the cataract knife, the lower the resistance, and the less important this requirement. However, if tissue sectility is poor (as when the globe is soft by either preoperative measures or premature aqueous drainage), observance of this rule will facilitate a smooth incision.

3.4 Cutting with Point Cutting Edges

Keratomes, cataract knives and other broad-bladed knives can in principle make incisions in one plane only. To produce more complex incisions, techniques are required in which only a very small blade width penetrates the tissue (see Fig. 51). The blade will then behave more or less as a point cutting edge and can be directed as needed to produce incisions of any shape desired (Fig. 233; see also Fig. 43).

Under these conditions, however, the blade can no longer seal the opening, and most of the incision must be made with the chamber opened, and thus with reduced tissue sectility. This places very high demands on the cutting ability of the instrument, but even with a very sharp blade, only *short* chamber openings can be obtained unless the tissue resistance is extremely low.[22]

With an unsealed opening the diaphragm will move forward on deformation of the globe (see Fig. 126). Centripetal force vectors therefore should be avoided during cutting and a small blade be guided strictly in a tangential direction (Fig. 254, see also Fig. 129).

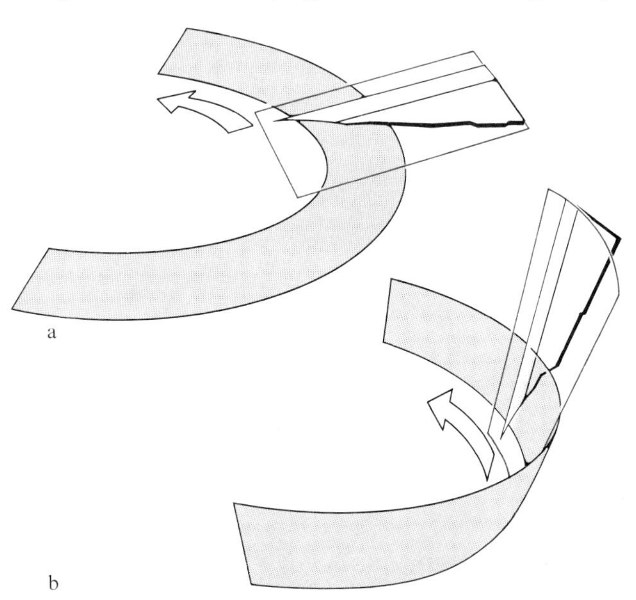

Fig. 233. **Opening the anterior chamber with a razor blade.** The manner of holding and guiding the blade determines the profile of the resulting incision.

a Plane incision by blade guided in one plane (imitating cataract knife or keratome incision).

b Perpendicular incision by blade held upright and guided along a conical surface

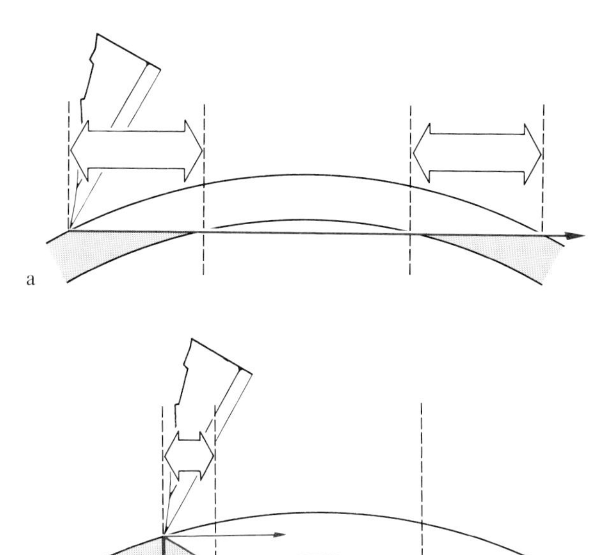

Fig. 234. **Opening the anterior chamber by tangential guidance of the blade**

a If the blade is directed tangentially, it must be applied far ahead of the planned inner opening due to the thickness of the tissue layer to be traversed. It must first pass through an intramural "lead segment" (arrow) before reaching the anterior chamber.

b If on the outside the blade is applied too near the planned inner opening, it must be guided with perpendicular vector components directed toward the interior of the globe

3.5 Cutting with Scissors

When scissors are used to cut the anterior chamber, the decrease in tissue sectility after the chamber is opened is of little consequence, since the scissors blades will hold the tissue and prevent shifting during the cut. Safety and precision can be increased by minimizing the size of the "danger zone" (see Fig. 60b) through the use of small blade apertures and the avoidance of swivelling motions (Fig. 235). The force vectors can be kept tangential, thereby providing an additional safety factor during cutting (Fig. 236b). Centripetal vectors are unavoidable only when the blade is introduced into the chamber (Fig. 236a).

The end of the penetrating blade is rounded to prevent inadvertant tissue lesions

[22] Such as after incision of a deep precut groove, when only a very thin lamella remains to be sectioned before the chamber is opened.

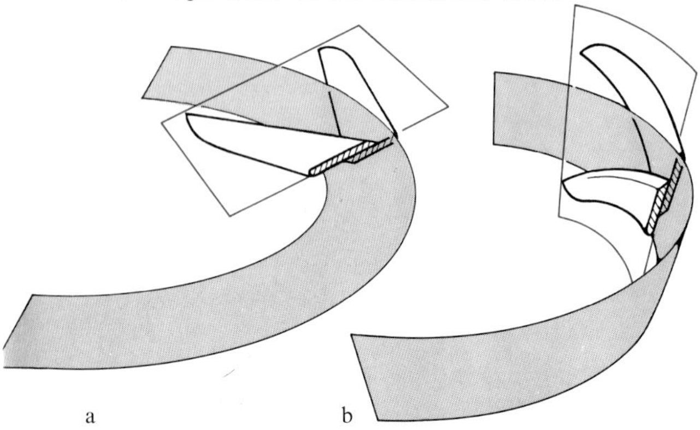

Fig. 235. **Special design features of corneal scissors:** curvature of the blades. If the shape of the blades is consistent with the desired shape of the cut (i.e. the guidance path congruent with the cut surface), the cut can be completed by simple closure of the blades.

a Straight blades are suited for making plane cuts parallel to the iris.

b Blades curved in accordance with the conical surface they must describe are used for making oblique cuts

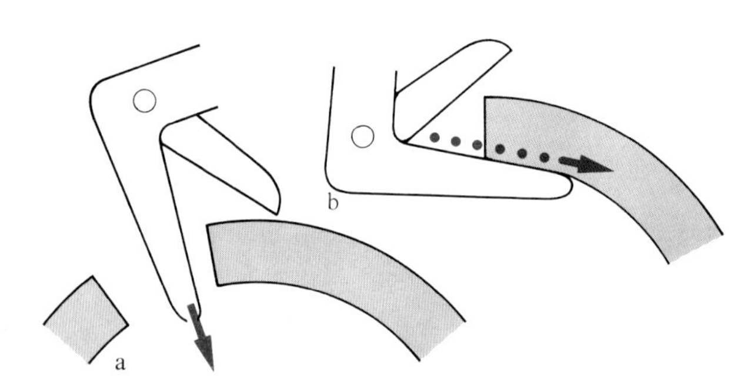

Fig. 236. **Force vectors of scissors**

a Centripetal vectors are inevitable when the blade is introduced into an opening.

b During cutting, the vector of the cutting point movement is parallel to the surface

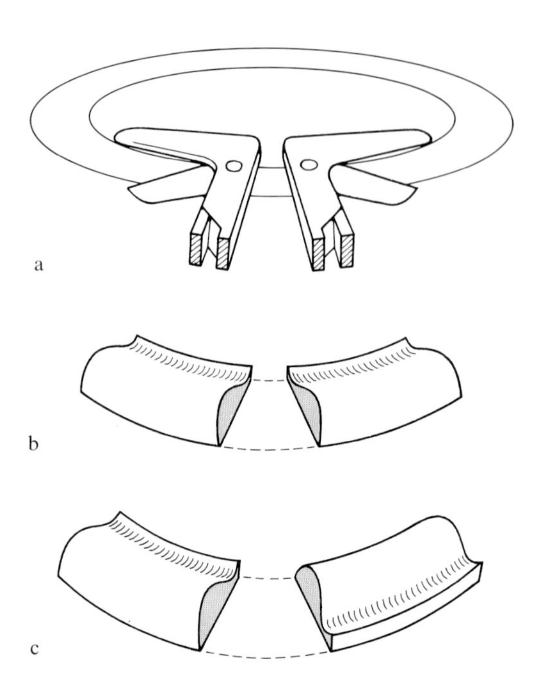

Fig. 238. **Special design features of corneal scissors: arrangement of blades.** To obtain identical S-shaped cut profiles when cutting in two directions, two scissors, each a mirror image of the other, are required.

a Mirror-image scissors for cutting in two direction.

b Continuous profile (see also Fig. 58) obtained with mirror-image scissors.

c Discontinuous profile made by using a single scissors to cut in both directions

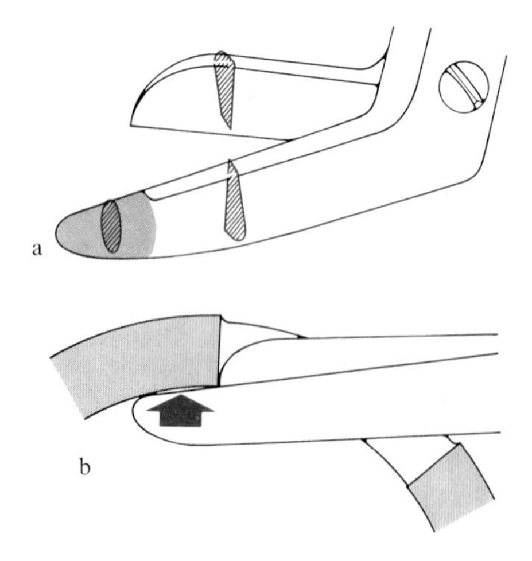

Fig. 237. **Special design features of corneal scissors: blade tips**

a If the blade introduced into the chamber is blunt-tipped and well rounded, it forms a kind of spatula (*gray*) which projects beyond the ground edges of the blade. *Red:* cross-section of cutting and blunt blade.

b The longer inner tip prevents the scissors from slipping out of the chamber during complete closure

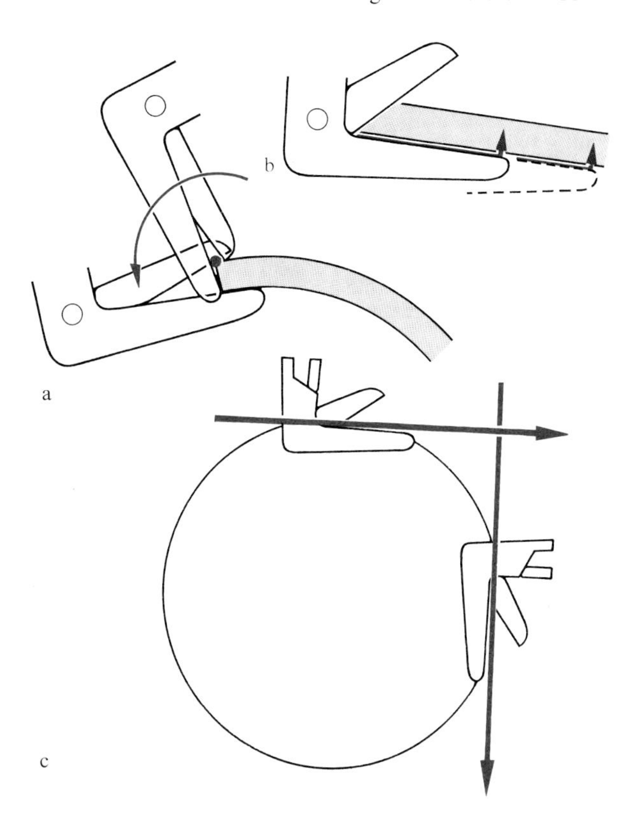

Fig. 239. **Cutting with scissors**

a Introducing the scissors: The scissors is almost closed when introduced to prevent internal structures from coming between the blades. An aperture just large enough to accomodate the corneal thickness will obstruct access to the interblade area. To prevent inadvertant entry into the chamber the outer blade is braced against the surface. The instrument is then rotated about the outer blade tip into the chamber (*red point:* center of rotation).

b Extending the cut: The inner blade is apposed firmly against the posterior corneal surface to guard against iris incarceration.

c Guiding the scissors: If the cutting point is to move tangentially to the cornea at all times, a 90° change of direction is required over each quarter-circle. If this is not guaranteed by the blade curvature, the handle must be moved in a broad arc during cutting

(Fig. 237). If the inner blade is made longer than the outer, *two scissors* are needed for cutting in two directions, each a mirror image of the other to ensure continuity of the cut profile (Fig. 238).

The main problem in cutting with scissors is to keep the *iris* away from the interblade "danger" zone. Thus, the blades are opened only slightly when passed into the chamber so that the enclosed corneal tissue will obstruct access to this zone (Fig. 239a). The depth of penetration can be limited by bracing the outer blade against the corneal surface. During cutting, the inner blade is pressed firmly against the inner corneal surface to prevent incarceration of underlying structures (Fig. 239b). The safety of the iris can be checked either by direct observation of the blades or indirectly by watching concomitant movements of the pupil (Fig. 240).

Disadvantages in the use of scissors are the high cutting resistance and complicated profile of the scissors cut. Both are correlates of the tissue thickness, however, and so these difficulties can be overcome by *preliminary thinning of the tissue layer* (see Fig. 59).

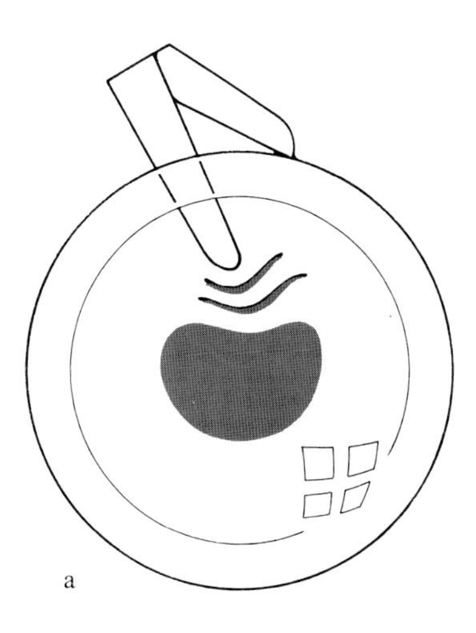

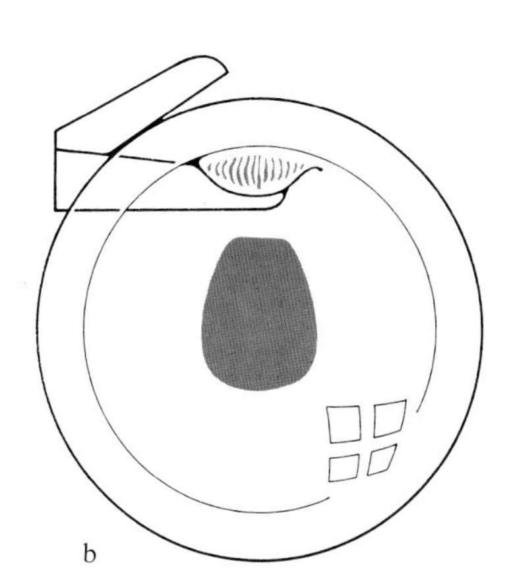

Fig. 240. **Monitoring the iris when cutting with scissors.** Deformations of the pupil are an indication that the iris has been caught by the blades.

a Inward dislocation of iris on insertion of spatula (→iridodialysis).

b Incarceration of iris between blade and cornea (→iridectomy).

3.6 Two-Plane Step Incision

If scissors are used to extend a precut groove (Fig. 241), a step is always formed. Its width can be controlled to some extent by the *inclination of the scissors* (Fig. 242), although this control is inexact due to the tendency of the tissue to shift in unpredictable ways.

Narrow steps cause few problems in this type of incision. But if the goal is a wide step, the tissue resistance rises with increasing step width (see Fig. 219c). Also, scissors held at an oblique angle pose the risk of desquamation of the corneal endothelium and Descemet's membrane.

3.7 Three-Plane Step Incision

In the three-plane step incision, the resistance on opening the chamber is independent of the step width. The intralamellar portion of the step is formed in a separate phase (Fig. 243); it can be made as broad as desired and placed at any depth.[23]

When opening the chamber, perpendicular vectors (directed toward the ocular interior) can be avoided by tenting the inner lamella with forceps (Fig. 243c) and then sectioning it with a purely "tangential" guidance motion.

The width of the step is controlled by *varying the guidance direction* (Fig. 244) – not by the inclination of the cutting instrument as in the two-step incision. This is advantageous in that cutting can always be done on a vertical, when tissue resistance is lowest.

[23] In unusual situations the step may be placed so deep that the inner lamella is actually transparent and affords a direct view into the chamber.

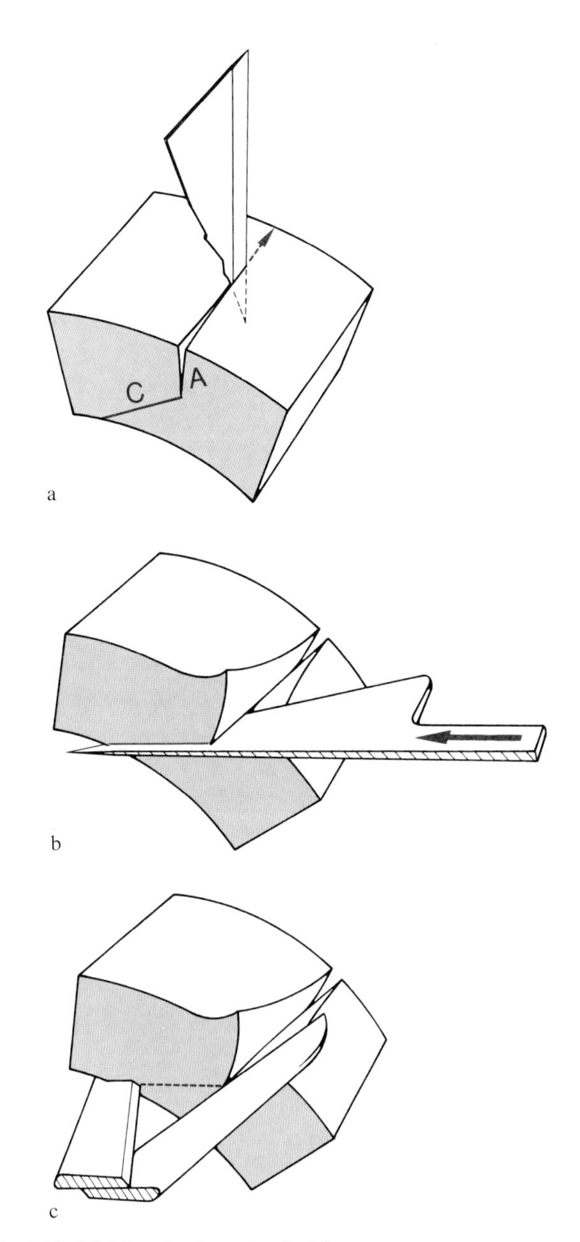

Fig. 241. **Making the two-step incision**

a A preliminary perpendicular incision is made in the sclera (*A*) (cf. Fig. 188).

b The chamber is opened at an angle to the preliminary groove (*C*) (here with a keratome).

c The incision is extended with scissors. The guidance path of the scissors is congruent with that of the knife used for opening the chamber (**b**)

→

Fig. 242. **Changing the step width.** The width of the step (segment *C* in Fig. 241a) is controlled by varying the inclination of the cutting instrument (*red:* guidance path of the blades)

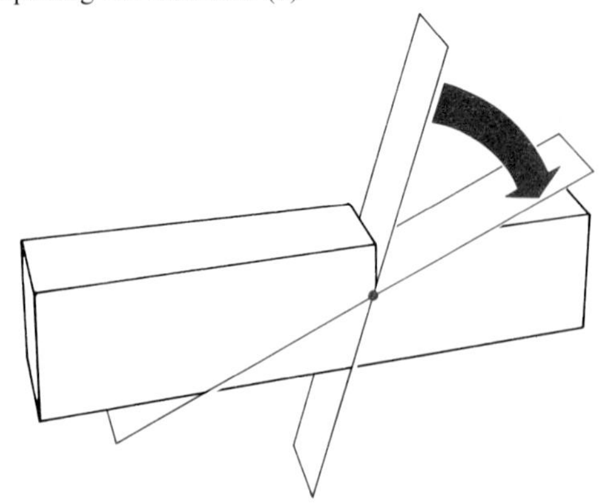

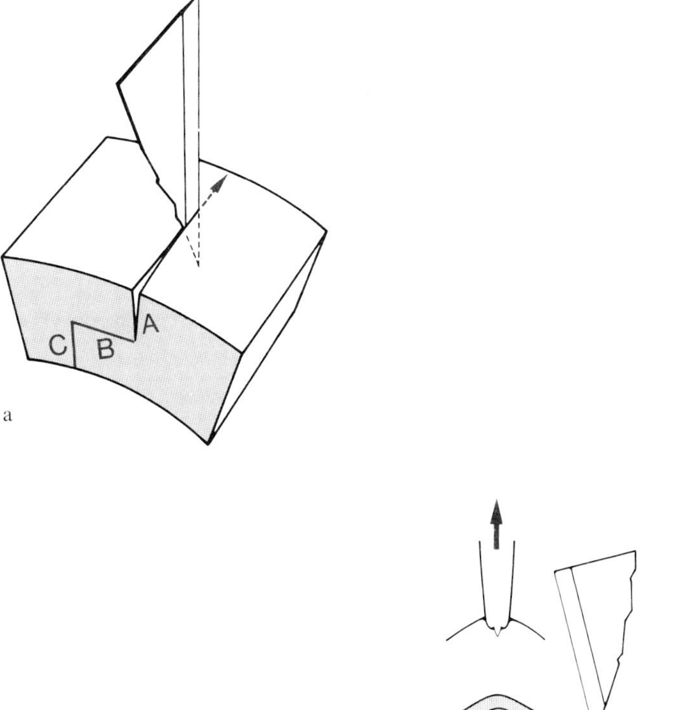

Fig. 243. **Making the three-step incision**

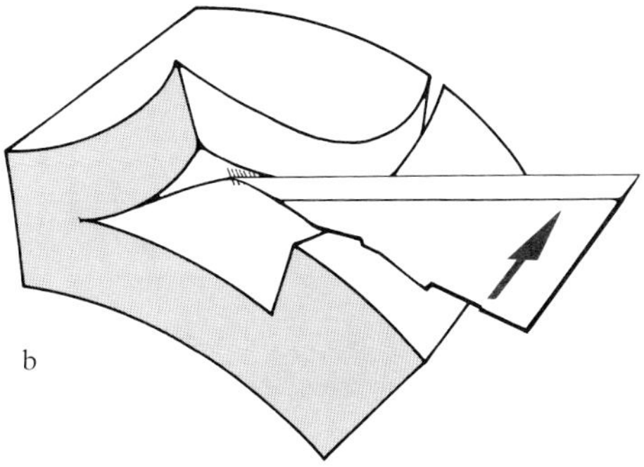

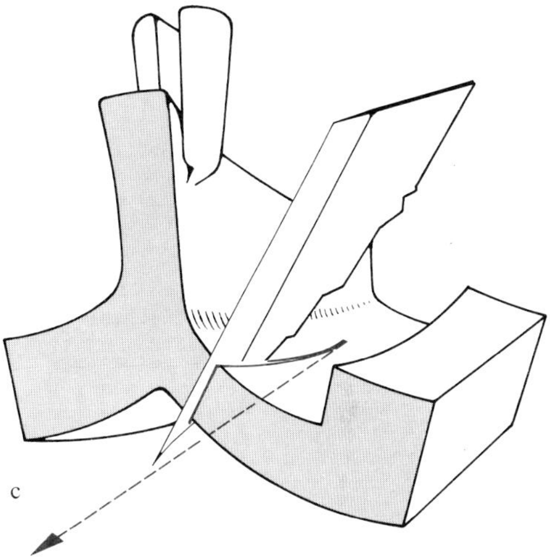

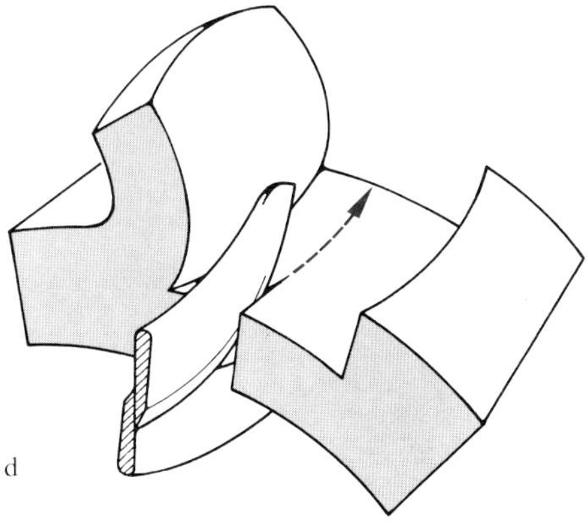

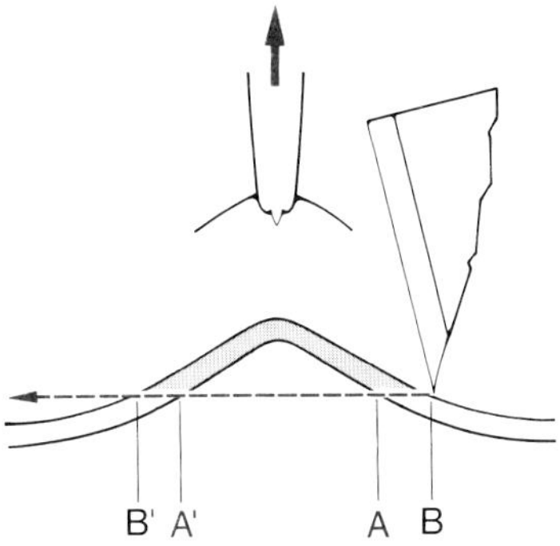

a A preliminary perpendicular incision (*A*) is made to the desired depth in the sclera.

b The intralamellar portion of the step is dissected back to the desired width (*B*) (see Figs. 190 and 191).

c The chamber is opened in a perpendicular direction (*C*). It is easier to maintain a tangential guidance direction if the inner lamella is tented with fixation forceps.

Inset: The lead distance *B-A* is again required but is smaller than in Fig. 234 due to the preliminary thinning of the cornea.

d The incision is extended with scissors

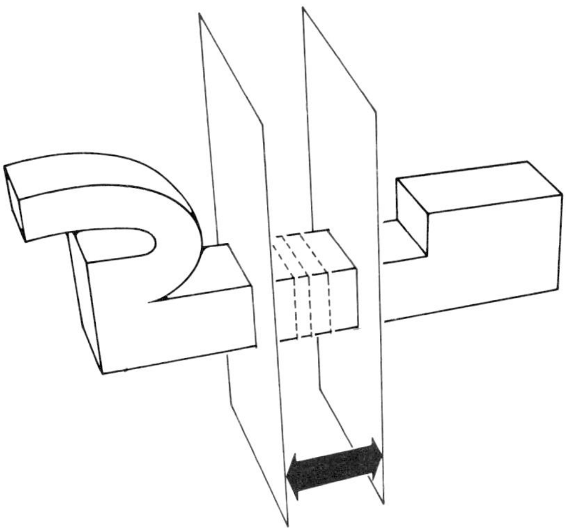

Fig. 244. **Controlling the step width.** The step width is varied by shifting the cutting instrument laterally, i.e., toward the limbus or toward the corneal center, as needed (*red:* guidance path of the cutting edge)

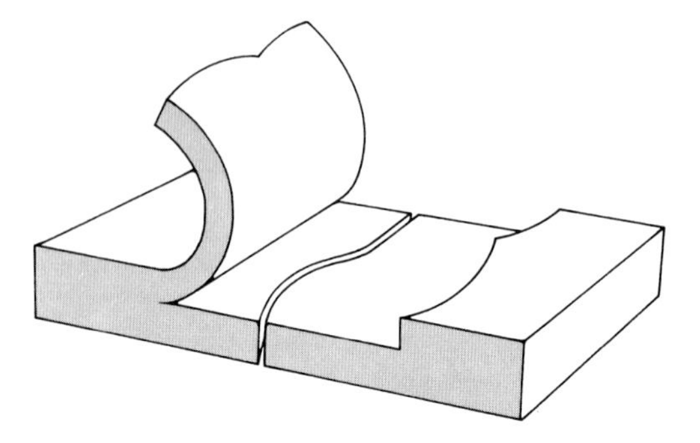

Fig. 245. **Irregularities in the step incision.** Irregularities in the course of the incision do not impair wound closure, since its valvular function remains intact

All step incisions, whether two- or three-plane, are easy to make because *corrections* are possible in each phase of the procedure. Small irregularities (Fig. 245) usually cause no harm, and a serration in the course of the surface groove can even provide a good landmark for apposing the wound edges. Variations in the step width also cause few problems, since the consequent change in the margin of watertightness can be compensated by appropriate suture placement according to the hinge rule (Fig. 266).

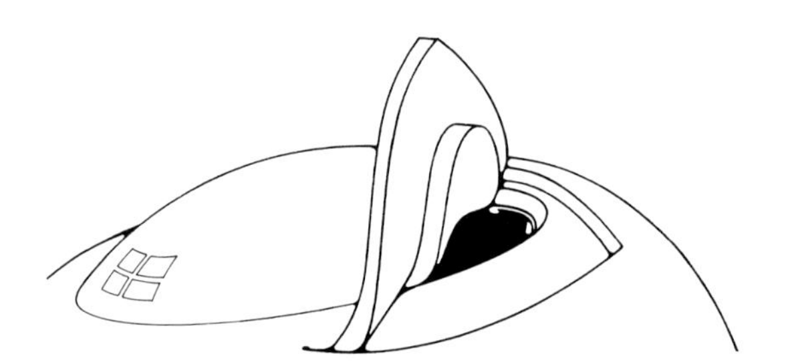

Fig. 246. **Different shaping of the outer and inner margins of the incision ("gothic arch" incision).** The outer wound margin consists of two intersecting segments of great circles and can be sealed with a single suture (see Fig. 214). The inner wound margin parallels the limbus in order to respect the anatomical structures

The mutal independence of the outer and inner wound margins in the three-step incision (see also Fig. 218b) can be utilized to achieve specific operative results. For example, the outer wound margin can be shaped to provide optimal closure while the inner margin is adapted to suit anatomic conditions (Fig. 246).

3.8 Trephine Incisions

Trephines are designed to produce circular incisions of a precisely-defined diameter and profile. However, the same trephine will not necessarily make the same incision in different eyes. This can occur only if the shifting tendency of the tissue is identical in each eye, which implies that all resistances are equal.

The resistance inherent in the *instrument* depends on the way the trephine is held and rotated. Motion is regular only with a motor-driven trephine; in hand-driven instruments it is unstable (Fig. 247b).

The resistance of the *tissue* depends mainly on its tension and can be influenced by creating equal intraocular pressures in both eyes. The shifting tendencies are minimal at a high intraocular pressure, but this condition is contrary to our general safety strategy which de-

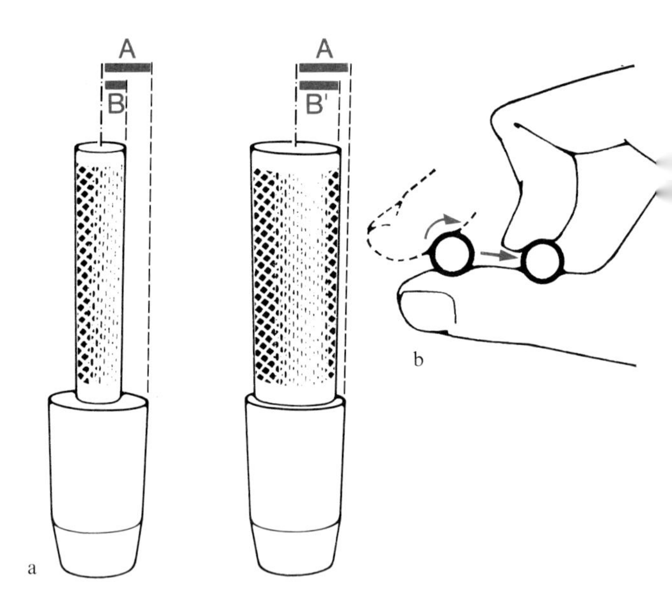

Fig. 247. **Hand-driven cylinder trephines**

a Effect of handle diameter on the extent of rotation. The circumference of the handle determines the number of revolutions made by the trephine when it is rolled between the fingers. The two trephines shown have the same cutting diameter (*A*), but the trephine with the smaller handle radius (*B*) will make more revolutions (= greater pull-through motion) when rolled than the thick-handled instrument.

b When rotated, the trephine rolls along the fingers. Rotation thus is unstable, since the trephine has a tendency to travel

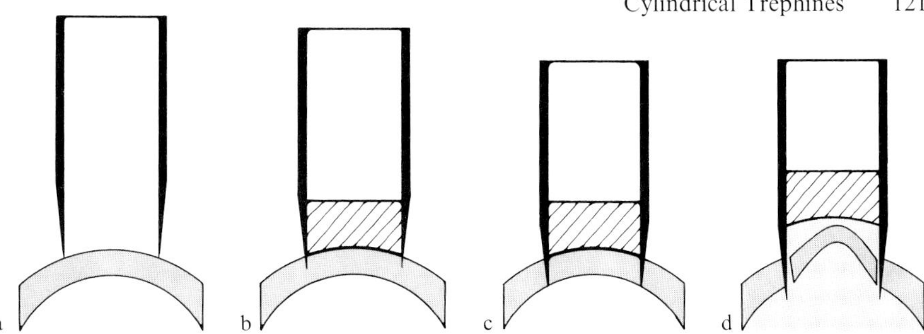

Fig. 248. **Regulating the depth of the trephine incision**

a Open trephine with no depth stop. The operative field is visible though the opening.

b Trephine fitted with stop. The stop limits the depth of the cut for lamellar keratoplasty.

c In penetrating keratoplasty, the stop prevents the cutting edge from passing too deeply.

d The stop seals off the aqueous space and prevents complete drainage of the anterior chamber during trephination of an irregularly-arched cornea

mands a soft eye. Good cutting conditions as well as a large safety margin result when prior to trephination the intraocular pressure is raised by filling the anterior chamber with a viscous substance in both donor and recipient eye. If the differences in tissue tension are anatomically determined (e.g. scars, keratoconus), however, the shifting tendencies cannot be equalized and the only recourse is to try to minimize them by increasing "sharpness".[24]

[24] That is, by cutting at high tissue tension and cutting mainly by a pull-through movement of the blade (=rotating the trephine)

[25] Note: The cavity of the trephine with a stop must be dry before use. Liquid residue hinders air escape from the cavity, causing the trephine to rotate on a cushion of air and slip off the corneal surface.

3.8.1 Cylindrical Trephines

Cylindrical trephines (Fig. 247) have a linear cutting edge. Open trephines allow the cutting edge to be viewed from the inside, but its entire length cannot be seen at one time owing to the parallel walls of the cylinder. To monitor the perpendicular position of the trephine blade from the outside, two observers are needed.

The depth of the cut can be limited by a stop[25] (Fig. 248). Lateral deviations of the cut are unlikely once the trephine has entered the tissue, owing to the three-dimensional preferential path of the cutting edge. However, the tissue may shift toward the trephine opening in the direction of thrust as a result of lamellar

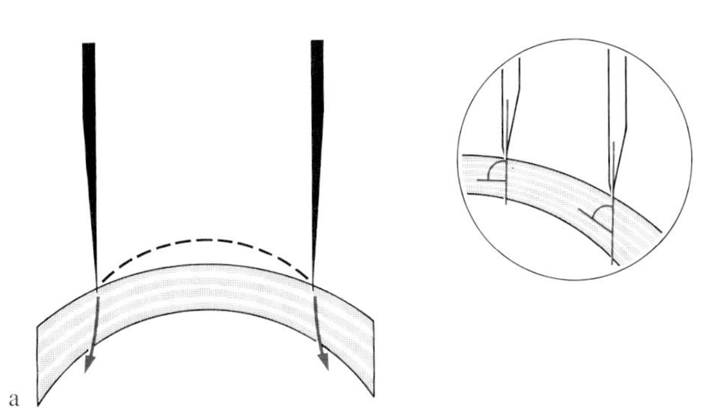

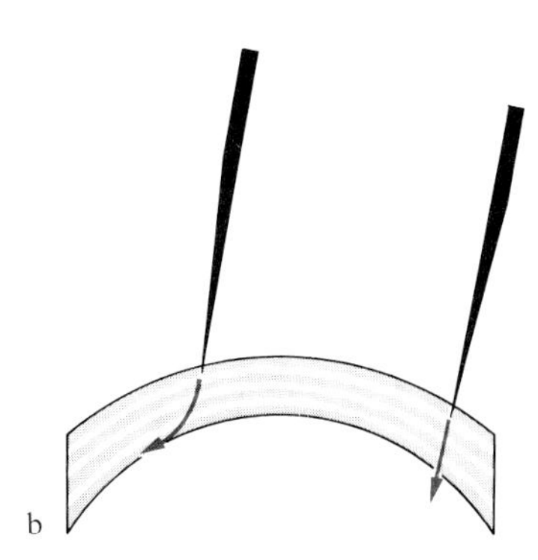

Fig. 249. **Angles of attack.** The tendency of the cut to deviate in lamellar tissue depends on the angle of incidence between the preferential path of the cutting edge and the corneal surface. This angle becomes more oblique with increasing trephine diameter (*inset*).

a Perpendicular position of the trephine. As the cut progresses, lamellar deflection causes the cornea to bulge, with a slight increase in the diameter of the excision in deeper layers.

b Oblique position of the trephine. If the trephine is not held strictly perpendicular, the lamellar deflection increases on one side and decreases on the opposite side

deflection. The latter depends on the angle of attack of the cutting edge, which is governed by the shape of the carrier. Lamellar deflection is particularly a problem when the trephine is not held strictly perpendicularly (Fig. 249). Lamellar deflection can be reduced by avoiding pressure in the direction of thrust and by cutting with maximum sharpness.[24]

3.8.2 Trephines with a Pointed Blade

The freedom of movement of a pointed blade allows a wide choice of attack angles, including oblique angles which allow the cutting process to be observed through the trephine opening (Figs. 250, 251). But this freedom also requires that the blade be very precisely guided by the carrier, which determines the angle of attack and depth of incision.

Lamellar deflection has little impact on the cut, since the cutting point is moved essentially along the lamellar surface. Moreover, a perpendicular attack angle can be chosen, thereby avoiding lamellar deflection altogether. But in contrast to cylindrical trephines, deviations can still occur in a lateral direction if differences in tissue resistance are encountered (e.g. scars, Fig. 252). To avoid this, the trephine and cornea must be in such firm apposition that the resistance is greater than the force causing the deviation.

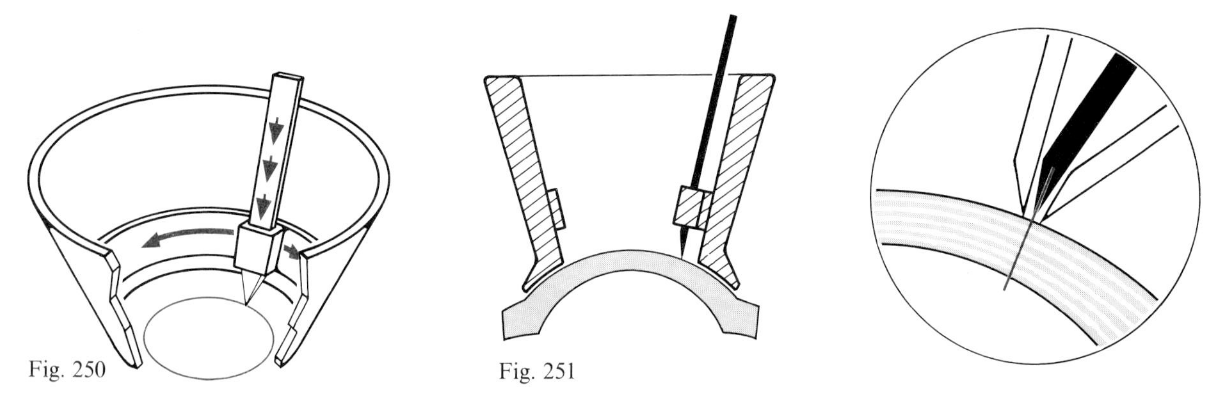

Fig. 250. **Trephine with a point cutting edge.** The point cutting edge moves along a conical carrier and is simultaneously advanced inward. Both motions require mechanical means for precise control

Fig. 251. **Angle of attack.** With cones of varying shapes, the angle of attack at the tissue can be chosen as needed (*inset*)

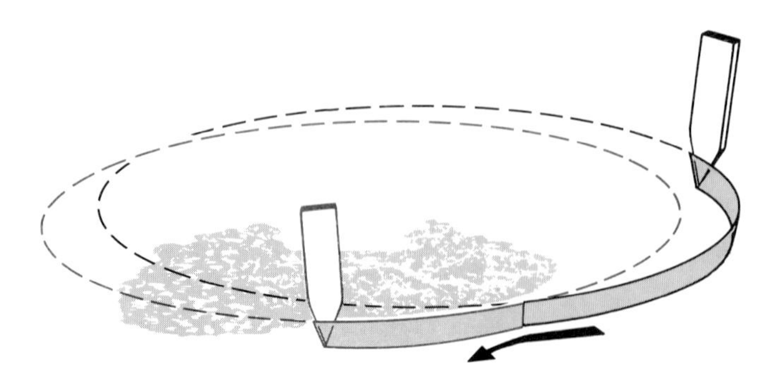

Fig. 252. **Lateral shifting tendency of the trephine.** If sites of increased resistance are present in the cornea (*gray*), the cutting edge will tend to avoid them. The cone may shift relative to the corneal surface, or the globe may shift relative to the cone if the resistance to this shift is smaller than its force. In contrast to cylindrical trephines, therefore, the cut may deviate (*red*) from the intended circular path (*black*)

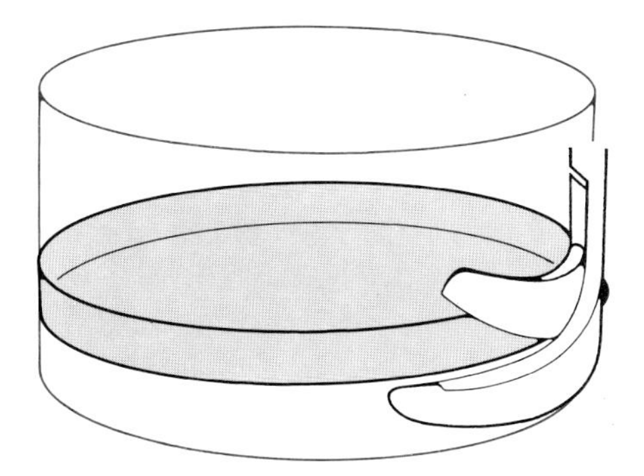

Fig. 253. **Completing the trephine incision with scissors.** If the radius of blade curvature equals the trephine radius, the cutting point will follow the trephine incision by a simple closing motion. The blades make no swiveling movements in the anterior chamber

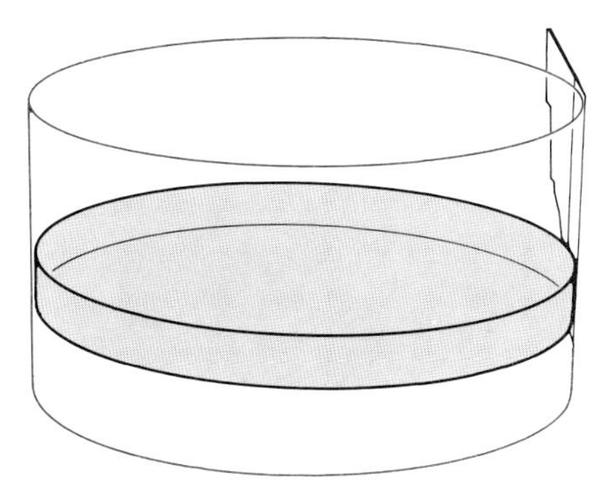

Fig. 254. **Completing the trephine incision with a sharp-pointed blade.** The cutting edge of the blade is guided carefully along the face of the trephined disk. It is held in the same plane as the trephine cylinder (i.e., vertically) and follows the circular line of the trephine incision exactly

3.8.3 Completion of the Trephine Incision

If aqueous fluid escapes, trephination can be continued only as long as the chamber retains a sufficient depth.[26] If the corneal disk has not been completely excised by trephination alone, the cut must be completed with a scissors or sharp-pointed blade. This always produces a step. To keep the step as narrow as possible, the cutting edge of the instrument is guided as carefully as possible along the cut surface already begun (guidance path = cut surface) (Figs. 253, 254). The position of bulky instrument parts (Fig. 255) and tissue deformations resulting from forceps traction (Fig. 256) must also be taken into account.

When the final lamella is divided, there is a danger of iris lesion. This danger is relatively slight as long as the iris can be freely displaced by the blade, because then it is considerably less sectile than the firm corneoscleral tissue (see Figs. 31b, 39b). However, concomitant movements of the iris are a warning sign and must be closely watched.

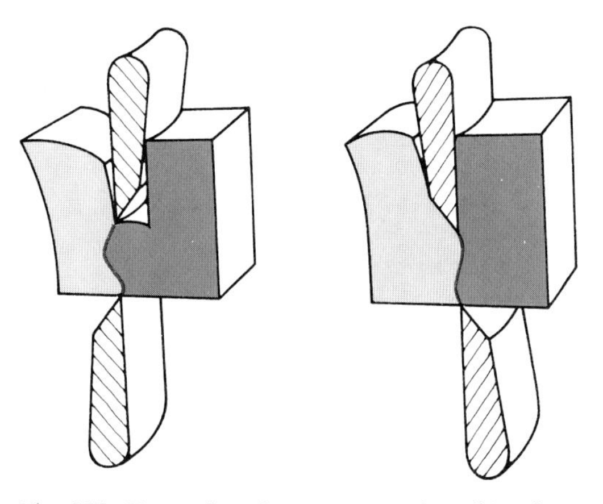

Fig. 255. **Formation of a step on cutting with scissors.** The position of the blades determines the size of the step on the host cornea (see Fig. 59). *Light area:* mobile disk. *Dark area:* less mobile host cornea

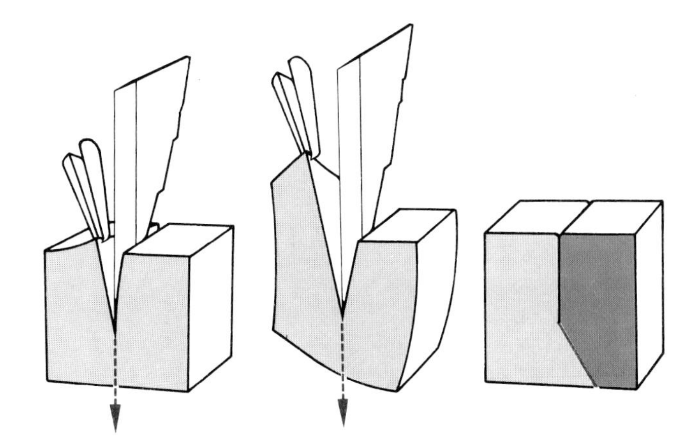

Fig. 256. **Formation of a step on cutting with a blade.** If the disk is scarcely deformed by the forceps prior to cutting, the blade can make an almost step-free incision *(left)*. But if the disk is pulled upward *(center)*, an inverse step (= defect) may form on the host cornea *(right)*

[26] This depth can be maintained longer if the chamber previously is filled with viscous aqueous substituents.

4 Suturation of the Cornea and Sclera

Extraordinary *precision* is required in suturation of the cornea and sclera. Due to the unyielding nature of the tissue, even small errors can impair the apposition and watertightness of a wound.

When cutting the suture canal, the **lamellar rule** applies. This means that the highest accuracy is achieved when the needle tip is passed either parallel or perpendicular to the lamellae (Fig. 257), and not obliquely (see also Fig. 187).[27]

The tissue deformation caused by the grasping forceps must be compensated for by adequate countermovements during passage of the needle (Figs. 258–260).

[27] Note: The lower the sectility of tissue, the lower the cutting ability of the needle, and the more important is this requirement.

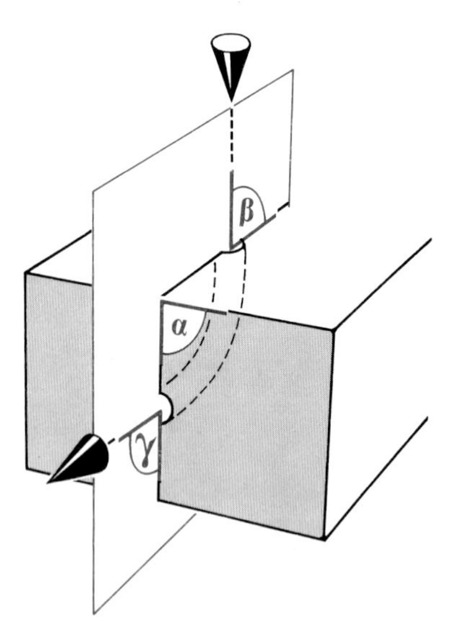

Fig. 257. **Suture characteristics.** A suture produces no vectors that shift the wound surfaces if:
- the suture plane is perpendicular to the tissue surface ($\alpha=90°$);
- the needle is inserted perpendicular to the tissue surface ($\beta=90°$);
- the tip emerges perpendicular to the wound surface ($\gamma=90°$)

Simple *apposition* sutures pose few problems, since they do not alter the tissue topography. However, tight sutures (e.g., *compression sutures*) shorten the suture canal and cause deformations which may interfere with wound closure. The nature of the deformation can be deduced from the **rule of suture tightening** (see Fig. 73). In *perpendicular incisions*, the internal wound edges begin to gape when su-

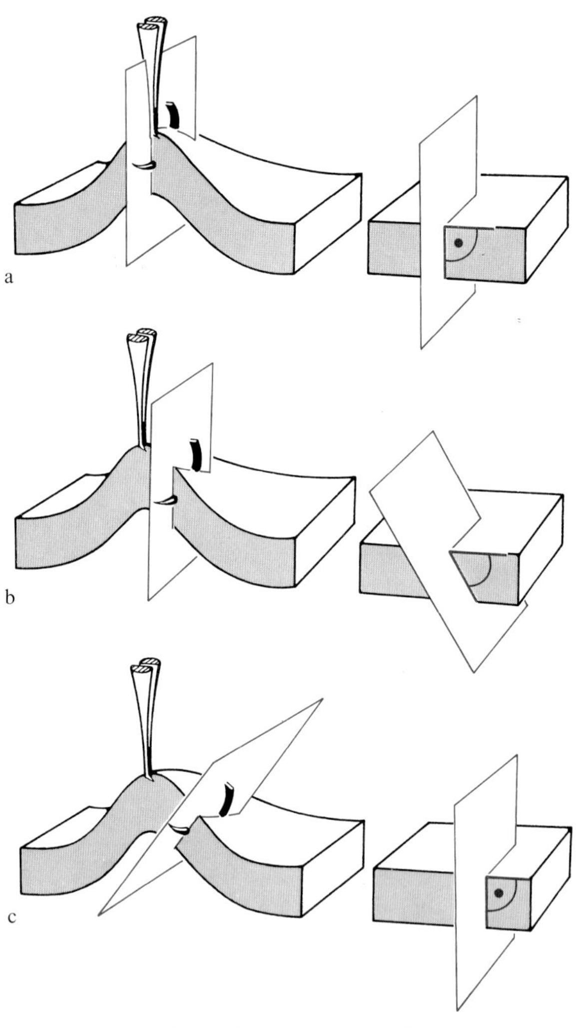

Fig. 258. **Vertical position of the suture plane**
Left: Tissue deformation by forceps.
Right: Position of suture plane after reversal of deformation

a If the needle is inserted vertically at the crest (beneath the forceps), the suture plane will also be vertical on release.

b If the needle is inserted "vertically" alongside the forceps, it is actually at an angle to the surface at that point.

c Compensatory slanting of the needle is necessary when it is inserted alongside the forceps

ture tension is increased (Fig. 261). In *single-plane oblique incisions,* the wound edges shift relative to each other and apposition is impaired (Fig. 262). In *step incisions,* apposition is retained in the external portion of the wound, but the valvular mechanism is destroyed internally (Fig. 263).

It must be borne in mind that a single *deforming suture* can impair wound closure for the full length of the wound due to the rigidity of the tissue (Figs. 264, 265). The surgeon should find and remove such faulty sutures at once if wound leak occurs on completion of a properly planned suture series. An attempt to improve the situation by applying countertension with additional corrective sutures restores watertightness only with great difficulty while raising the danger of large astigmatism.

Due to the difficulties that arise when sutures are tightened in rigid tissue, it is best to choose incisions which can be made watertight with simple apposition sutures *(valvular incisions)*, and avoid those requiring compres-

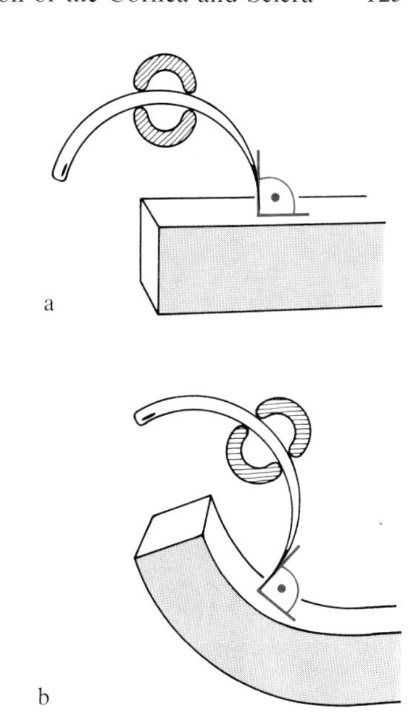

Fig. 259. **Inserting the needle perpendicular to the tissue surface**

a If the tissue surface remains undeformed, the needle shaft must be rotated back to insert the tip vertically (note position of needle holder).

b If the tissue surface is curved upward by the forceps, the needle position must be adjusted accordingly. The shaft is now in a more upright position

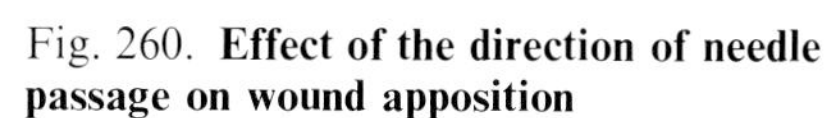

Fig. 260. **Effect of the direction of needle passage on wound apposition**

a Passing the needle through the wound interspace parallel to the surface creates an equal suture depth in the two wound edges *(A)*, regardless of the distance *(D)* between them at the time of passage.

b Passing the needle obliquely creates a difference in suture depths *($A \neq B$)* which increases with the distance *D*.
A step is formed whose size is independent of the degree of suture tension *(bottom left)*. If the wound lips are pressed together during oblique passage of the needle *($D = O$)*, the suture depth is constant *($A = B$)*, but the suture is asymmetrical *(bottom right)*. The wound remains apposed at low suture tension, but a step will form when tension is increased (see Fig. 76c)

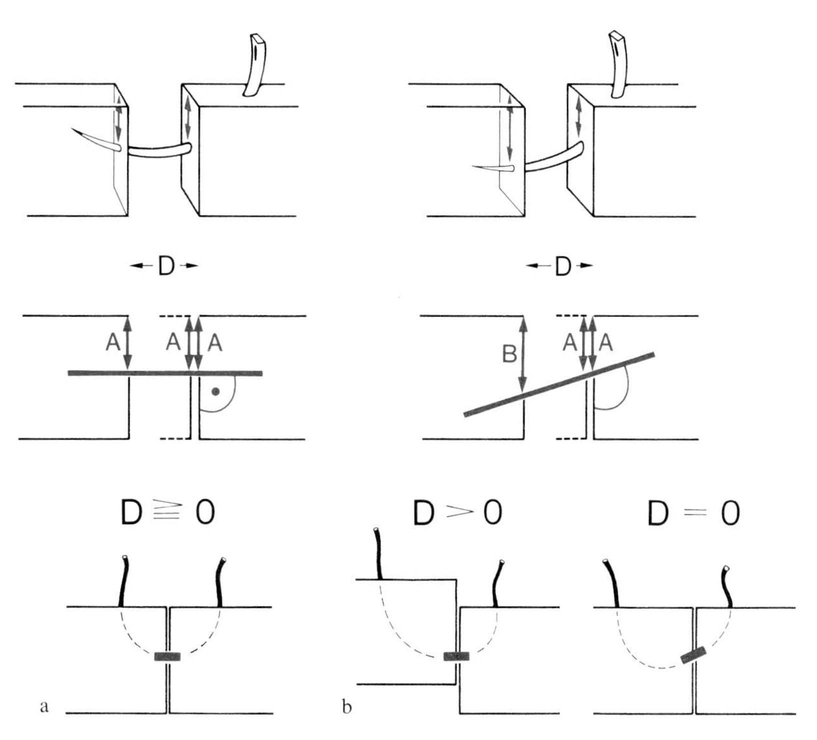

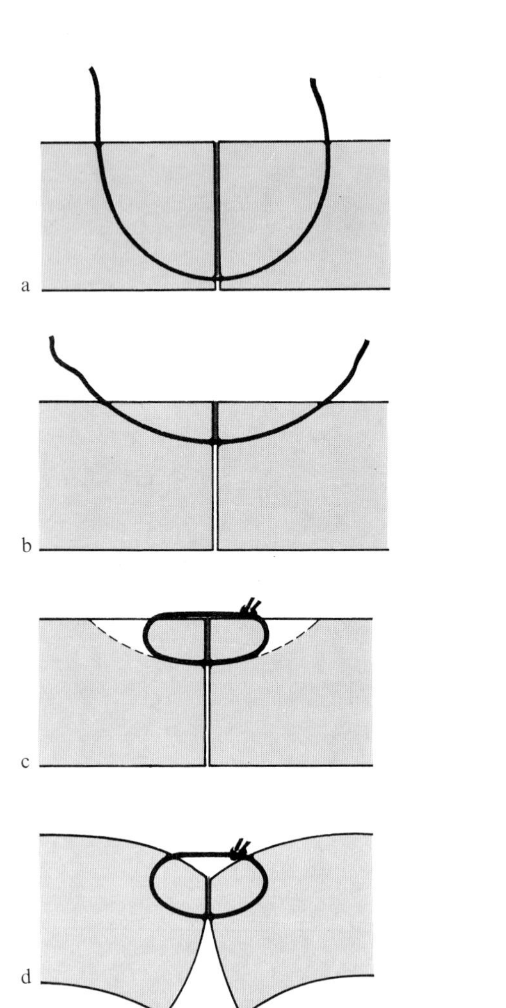

Fig. 261. **Suture problems in the perpendicular incision.** Comparison of sutures with entry and exit points equidistant from the wound line.

a Deep semicircular suture: produces a large compression zone. The possibility of placing the suture near the inner surface is limited by its tissue compatibility (inflammatory canal, see Fig. 93).

b Superficial suture: compresses only a small part of the wound surface. Contact in the uncompressed zone is maintained only if the tension does not shorten the suture canal.

c The thin surface lamella may tear when the suture is tightened. This places the suture closer to the wound line than planned.

d If the tissue does not tear, the contact area is diminished when the suture is tightened. Aqueous fluid can rise to the suture canal. Contrary to expectations, the more the suture is tightened, the greater the danger of fistula formation

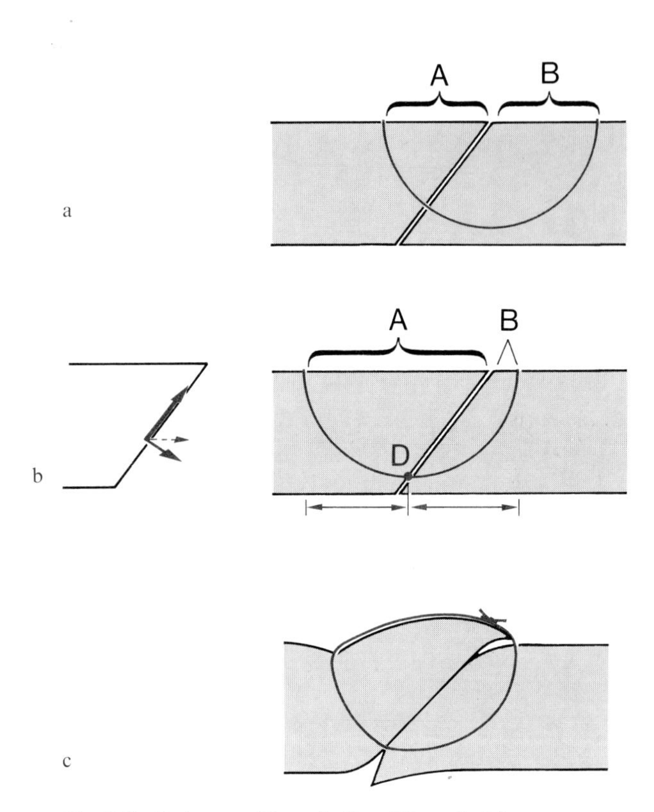

Fig. 262. **Suture problems in the oblique incision**

a If the entry and exit points are symmetrical with respect to the superficial wound line *(A = B)*, the suture is asymmetrical in the tissue and includes only a small part of the overlapping wound lip.

b If the entry and exit points are equidistant from the point of deep suture passage *D*, the suture is asymmetrical on the tissue surface *(A > B)*.

c When the suture is tightened, a vector component acts along the oblique wound surface to shift the wound edges relative to each other *(inset)*. The wound remains watertight, but apposition is faulty

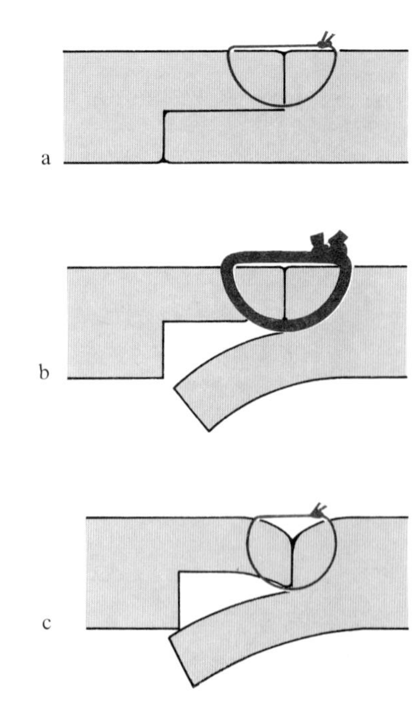

Fig. 263. **Suture problems in the step incision**

a The outer step is fixed for its full thickness.

b Valvular function is impaired by thick threads in the interlamellar layer.

c Valvular function is impaired by excessive suture tension. The entire valve is deformed and may leak due to shortening of the outer step

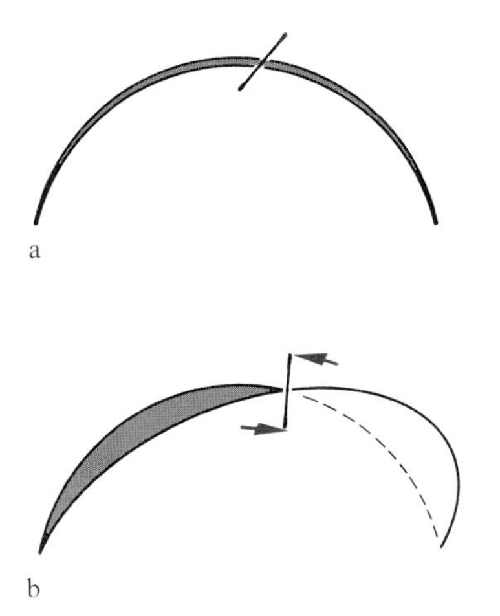

Fig. 264. **Tightening of obliquely-placed sutures**

a When loose, an obliquely-placed suture does not impair apposition.

b When the suture is tightened, the wound edges are shifted, and wound leak develops not only at the site of the suture, but along the entire wound

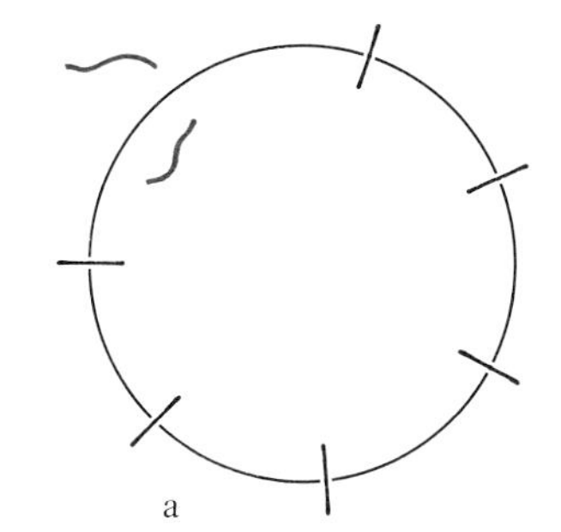

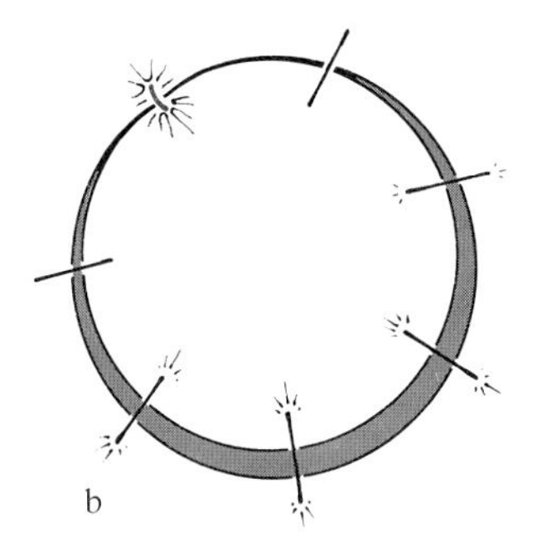

Fig. 265. **Tightening of sutures placed perpendicular to the wound margin**

a If suture tension is uniform, the wound edges are pressed together uniformly about their circumference, and the wound remains closed.

b If even one suture is overtightened, the remaining sutures become in effect loose, and the wound gapes

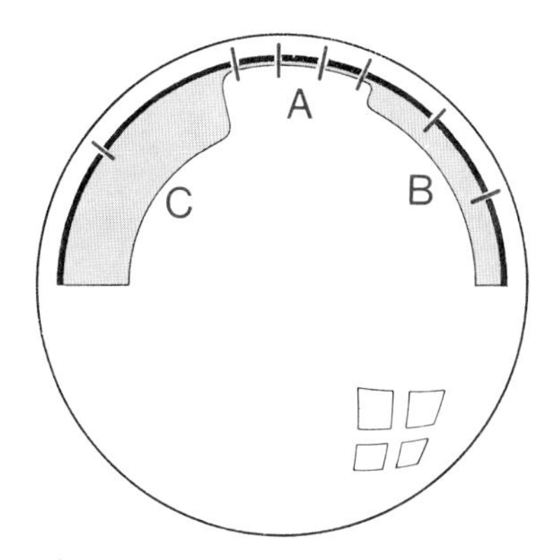

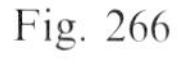

Fig. 266

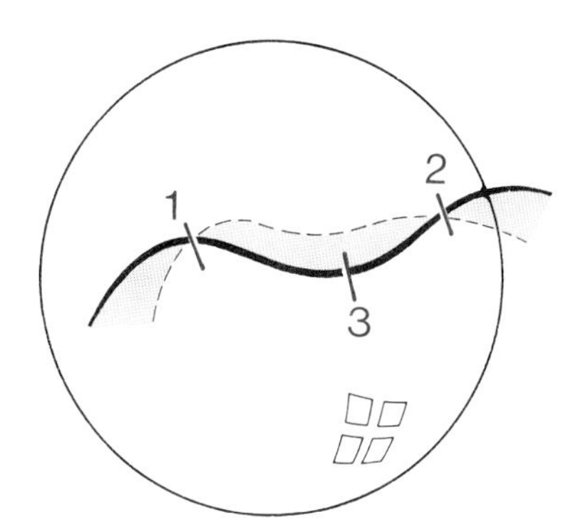

Fig. 267

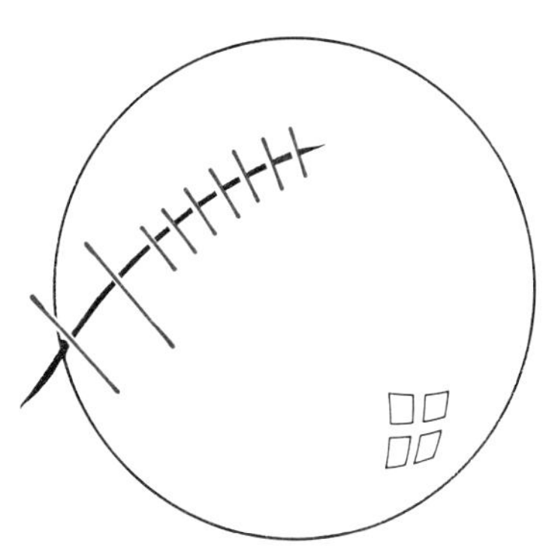

Fig. 268

sion sutures to effect closure *(perpendicular incisions)*. In cases where an irregular incision has resulted (Fig. 266) or in traumatic wounds, the surgeon must confront the given situation and adjust his suturing technique accordingly. Optimal solutions can be deduced from the valve and hinge rules, as well as from the rules on suture tightening. Examples of their application are shown in Figs. 266–270.

Fig. 266. **Sutures in an irregular incision.** Pictured is a curved surgical incision which is quite steep at its origin *(A)* but formed irregular valves *(B* and *C)* when extended on both sides. The suture placement derives from the hinge rule and depends on the width of the wound surface as projected onto the ocular surface (see Figs. 210 and 213)

Fig. 267. **Suturing a traumatic wound of irregular curvature.** The S-shaped wound is first sutured at the points where the wound surfaces are perpendicular *(1* and *2)*. The intervals, which form valvular openings, are managed according to the hinge rule *(3)*

Fig. 268. **Applying the distance rule in closing a linear corneal wound.** In the optical region, the sutures are placed at a small distance from the wound edges to minimize the width of the scar zone and are correspondingly closely spaced (see Fig. 75). In the marginal region they are spaced farther apart to allow access to the chamber for restorative measures with a cannula. They are correspondingly longer

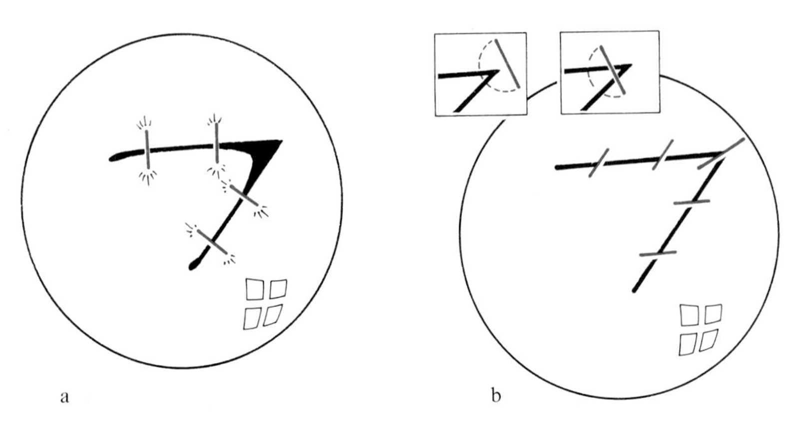

Fig. 269. **Suturing a triangular flap**

a Compression sutures on the lateral wound edges cause the apex of the flap to retract.

b The apex is secured first, therefore. This can be done by direct suture if sufficient tissue is present, i.e., if the flap angle is sufficiently large. If it is small, the loop can be passed through the apex intramurally. In the inset at *upper left*, the apex will have a tendency to rise; in the inset at *upper right* this is prevented by the overlying loop. On the lateral wound edges the sutures are placed at an angle to the wound line to relieve tension on the apex

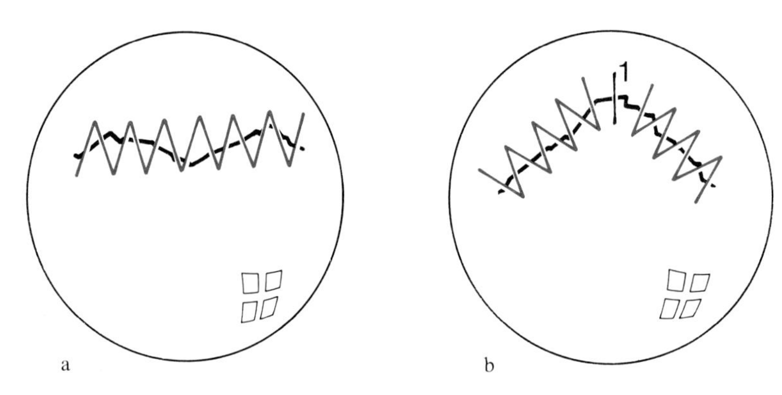

Fig. 270. **Running sutures on irregularly-shaped wounds**

a Running sutures tend to linearize the area encompassed by them (see Fig. 84b). The irregularities of the wound are not followed by the suture, therefore, but the entire wound area is treated as a linear compression zone.

b If the wound line is too irregular to permit this, loop sutures *(1)* are used to subdivide the wound into segments, which are then managed in accordance with **a**. (*Note:* High suture tension tends to flatten the corneal dome, see Fig. 84a)

VI Operations on the Iris

1 General

The tissue of the normal iris is extremely mobile and distensible. This reduces its sectility and proneness to injury despite its delicate structure. The *normal iris* is elastic and has a tendency to reassume its original shape even after extensive distortion (Fig. 271). In contrast, the *pathologically altered iris* ruptures easily and is very difficult to reposition, especially if the tissue has undergone structural changes in an abnormal position.[1]

If the iris is to possess its **normal mobility,** it must be surrounded on all sides by a *fluid cushion,* since its elasticity and the forces of the pupil-regulating muscles (Figs. 272, 273) are too weak to withstand even a slight frictional resistance. If the anterior chamber has drained completely or if the watery aqueous has been replaced with viscous material, the iris loses its normal mobility and will not respond to medication until the chamber has been refilled with watery fluid.

Injuries of the iris do not cicatrize as long as the openings are perfused with aqueous fluid. **Cicatrization** occurs only if the passage of fluid is obstructed by suturing or by contact with adjacent tissue structures. Openings which are to ensure the free circulation of aqueous are therefore placed at the base of the iris, where there is little likelihood of such contact (Fig. 274).

[1] Anterior synechiae, which are easily corrected if promptly attended to, may be extremely difficult to cure later on. If structural changes have taken place, especially if they have spread to the iris root (e.g., anterior synechiae near the base of the iris following keratoplasty, traumatic synechia formation), the tissue tends to return to its former position (adhesion) after dissection. This tendency is not counteracted by the restoration of the chamber with fluid. To prevent the recurrence of synechiae, viscous substances can be used to keep the interspace open.

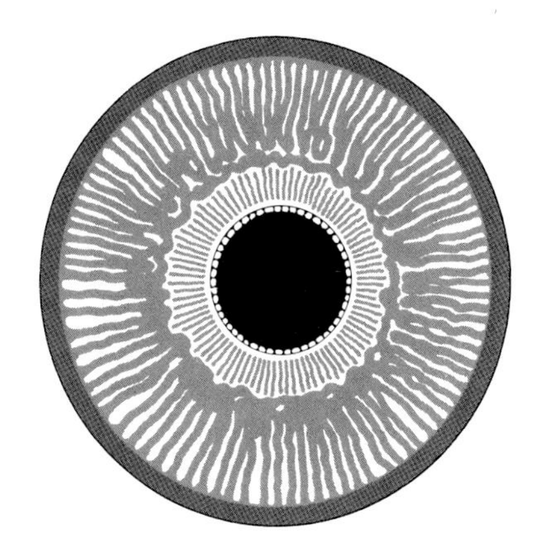

Fig. 271. **Normal iris position.** The criteria for a normal iris position are a centered pupil and radially-directed trabeculae. The base of the iris is separated from the sinus of the anterior chamber by the anterior face of the ciliary body *(pink)*

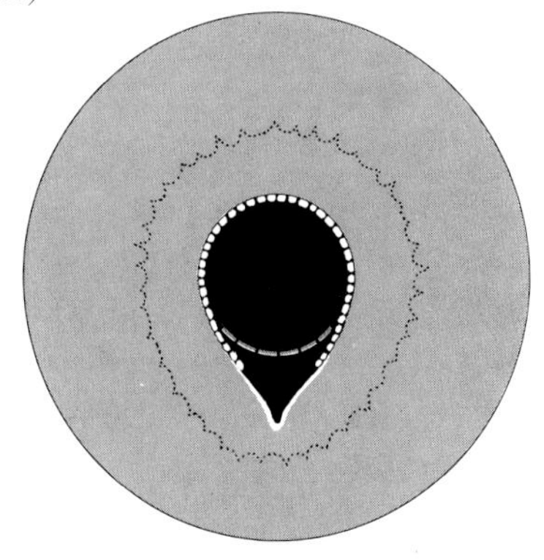

Fig. 272. **Disturbance of muscle balance: sphincterotomy.** The pupil is enlarged by surgical lesion of the sphincter pupillae

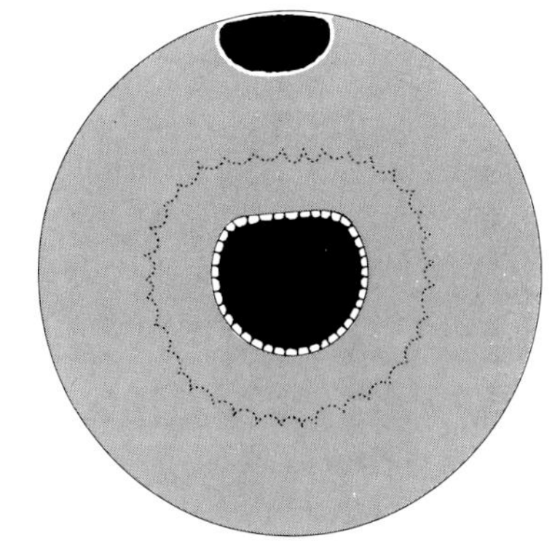

Fig. 273. **Disturbance of muscle balance: basal iridectomy.** Through a circumscribed lesion of the dilatator pupillae, the pupil is narrowed in the region of the iridectomy and appears "flattened"

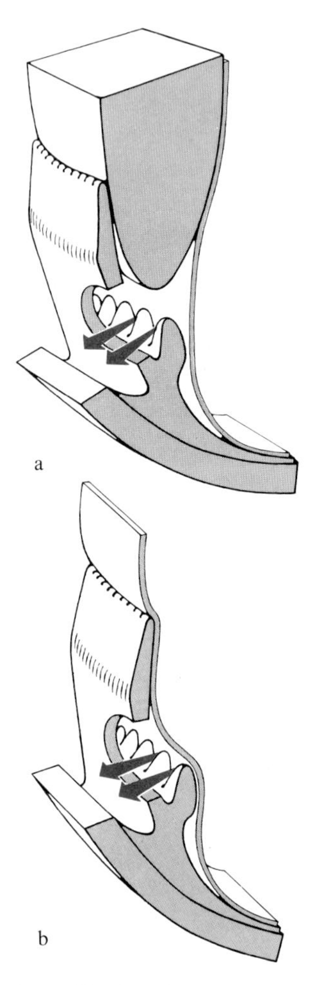

Fig. 274. **Openings for aqueous circulation (basal iridectomy).** If the opening lies directly anterior to the ciliary processes, contact with adjacent tissues is unlikely in both the normal **(a)** and aphakic eye **(b).** The ciliary processes act as a rake to hold back posterior structures (lens, anterior hyaloid) while allowing aqueous to circulate between them

The iris can be surgically **approached** in its normal anatomic position *(intrabulbar iris operation)* provided the corneal opening is long enough[2] and the margin of deformation large enough that a flap can be raised (Fig. 275).

If the corneal opening is small, the mobility of the iris is utilized to bring it out of the wound and operate on it there *(extrabulbar iris operation)*.

The iris can be either expressed by raising the intraocular pressure (Fig. 276), or drawn out with a small hook or forceps.[3]

When the iris is *prolapsed*, the exact topographic relations are difficult to assess due

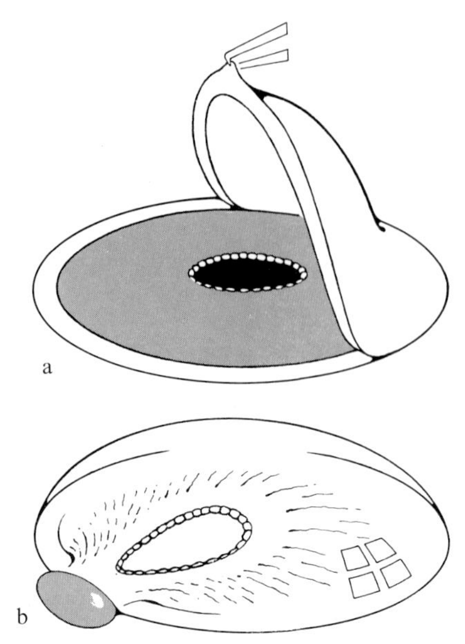

Fig. 275. **Approaches to the iris**

a If the corneal wound is large enough to open as a flap, the iris can be approached in its normal anatomical position *(intrabulbar iris operation)*.

b If the opening is small, a portion of the iris must be exteriorized as a prolapse and operated on outside the eye *(extrabulbar iris operation)*

to the shifting and stretching of the tissue. The best information is obtained by observing the parts of the iris still within the chamber, because they are less deformed. The position and shape of the pupil are especially helpful in assessing iris topography (Fig. 277).

[2] Example: Iris operations combined with other operative goals which require a large opening (e.g., cataract operation).

[3] Hooks open the corneal wound less than forceps; the latter causes the anterior chamber to drain as soon as the blades are opened.

Fig. 276. **Expression of the iris**

a Two blunt expressors (e.g., spatulas) are applied to the wound edges. By pressing on the upper expressor, which simultaneously seals the wound, the intraocular pressure is increased.

b If then the lower expressor is also slightly depressed, the valvular wound will open and the iris will be pushed outward by the intraocular pressure.

c If directly apposed to the wound, the iris behaves as part of the chamber wall. If the intraocular pressure rises, the iris will stretch more than the cornea (due to its greater distensibility) and will be displaced outward. The prolapse is a part of the pressure chamber.

d Incising the prolapse destroys the pressure chamber. Once the prolapse has collapsed, the iris cannot be expressed further by an additional pressure increase. Instead, the valvular mechanism becomes active again and incarcerates the iris tissue

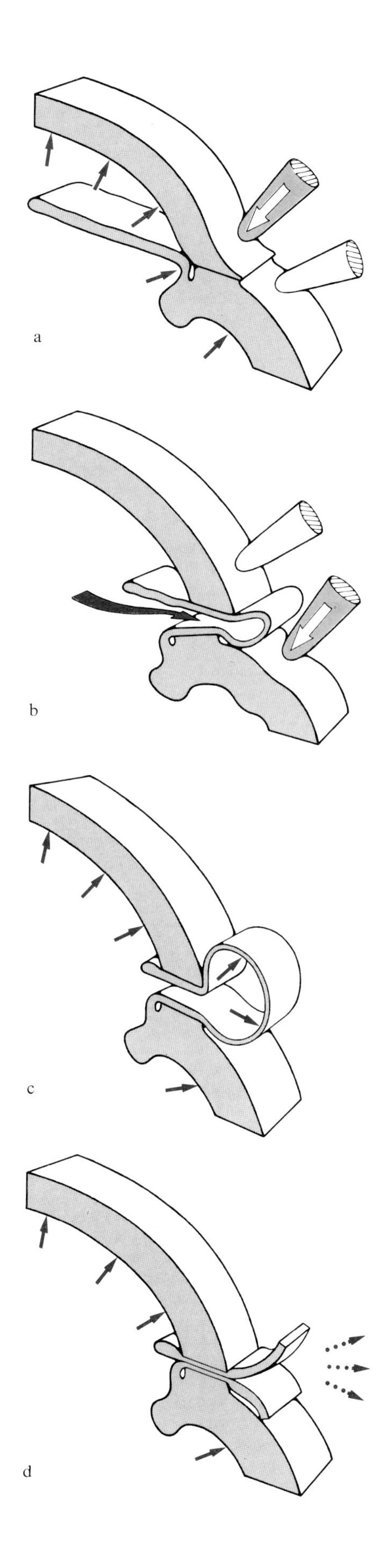

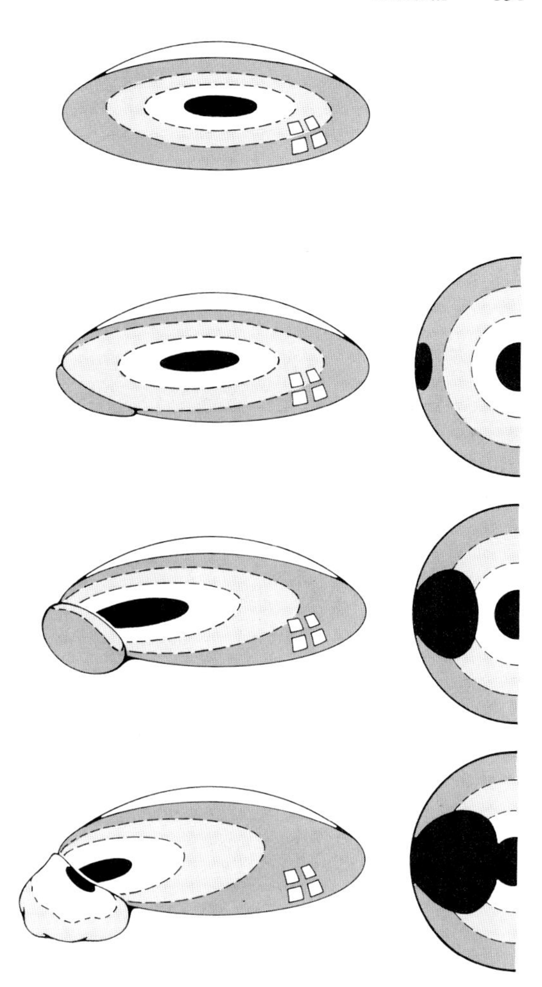

Fig. 277. **Topographic conditions in extrabulbar iris operation.** Due to stretching of the tissue, it is difficult to judge how much iris tissue is contained in the prolapse by its size. This can be better judged from the position of the iris tissue still in the eye. In the illustrations, the iris is divided into zones with different shades of gray to show the extent of the prolapse. The drawings on the left show various degrees of prolapse. Those on the right show the size of the iridectomy which results when the prolapse is sectioned directly at its base

2 Iridectomies

Due to its extreme mobility, the iris is strongly deformed and displaced when handled. This can impair the precision of iridectomies with respect to their shape and extent. However, if the surgeon is familiar with the behavior of the iris when it is grasped, pulled and cut, he can exploit this knowledge to achieve precise results.

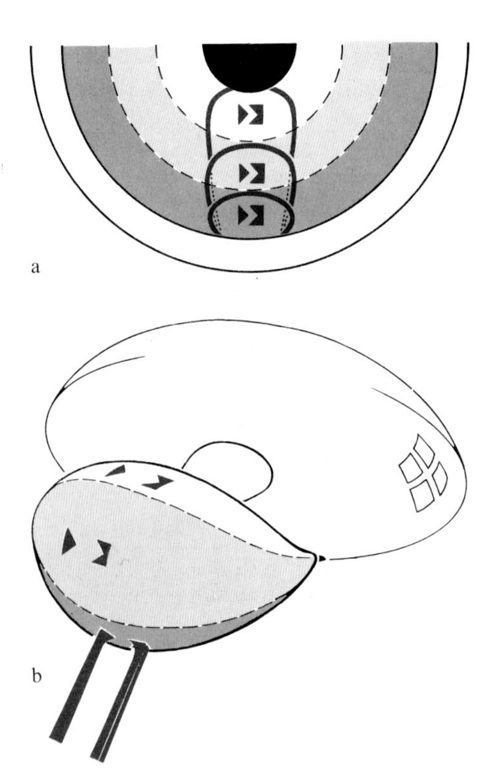

Fig. 278. **Effect of grasping on the minimum distance of the iridectomy from the base.** If the cut is made basalward below the forceps, the margin of the iridectomy can be no closer to the base than the site of forceps application.

a In intrabulbar iridectomy the topographic relations are clearly visible. *Red triangles:* Site of forceps application, *red outline:* margin of iridectomy.

b In extrabulbar iridectomy the topographic relations are difficult to judge from the prolapsed tissue (see also Fig. 277). If a small basal iridectomy is desired, the tissue is grasped as close as possible to the basal lip of the wound (the position of the forceps in the dark grey area)

With the **grasping motion** of the forceps, certain quantities are already established,[4] such as the *minimum size* of the iridectomy (Fig. 279), its *minimum distance* from the base or the pupil (Fig. 278), and its *width at the base* (Fig. 280).[5]

Traction with the forceps creates a "pyramid" of tissue. The **degree and direction of traction** determines not only the shape of the pyramid, but also the tension of the tissue and thus its sectility. The segment between the forceps and the iris root *(basal segment)* becomes tense; if traction is increased, the tissue tension in this area is increased, but the quantity of tissue contained in the segment remains unchanged. The segment between the forceps and pupil, on the other hand *(pupillary segment)*, remains lax; increased traction causes no change of tension in this area,[6] but does draw more tissue into the pyramid (Fig. 281).

Thus, in the *tense* basal segment, an *increase of traction* increases sectility and ensures a more precise cut;[7] owing to the retractile tendency, moreover, an iridectomy will be brought closer to the base and reduced in area. In the *lax* pupillary segment, on the other hand, the iridectomy becomes larger with increasing traction, and its edges are rounded as a result of tissue shifting (Fig. 282).

When cutting, the surgeon can exploit the variations in sectility and in the shifting and retractile tendencies by selecting the most favorable segment on the iris pyramid to influence the shape and size of the iridectomy. Intra- and extrabulbar operations differ in the way in which this selection is made. In *intrabulbar* iridectomy the angle between the scissors

[4] We are assuming the customary technique in which the iris is seized with a forceps and sectioned below it (the tissue traumatized by the forceps being excised with the rest). Other techniques can easily be derived from the criteria presented here.

[5] Note: The maximum attainable width is limited by the width of the corneal opening.

[6] Unless its mobility is restricted (e.g., by friction at the wound lips in extrabulbar iridectomies).

[7] The resulting cut corresponds more accurately to the geometric section of the guidance path of the cutting instrument. Thus, straight-blade scissors produce an iridectomy with straight edges.

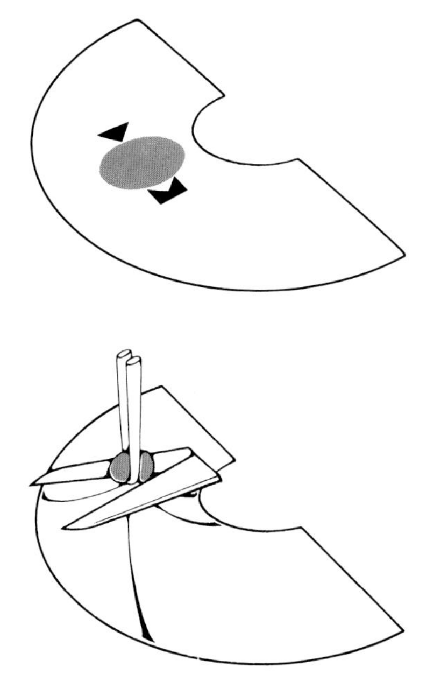

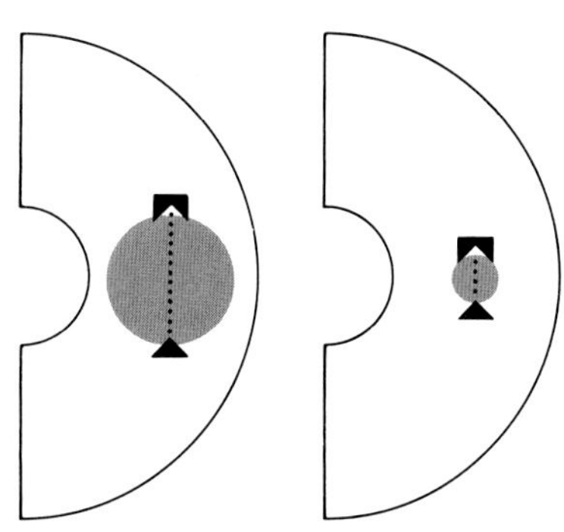

Fig. 279. **Effect of grasping on the minimum size of the iridectomy.**
Left: The blade spacing determines the minimum size of the iridectomy *(top)*, for the iridectomy can be no smaller than the area grasped between the blades *(bottom)*.
Right: Examples of minimum iridectomy size for various blade spacings

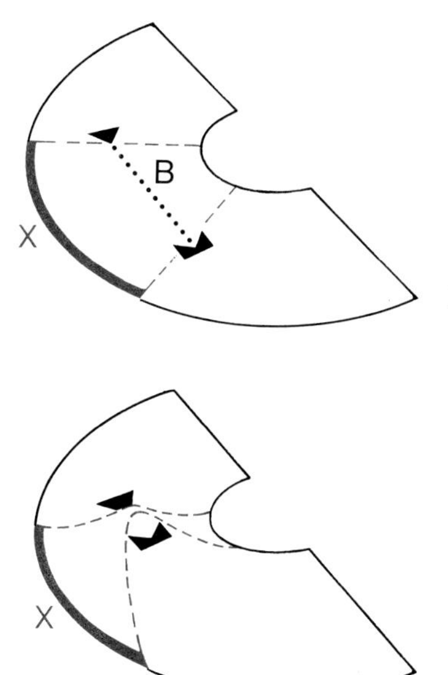

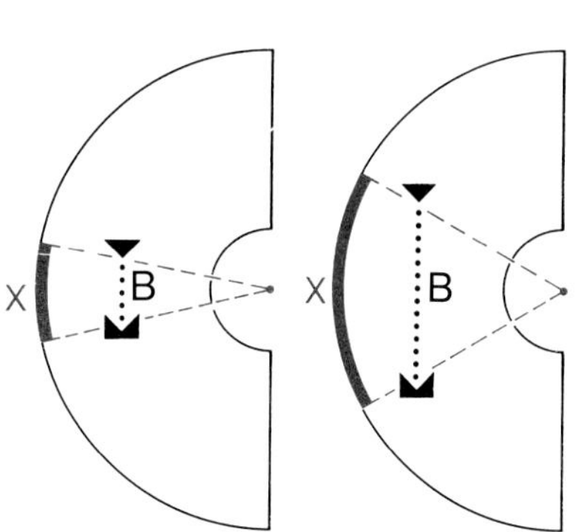

Fig. 280. **Effect of grasping on the basal width of the iridectomy.** At a given distance from the base, the blade spacing *(B)* determines the basal width *(X)* of the "pyramid" of iris and thus, after its dissection, the basal width of the iridectomy *(left)*. *Right:* Examples of basal widths for different blade spacings

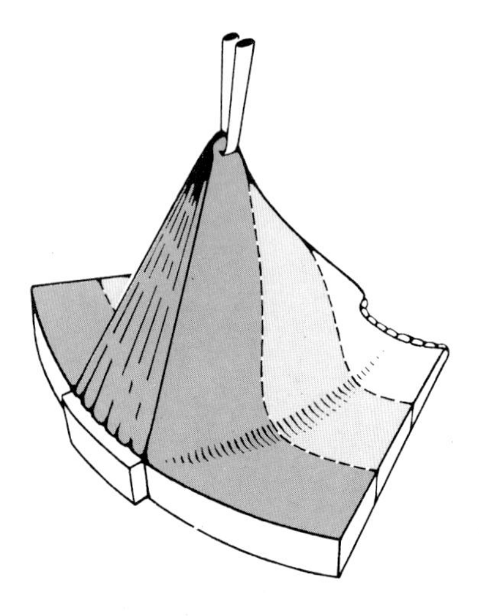

Fig. 281. **Effect of traction on the iris.** If the iris is raised, a pyramid of tissue is formed. The tissue tension is unequal at its lateral surfaces, because the portion between the forceps and base is more tense than that between the forceps and pupil. Being stretched, the *basal portion* of the pyramid contains less tissue per unit area than the lax *pupillary portion*, as shown in the drawing by the distribution of the gray-shaded zones: The basal portion contains only material from the dark-gray zone, while the pupillary portion contains material from all three zones (zonal divisions as in Fig. 277)

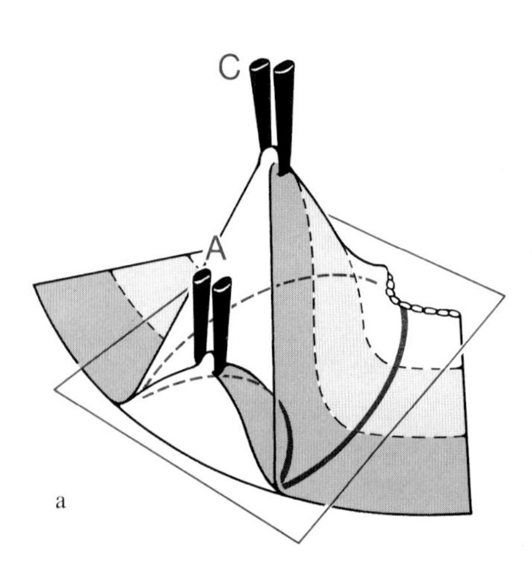

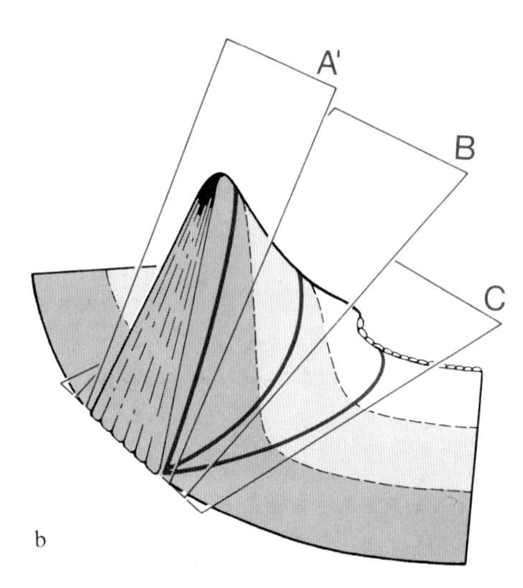

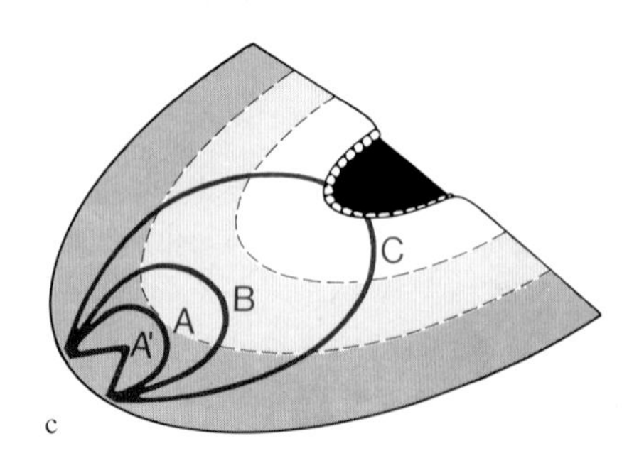

Fig. 282. **Controlling the size of the iridectomy**

a Control by degree of traction: If the position of the iris scissors (shown by its plane guidance path outlined in red) is kept constant, the shape of the iridectomy is controlled by forceps traction. If upward traction is increased, the pyramid is raised higher above the guidance plane of the scissors, and a larger iridectomy is obtained *(C)*.

b Control by varying the inclination of the scissors: If the forceps is held steady, the size of the iridectomy can be regulated by varying the inclination of the scissors (plane guidance paths *A′*, *B*, *C*).

c Resulting shapes of iridectomy from a and b: If the size is controlled by varying the scissors inclination, small iridectomies are cut in a region of high tissue tension, and straight edges result *(A′)*. In control by forceps traction, small iridectomies are cut in lax tissue, and the iridectomy becomes larger due to tissue shifting and has rounded edges *(A)*. In large iridectomies cut far from the forceps, the two control methods differ little *(B, C)*

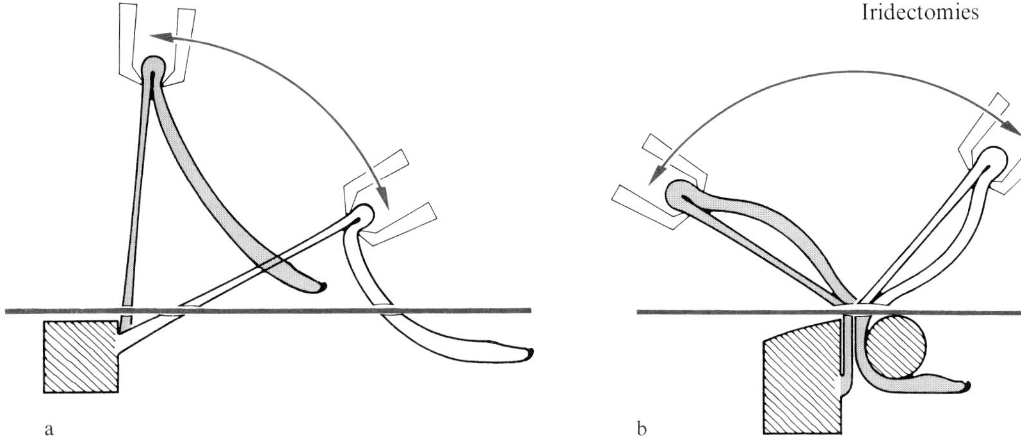

Fig. 283. **Effect of changing the direction of traction in intra- and extrabulbar iridectomy**

a In intrabulbar iridectomy, new tissue is brought above the guidance plane of the scissors *(red)* when the direction of traction is changed; this alters the shape of the iridectomy.

b In extrabulbar iridectomy, merely changing the *direction* of traction does not affect the portions of iris lying above the guidance plane. Thus, the shape of the iridectomy depends on the *degree* of traction rather than its *direction*

blades and pyramid is varied mainly by *forceps traction,* while in *extrabulbar* iridectomy it is varied by the *inclination of the scissors* (Figs. 283–285).

The various shifting tendencies of compliant and resilient tissue (see Figs. 39, 40) play an important role during **cutting.** For example, the *forward shifting tendency* drives the tissue toward the ends of the blades. If the iridectomy is to be cut with a single snip of the scissors, therefore, the blades must be held so that they extend well beyond the desired endpoint of the iridectomy (Fig. 286). The *lateral shifting tendency* causes the tissue to shift toward its point of fixation: toward the base of the iris or toward the iris forceps. *Lamellar deflection* is also a factor in iris operations, because the trabeculae behave as lamellae due to the regularity of their arrangement and cause the cut to deviate in their direction (Fig. 287).[8]

Iridectomies tend to be *oblong* in shape, because the pyramid is pressed together between the blades. The direction of the long axis of the oval is determined by the position of the scissors (Figs. 288a, 289a).

The **control of iridectomies** is facilitated if the cut is made *toward the base:* The maximum pupillary extent of the iridectomy is then determined by the point at which the scissors is applied, and lateral shifting is limited by the high tissue tension in the basal portion of the pyramid as well as by the direction of the cut parallel to the trabeculae (Fig. 288). If the cut is made *parallel to the base,* however, the shifting tendencies of the tissue will produce iridectomies which are larger than planned: The pupillary extent of the iridectomy is not limited by the site of application of the scissors, then, but depends chiefly on the mobility of the tissue. This will tend to shift continuously from the lax pupillary part of the pyramid toward the forceps or the base, this tendency being reinforced by the crosstrabecular direction of the cut (Fig. 289). Thus during cutting, the excision extends farther and farther toward the pupil and may result in an unintentional sector iridectomy if the cut then crosses the pupillary margin. To recognize this danger promptly, pupillary movements must be closely watched during the iridectomy. To prevent the danger, iris mobility can be reduced by incising the pyramid to drain the fluid below it (Fig. 276d).

Some examples will show how the interplay of all these factors can be utilized to achieve specific operative goals.

---

[8] In other words: The lateral shifting tendency decreases when the cut parallels the trabeculae.

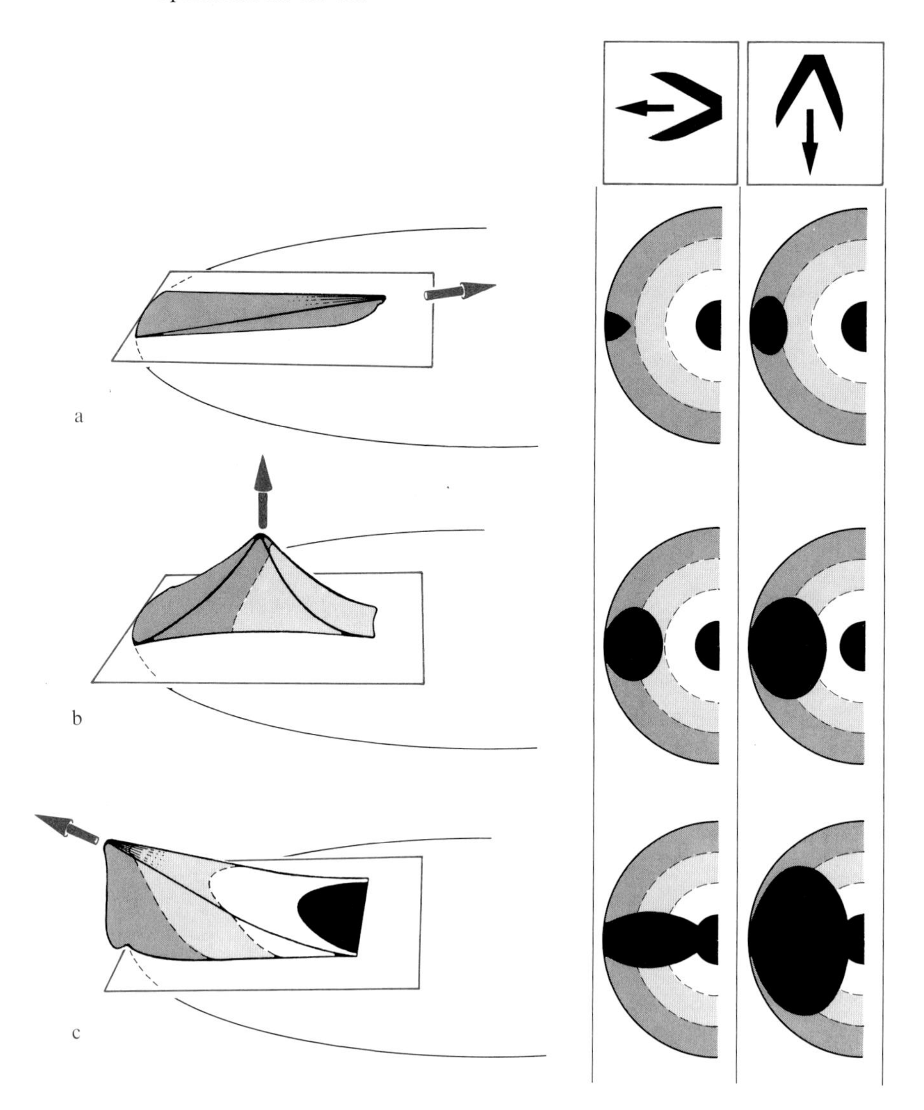

Fig. 284. **Controlling the shape of the intrabulbar iridectomy.** *Left:* The pyramid of iris above the scissors guidance plane. *Center:* Resulting shape of iridectomy for a basalward cut (see also Fig. 288). *Right:* Shape of iridectomy for a base-parallel cut (see also Fig. 289).

a Traction *toward the pupil* brings the cut selectively into the basal portion of the pyramid, and a small basal iridectomy is obtained (with straight edges if cut is basalward).

b Traction *upward* raises more tissue from the pupillary portion and produces a larger iridectomy with rounded edges.

c Traction *basalward* pulls the pupillary margin above the guidance plane of the scissors, and a sector iridectomy results

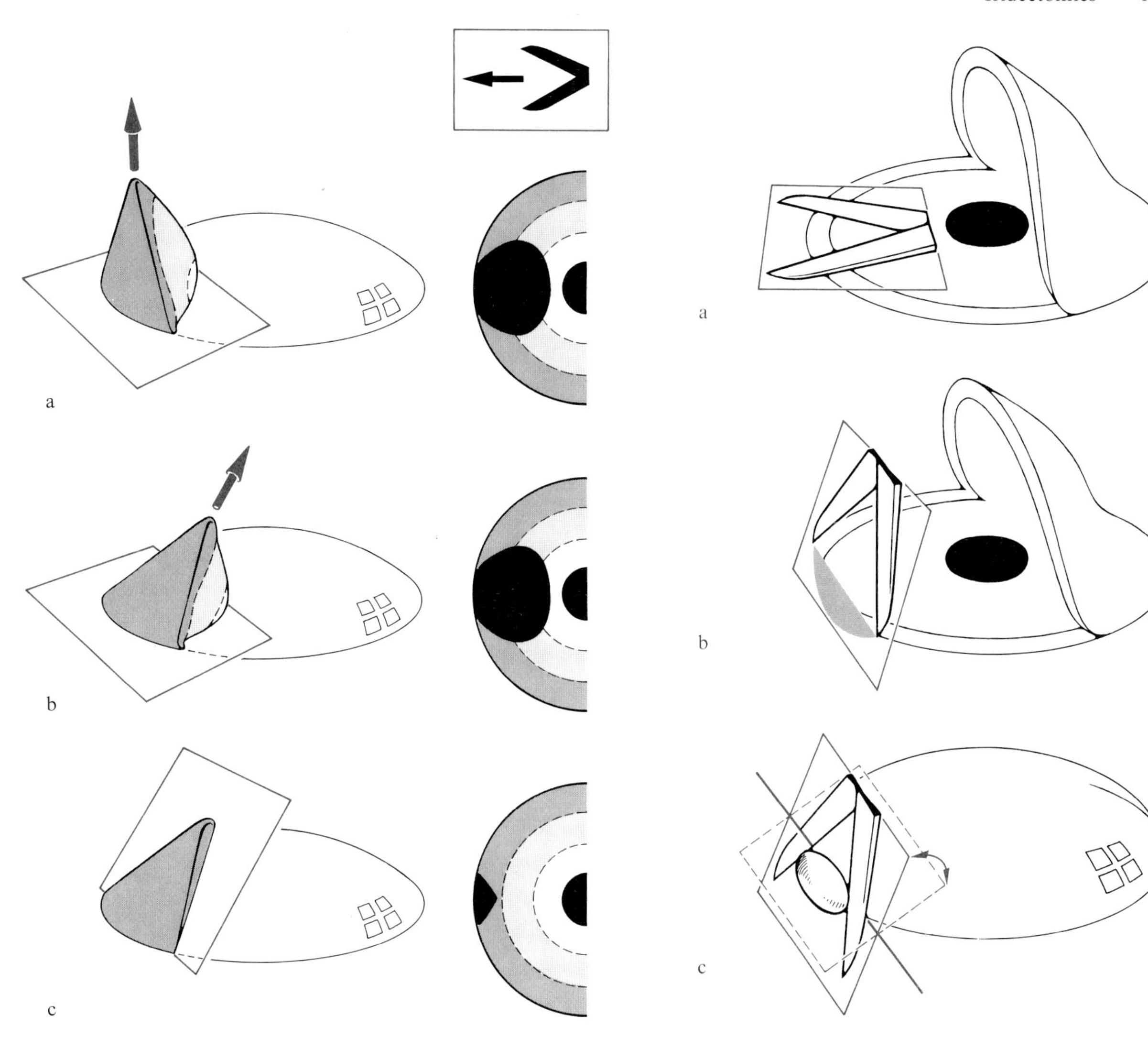

Fig. 285. **Controlling the shape of the extrabulbar iridectomy**

a A tangential guidance plane produces an iridectomy with rounded edges whose size depends on the degree of traction.

b Changing merely the direction of traction does not alter the shape of the iridectomy.

c The shape of the iridectomy is changed by varying the application angle of the scissors (see also Fig. 282 b)

Fig. 286. **Position of scissors for performing an iridectomy with a single snip**

a In *intrabulbar* iridectomy, the blades may extend beyond the base of the iris if the blades are parallel to the iris.

b If in intrabulbar iridectomy the blades are at a steep angle to the iris plane, their tips cut into deeper tissues and thus cannot be extended beyond the iris base. A basal iridectomy would require several cuts.

c In *extrabulbar* iridectomy, the blades are in open space even beyond their contact with the prolapsed iris, and a basal iridectomy can be cut with one snip at various scissors inclinations

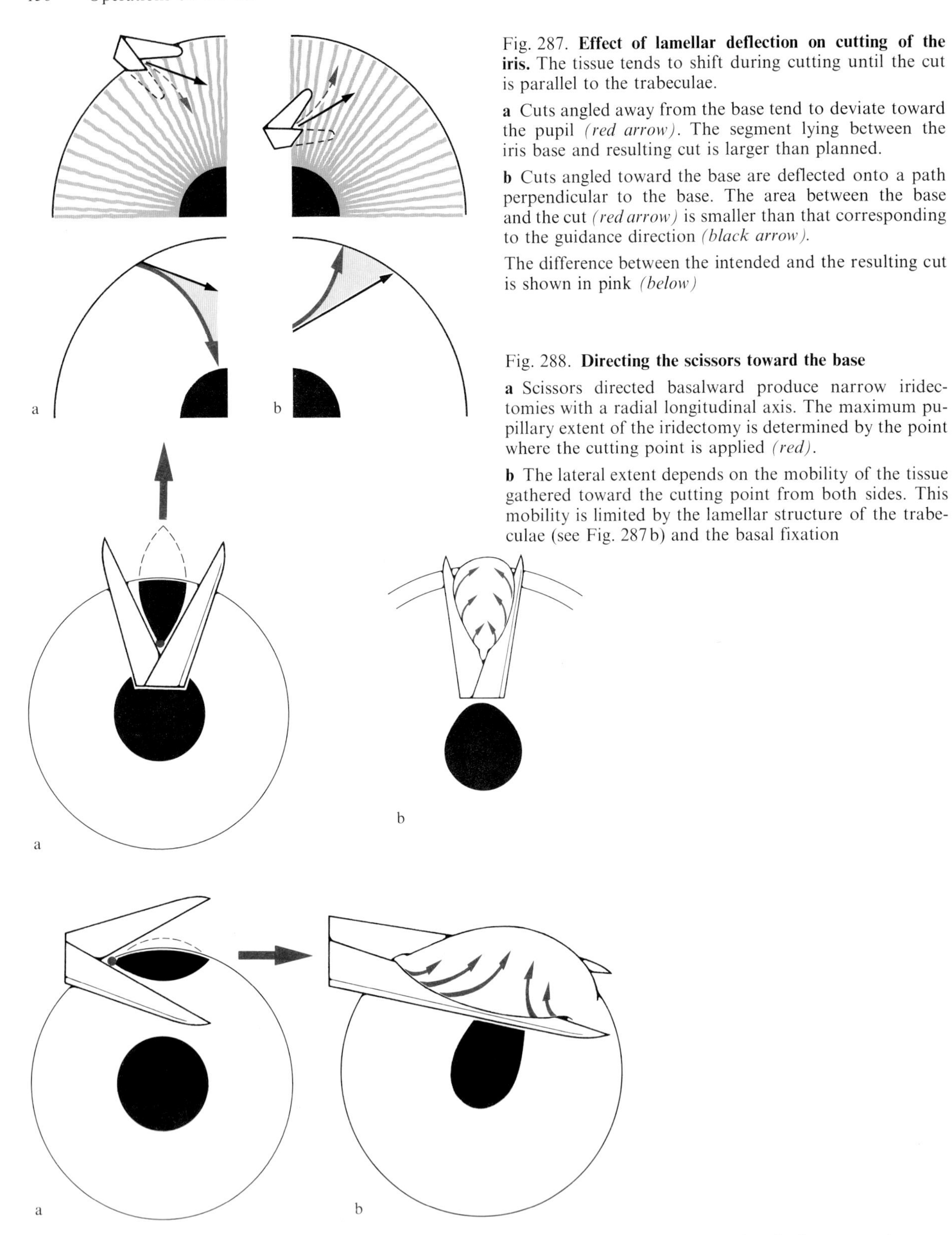

Fig. 287. **Effect of lamellar deflection on cutting of the iris.** The tissue tends to shift during cutting until the cut is parallel to the trabeculae.

a Cuts angled away from the base tend to deviate toward the pupil *(red arrow)*. The segment lying between the iris base and resulting cut is larger than planned.

b Cuts angled toward the base are deflected onto a path perpendicular to the base. The area between the base and the cut *(red arrow)* is smaller than that corresponding to the guidance direction *(black arrow)*.

The difference between the intended and the resulting cut is shown in pink *(below)*

Fig. 288. **Directing the scissors toward the base**

a Scissors directed basalward produce narrow iridectomies with a radial longitudinal axis. The maximum pupillary extent of the iridectomy is determined by the point where the cutting point is applied *(red)*.

b The lateral extent depends on the mobility of the tissue gathered toward the cutting point from both sides. This mobility is limited by the lamellar structure of the trabeculae (see Fig. 287b) and the basal fixation

Fig. 289. **Directing the scissors parallel to the base**

a Scissors directed parallel to the base produce broad iridectomies in the form of a transverse oval. The site where the cutting point is applied *(red)* determines the position of one lateral edge of the iridectomy, but the maximum pupillary extent and endpoint cannot be accurately predicted.

b The tissue is displaced toward the base by the advancing cutting point. The resulting iridectomy extends farther pupilward than the blade position would suggest. There is a danger of a "total" sector iridectomy

Fig. 290. **Objective: Basal iridectomy of minimal size**
Grasping: Blade spacing *(A)*: small; distance from base *(B)*: small.
Traction: Firm in direction of cutting point (see Fig. 284a).
Cutting: Position of guidance plane: in tense portion of pyramid, i.e., just below forceps, close to traction fold, close to base. Guidance direction: basalward.

a Diagram of planned shape of iridectomy.

b, c Extrabulbar iridectomy: Selection of tense portion by inclining the scissors. If the tips may not extend beyond the base, the iridectomy is cut in two phases.

d Intrabulbar iridectomy: Selection of tense portion by directing traction just above the scissors blades. Since the blades of the scissors are parallel to the iris, they may extend beyond the base; the excision is done with one snip of the scissors (see Fig. 286a)

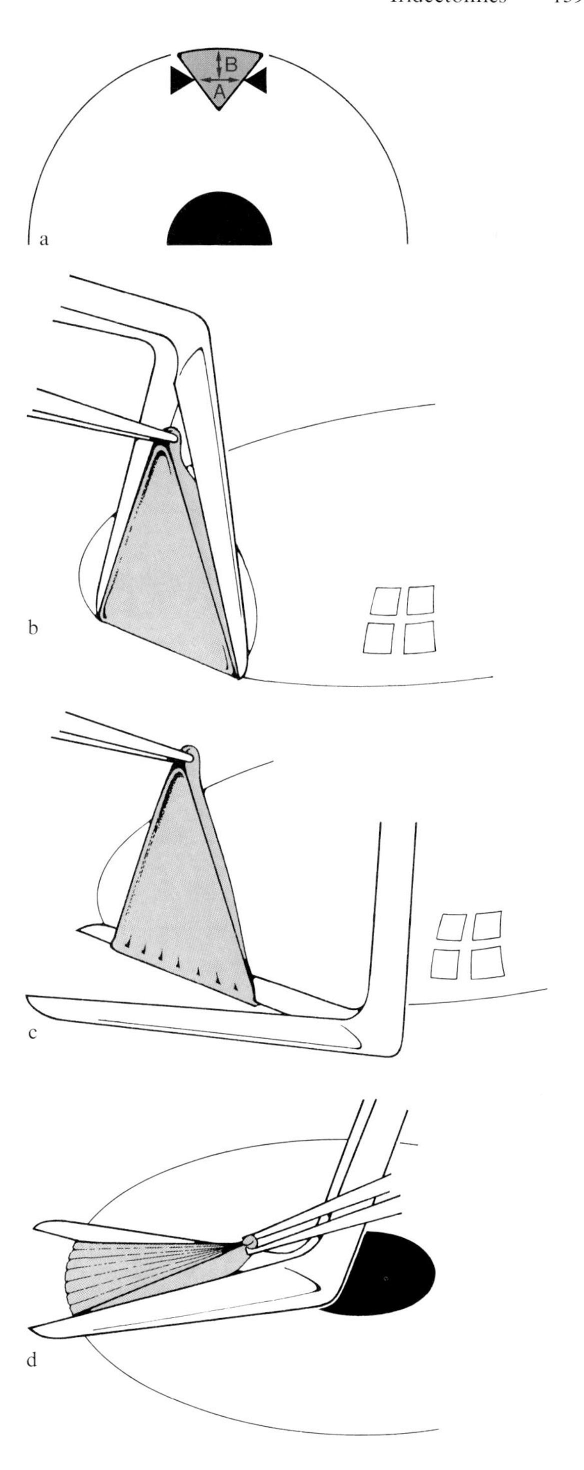

A **basal iridectomy** which is to be of *minimal size* (Fig. 290) is cut primarily in the tense portion of the pyramid in order to exploit the retractile tendency of the tissue to bring the cut nearer the base. Also, the cut is directed basalward so that the maximum pupillary extent is defined from the outset, and lateral shifting is limited (see Fig. 288).

If it is necessary to cut a basal iridectomy which is somewhat *larger than a given excised corneal opening,*[9] the principle of cutting under low tissue tension is utilized to bring more tissue between the cutting blades (Fig. 291). The degree and direction of traction depend mainly on the extent to which the size of the pyramid has been influenced by other factors (spontaneous prolapse, Fig. 277; application of forceps, Figs. 279, 280). The scissors is directed along the longitudinal axis of the corneal opening (Fig. 289a).

If a **sector iridectomy** ("total" iridectomy) is to be performed with a *single snip of the scissors* (Fig. 292), its edges will always be rounded, because a large part is cut in tissue which is not under tension.[10] If the goal is a *sector iridectomy with straight edges,* the cut must be made in *several steps* (Fig. 293).

[9] Example: In "fistular openings" by trephination or excision (trabeculectomy) the iridectomy may be made larger than the corneal opening to prevent synechiae with the wound margin.

[10] If, to avoid this, the forceps is applied at the pupillary margin, the resulting iridectomy will be triangular in shape, i.e., narrower at its base than at the pupil.

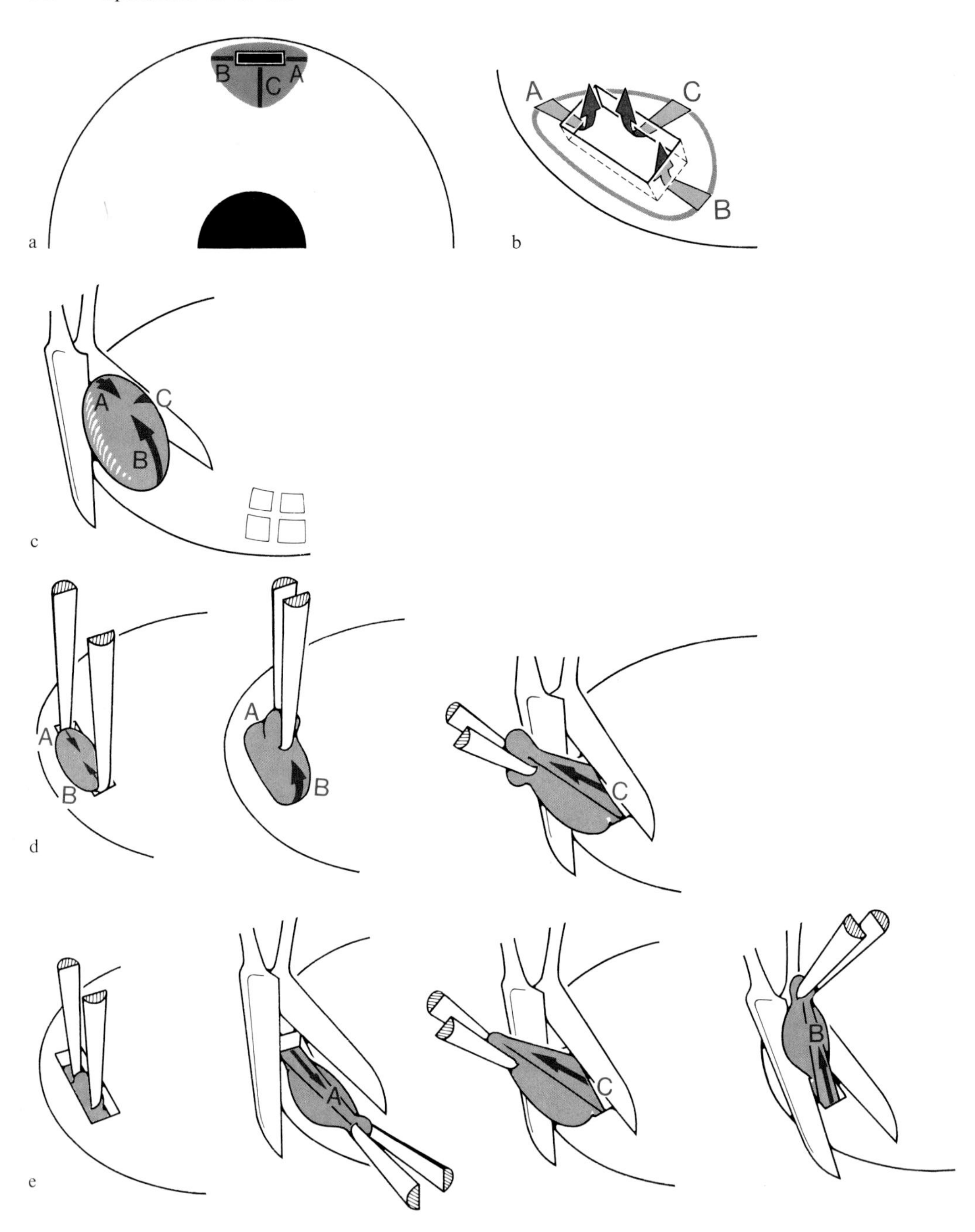

Fig. 291. **Objective: Basal iridectomy which is larger than a given excised corneal opening**

a *Diagram of the planned shape of iridectomy:* The edges of the iridectomy are to lie at distance ABC from the edges of the corneal opening (black rectangle).

b *Task:* Tissue segments must be exteriorized from the area corresponding to ABC.

c *First method:* Segments ABC are exteriorized by spontaneous prolapse. Control is difficult, and the effect is hard to judge due to stretching of the tissue (see Fig. 277).

d *Second method:* Segments A and B are exteriorized by closure of the forceps. If the forceps grasp the edges of a small spontaneous prolapse, segments A and B are both exteriorized by closure alone. Segment C is exteriorized by additional forceps traction in a basal direction.

e *Third method:* Segments *ABC* are exteriorized purely by forceps traction. If the iris is grasped in situ, closure of the forceps produces only a small tissue displacement. Segments *A*, *B* and *C* are exteriorized by consecutive traction toward the scissors tip, iris base, and cutting point

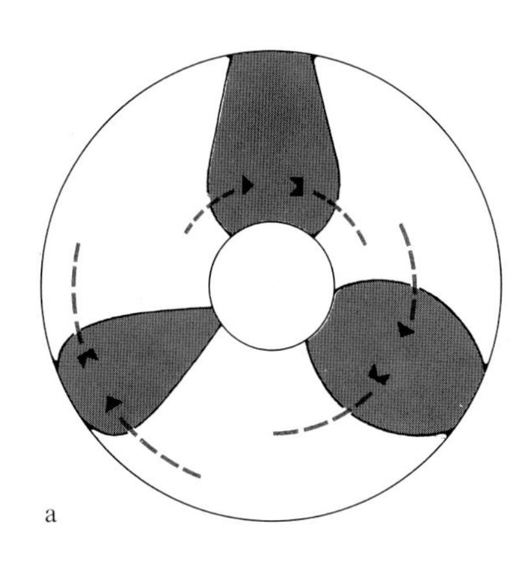
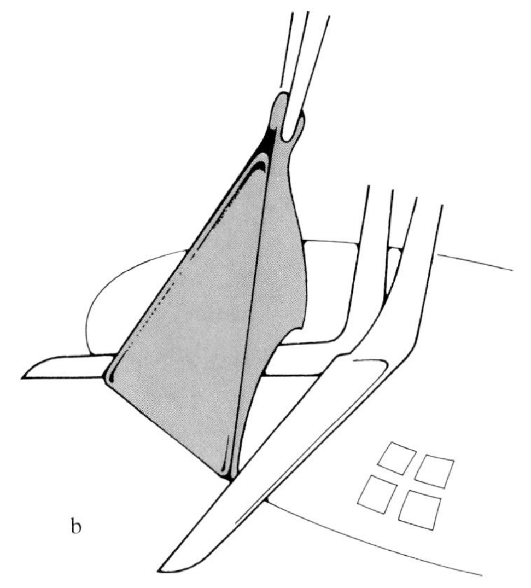

Fig. 292. **Objective: Total sector iridectomy with a single snip of the scissors**

Grasping: Blade spacing determines the minimum width. The distance from the base determines the point of greatest width.

Traction: The direction and degree of traction depend on the point of forceps application. Object of traction: to bring the pupillary margin above the scissors blades.

Cutting: Position of blades: parallel to the iris plane so that the blade tips can overhang the iris base. A basalward cut produces an upright ellipse according to scheme **a.** A cut parallel to the base produces a transverse ellipse with a large stromal excision for similar pupillary and basal widths (see Fig. 284c, right).

a Shape of iridectomy: At a defined interblade distance, it is the distance of the forceps from the base which determines the width of the iridectomy at the base and pupillary margin. The edges of the iridectomy are rounded.

b Criteria for controlling traction: Firm traction exploits the retractile tendency to bring the iridectomy close to the iris root. In sector iridectomy, it is essential that the pupillary margin be pulled above the plane of the blades

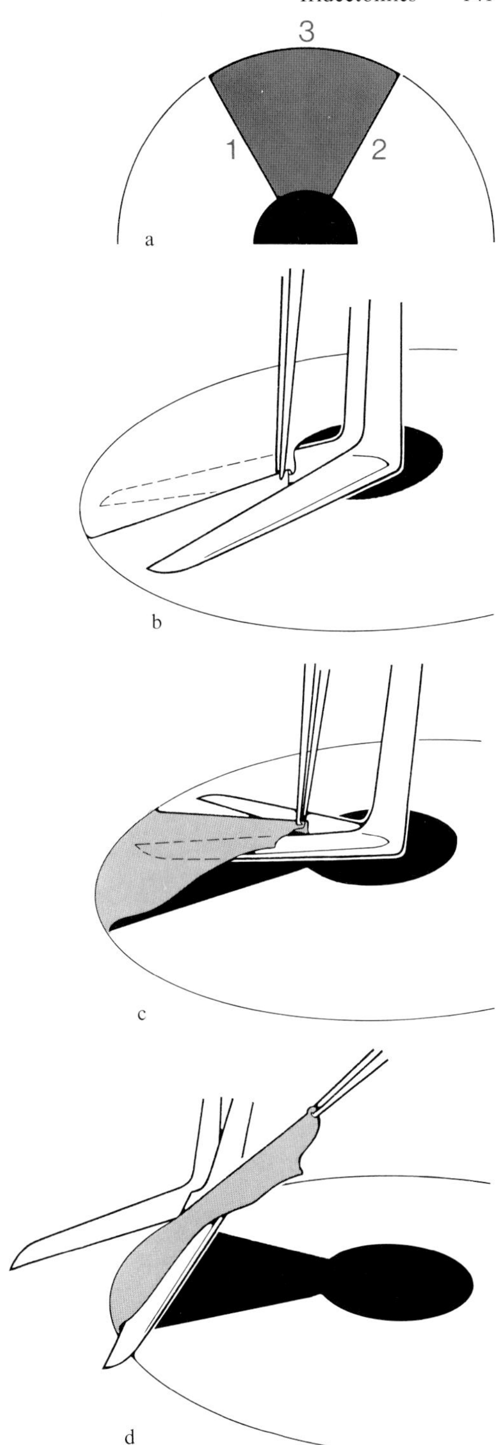

Fig. 293. **Objective: Sector iridectomy with straight edges ("keyhole" iridectomy)**

a Scheme of iridectomy (with three snips of scissors).

b Step 1: The pupillary margin is grasped at one corner of the planned iridectomy. The cut is made along the traction fold (for least deviation).

c Step 2: A similar cut is made from the other corner.

d Step 3: Excision parallel to base. Retractile tendency is utilized by applying firm tension

3 Enlarging the Pupil

If the pupil is too narrow for the passage of solid ocular structures (lens), it must be surgically enlarged. **Posterior synechiae** can be separated bluntly in most cases by directing the spatula so as to maximize sectility (by increasing tissue tension) and minimize resistance (by passing the spatula perpendicularly into the zone of adhesions, Fig. 294).[11]

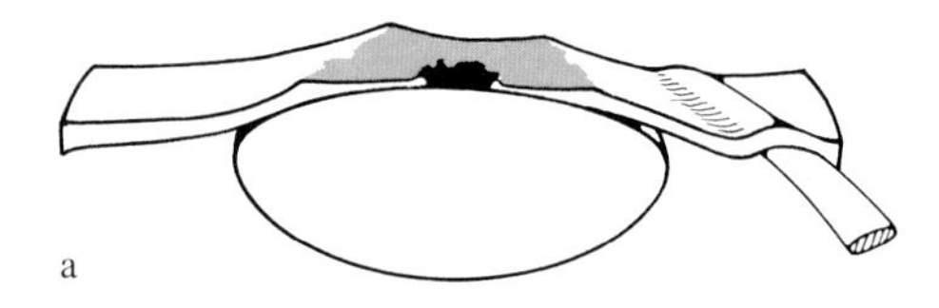

a

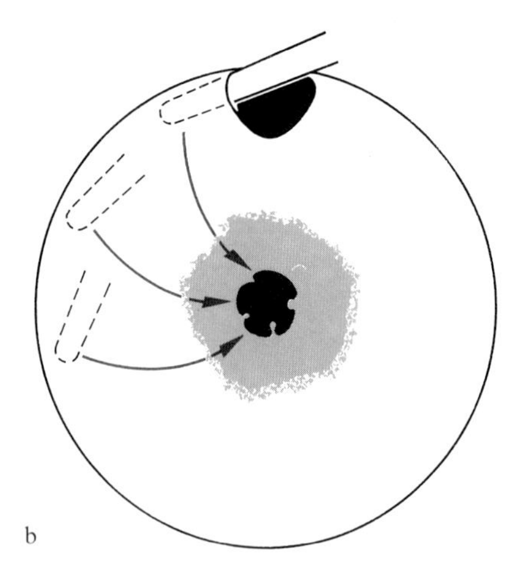

b

Fig. 294. **Separation of posterior synechiae**

a The spatula is advanced in the space with lowest adhesive tendency, i.e., the space peripheral to the lens margin. The position of the spatula is indicated by a bulge in the iris, which can be increased if necessary by slightly raising the spatula without advancing it (see footnote 2, p. 3).

b To separate the synechia, the spatula is swept in a centripetal direction, i.e., the direction in which the greatest tissue tension is produced (shortest path to fixation point at base of iris) and resistance is minimal (shortest diameter of adhesion zone, *gray*)

Retraction of the pupillary margin can be achieved simply by pulling the iris aside, provided the tissue is sufficiently distensible. *Retracting hooks* passed over the pupillary margin (Fig. 295) must be pushed back toward the pupil when removed. Easier to remove are *retractors*, which retract the iris while in direct contact with the lens surface (Figs. 296, 297).

If the pupillary sphincter is too rigid, it must be sectioned. This is done either by including the pupillary margin in an iridectomy *(sector iridectomy)* or with a simple radial incision *(sphincterotomy)*. In a **sphincterotomy** (Fig. 298), the pupillary margin must be brought between the blades of the scissors; inadvertant lesions are avoided by leading all guidance movements with the blunt parts of the blades (Fig. 298b). The *forward shifting tendency* of the rigid sphincter tissue will result in a shorter cut than the position of the blade tips would indicate. It can be reduced either by exploiting tissue inertia (i.e. by making the cut with a rapid snip)[12] or, for better control, by increasing tissue friction at the blades (i.e. by tipping the scissors to the side) (Fig. 298c).

[11] Note: Anterior synechiae, on the other hand, often adhere strongly at the pathologic fixation site. If blunt dissection is attempted, the tissue may tear more easily at the iris root than at the adhesion: Iridodialysis.

[12] See p. 15.

Fig. 295. **Iris retraction by means of broad and slender hooks**

a Slender hook is very mobile but exposes only a small field.

b Broad hook achieves broader retraction; its concave back conforms to the anterior lens surface to avoid lesions.

c Handle at right angles to the axis of curvature of the hook. To remove, the hook must be pushed back toward the pupil.

d Handle parallel to axis of curvature: The hook is removed by simple rotation of the handle

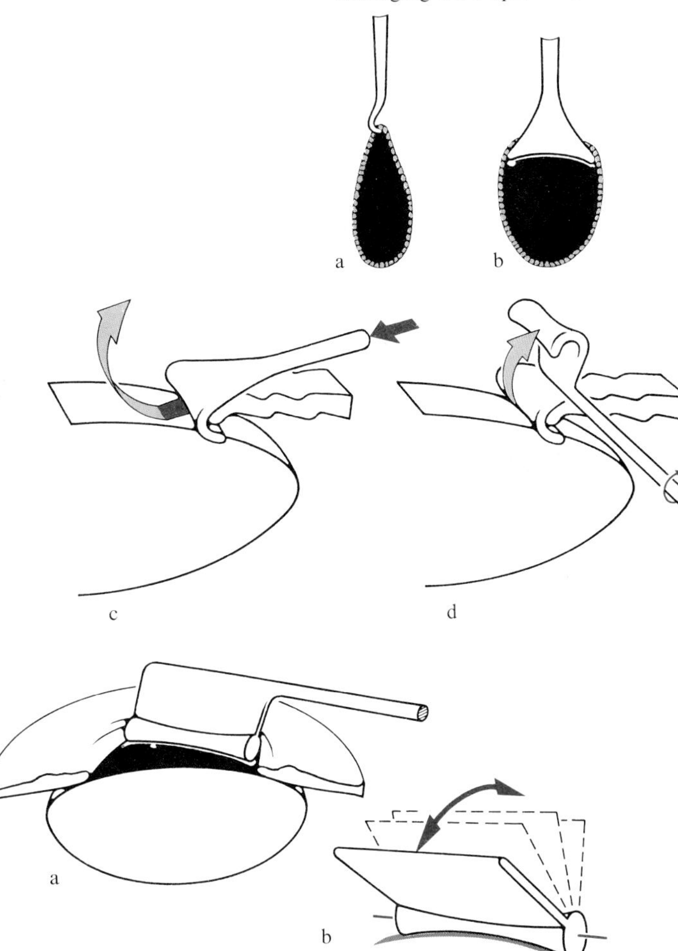

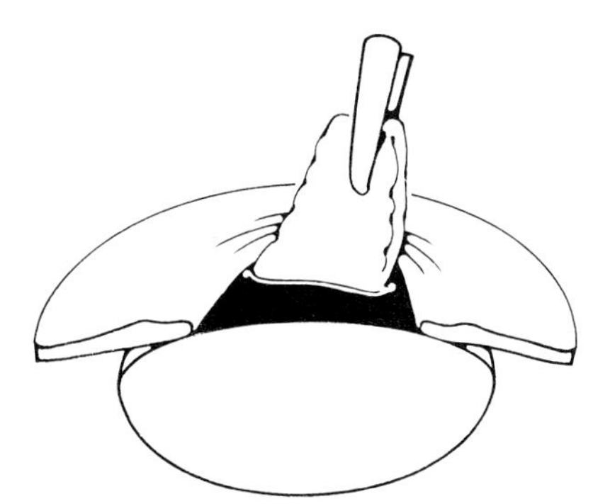

Fig. 296. **Foam swab as an iris retractor.** Foam swabs conform to the anterior lens surface when moist. They also adhere to iris tissue by suction and can thus be used to retract it. If the swab absorbs aqueous, it increases in size and endangers the corneal endothelium. If it becomes soft, its efficiency as a mechanical tool decreases

Fig. 297. **Rigid instruments for retracting the iris**

a Rigid instruments occupy a small and constant space. The curvature of their undersurface corresponds to that of the anterior lens surface.

b The blade is fashioned as a concave roller so that its contact surface remains constant at any angle

Fig. 298. **Sphincterotomy: Controlling friction**

a Friction and tissue tension are varied by tipping the scissors laterally.

b If the blades are not in contact with the tissue, no friction is created. This is the position assumed during guidance motions of the scissors when advancing to the point of incision; all motions are led with the blunt parts of the blades to avoid lesions.

c If the scissors is tipped to the side, the blades and the tissue will come into contact. Further tipping increases friction by raising tissue tension. This is the position assumed during the working motion (closure of scissors)

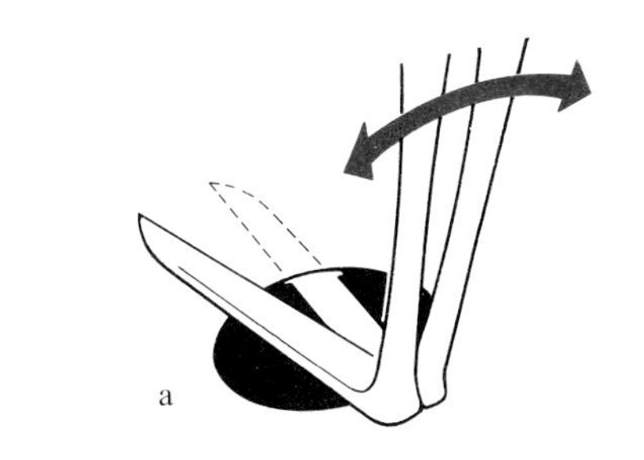

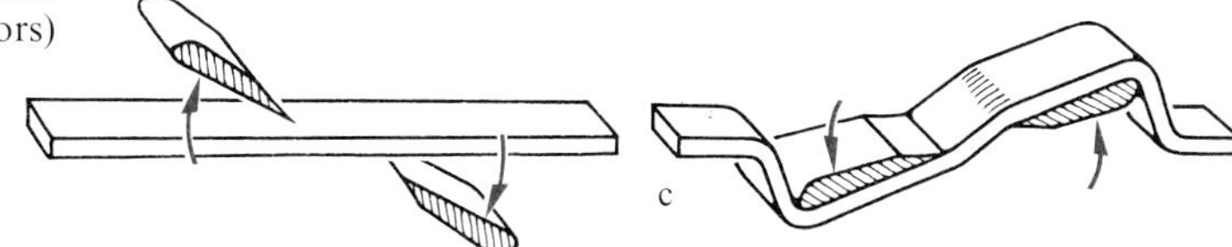

4 Repositioning of the Iris

If reposition does not occur spontaneously (Figs. 299, 300), all resistances must be eliminated, and iris mobility is assisted if need be by additional forces.

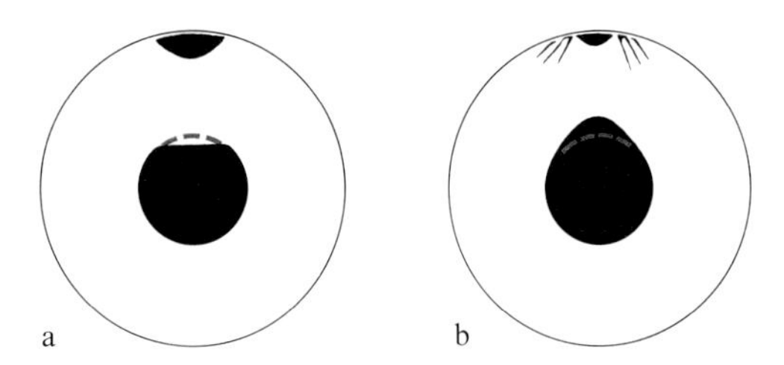

Fig. 299. **Iris incarceration in basal iridectomy**

a The criterion for successful reposition of the iris is a flattening of the pupil in the region of the iridectomy.

b A round pupil or a bulge in the direction of the iridectomy indicates incarceration of iris tissue

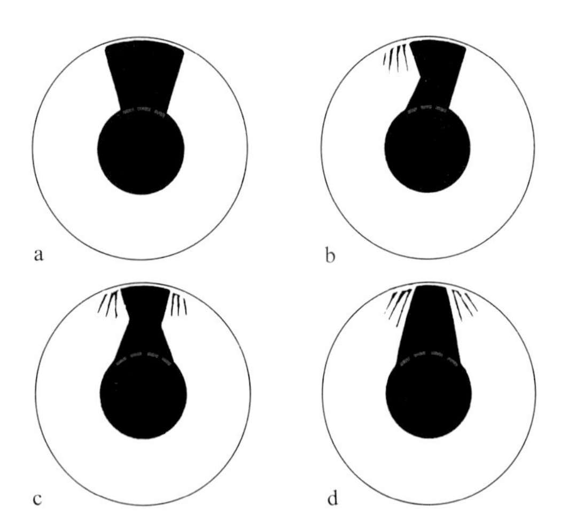

Fig. 300. **Incarceration in sector iridectomy**

a The criterion for successful reposition is a centered pupil. The pupillary margin is everywhere equidistant from the base, the sides of the iridectomy are of equal length, and its corners are well formed.

b Partial unilateral incarceration: The pupillary margin is displaced upward, one corner is blunted.

c Partial bilateral incarceration.

d Total bilateral incarceration. The iridectomy has no clear corners, and the pupillary margins pass into the wound

The **frictional resistance** is reduced first by refilling the anterior chamber with watery fluid (Fig. 301). If iris tissue is incarcerated in the wound, the friction there is reduced by slightly reopening the wound. To prevent the prolapse of internal structures, inertia is exploited by keeping the wound open only momentarily (Fig. 302). The repositioning forces can be increased by the injection of miotics,[13] which supplement the friction-reducing effect of the fluid. If this is not sufficient, forces can be transmitted to the iris with

[13] For example, 0.1–0.5% acetylcholine.

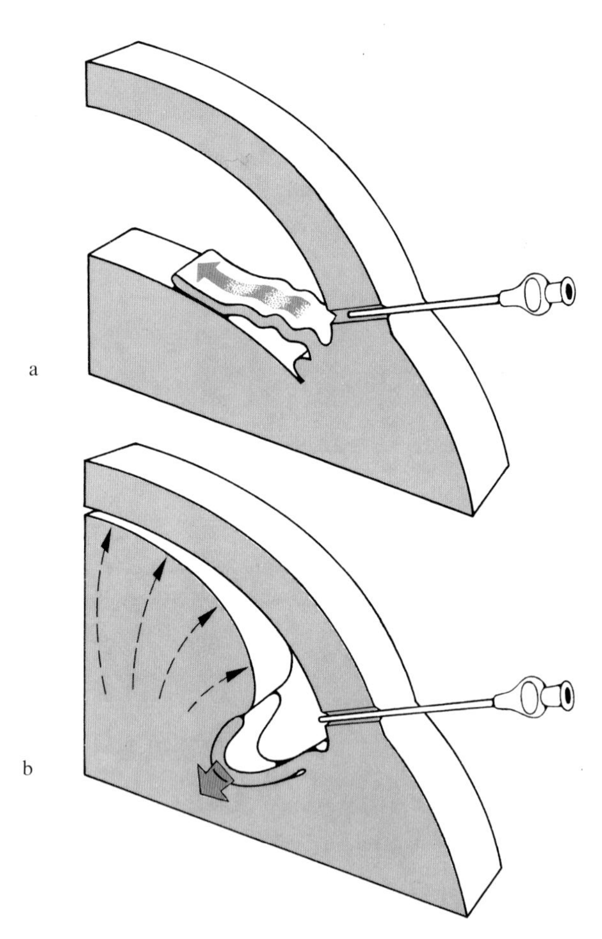

Fig. 301. **Repositioning the iris by refilling the anterior chamber**

a Fluid is injected, along with a miotic if desired, in a gentle stream to restore iris mobility and promote spontaneous repositioning.

b If the iris is pressed downward by a direct jet of fluid, the compensatory rise of vitreous forms a "mushroom" which hinders pupillary contraction (to prevent this, the pressure chamber must be restored, see Fig. 342)

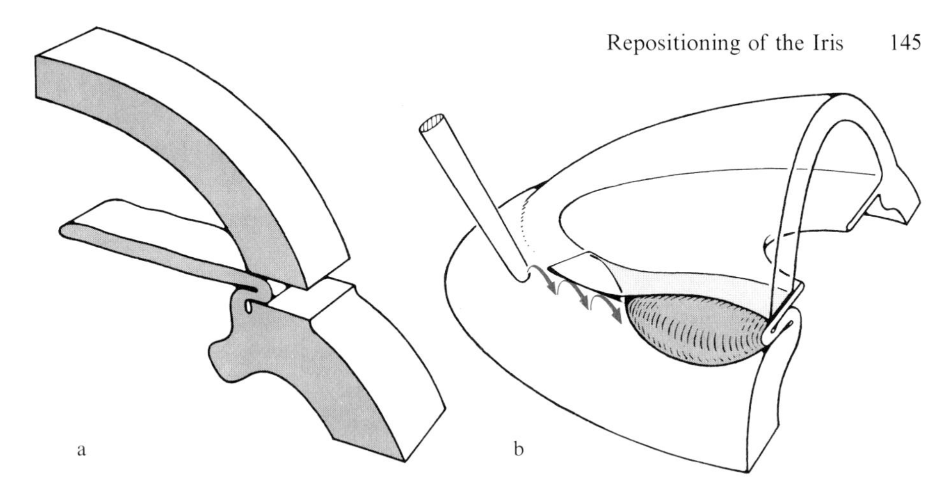

Fig. 302. **Repositioning the iris by tapping the wound**

a Incarceration of iris in the wound.

b Iris mobility can be restored by momentarily reopening the wound (tapping the lower wound lip). This is begun far from the outwardly-visible prolapse, since the incarceration zone is considerably larger internally *(light gray)* than its external appearance *(dark gray)* would suggest

instruments. Spatulas are used so as not to open the corneal wound.[14] The spatula makes contact with the iris through friction with the trabeculae, and the end of the spatula is moved centripetally away from the site of incarceration (Fig. 303). Spatular movements which go beyond the stroma into the pupil or iridectomy do not improve the effect and actually endanger structures located behind these openings.

Failure of all these repositioning maneuvers is indicative of **other obstructions** such as an incarcerated lens capsule or vitreous. Their correction exceeds the bounds of simple iris repositioning and implies far-reaching surgical measures adapted to the properties of the other tissues involved.

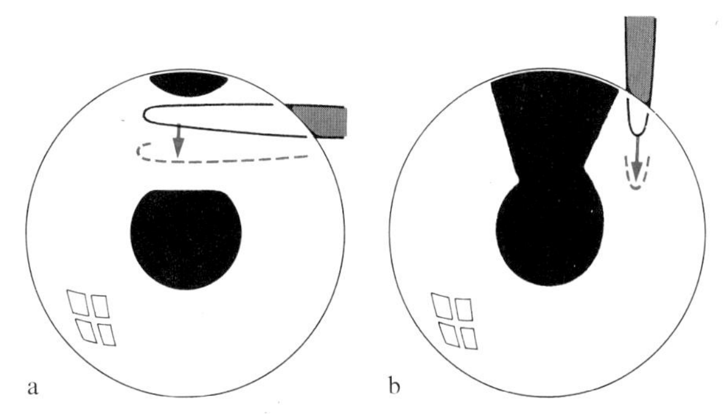

Fig. 303. **Repositioning the iris by stroking the stroma.** The spatula is stroked over the stroma, touching neither the pupil nor iridectomy.

a Stroking in basal iridectomy. The spatula is inserted beneath the iridectomy from the side and stroked toward the pupil with its long (=blunt) side.

b Guiding the spatula in sector iridectomy. Guidance vectors in the direction of the iridectomy or pupil are avoided if possible

[14] The center of rotation for all maneuvers lies at the corneal opening; any raising, lowering or tipping of the spatula will cause the wound to open.

5 Suturation of the Iris

Suturation of the iris poses few problems in itself, since the tissue is quite soft and pliable. Moreover, the sutures need withstand only small forces. The main problem is correct anatomical apposition, which requires adequate visibility.

Suture forms suitable for stitching iris to iris (iridotomies) or iris to the rigid ocular wall (irododialysis) can be derived from the descriptions in the general chapter on sutures (p. 37ff).

VII Operations on the Lens

1 General

The lens (Fig. 304) consists of an elastic capsular bag with more or less fluid contents and thus has the properties of a **pressure chamber** (Fig. 305). The influence of applied forces is primarily local in extent as long as the capsule is under little tension. However, if deformation has produced a *generalized* wall tension in the pressure chamber, the action of forces – regardless of their point of application – is transmitted to the entire system including the zonule.[1]

If the capsule is ruptured, the lenticular pressure chamber is destroyed. Applied forces then have only a *local* effect and are transmitted to the zonule only if applied close to its attachment.

The **contents of the capsular bag** are usually inhomogenous in case of cataract. The surgical procedure employed depends largely on the *water content* of the lens. In intracapsular extraction, lenses with fluid contents are easily deformed, but ice is slower to form in them than in hard lenses due to their higher thermal conductivity. In extracapsular extraction the material with a high water content can be aspirated through cannulas, while hard material must first be emulsified for such a procedure.

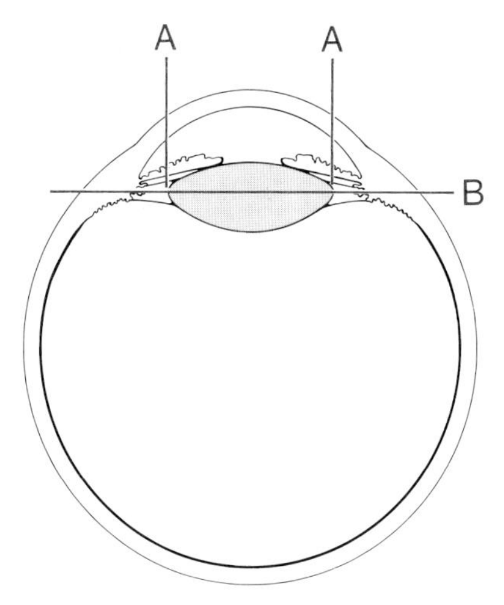

Fig. 304. **Topography of the lens.** The diameter of the lens is about 9 mm and is thus smaller than that of the cornea (see Fig. 186). Thus, an anterior projection of the lens border *(A)* lies within the cornea and cuts the iris approximately in half (at a mean pupillary diameter). The equatorial plane of the lens *(B)* intersects the ocular wall rather far posteriorly (4–6 mm behind the limbus, depending on lens position). Instruments which are to pass behind the lens border must be directed correspondingly far posteriorly. In case of cataract the thickness of the lens may change considerably, and sometimes its diameter as well

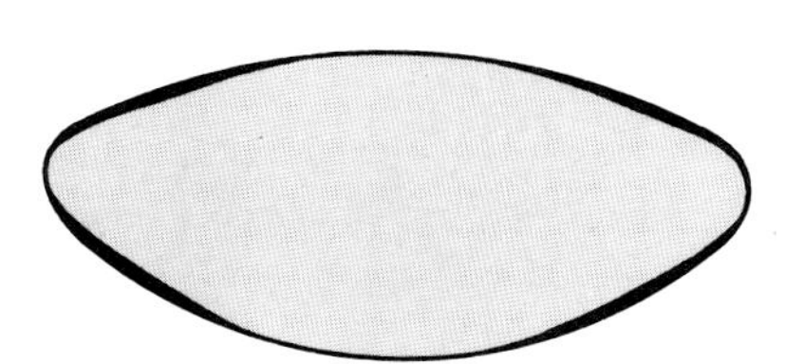

Fig. 305. **The capsular bag of the lens.** The lens capsule is thickest in the preequatorial region. In that area it is most easily grasped but is most difficult to cut or tear

[1] If the surface area is minimal from the outset, as in intumescent cataract, no further deformation is possible without raising the intralenticular pressure. Any deformation (such as an attempt to grasp the lens with forceps) poses the danger of capsule rupture.

2 Intracapsular Lens Delivery

Intracapsular lens delivery is in principle a precisely-controlled lesion of the diaphragm in which only the zonule is destroyed while the lens capsule and hyaloid membrane are left intact. The manipulations consist basically of the separation of the zonule *(zonulolysis)* and the passage of the lens through the pupil and corneal wound *(locomotion)*. There is no strict division between the two manipulations, because every movement of the lens has both a zonulolytic and locomotive effect.

The **forces or "motors" for lens delivery** may be either *pressure* (expression, Fig. 306) or *traction* (extraction, Fig. 307). In **expression,** the pressure in the vitreous chamber is increased, thereby pressing the diaphragm forward and expelling the lens from the eye. It does not matter, in terms of the *pressure increase,* where the instruments (expressors) are applied (Fig. 306a); their placement is governed entirely by the requirements of *control.* This control consists in minimizing the resistance in front of the part to be expressed (lens) and maximizing it in front of all the other parts

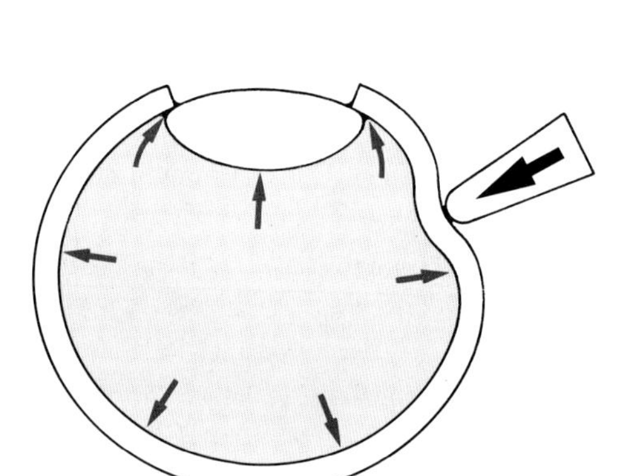

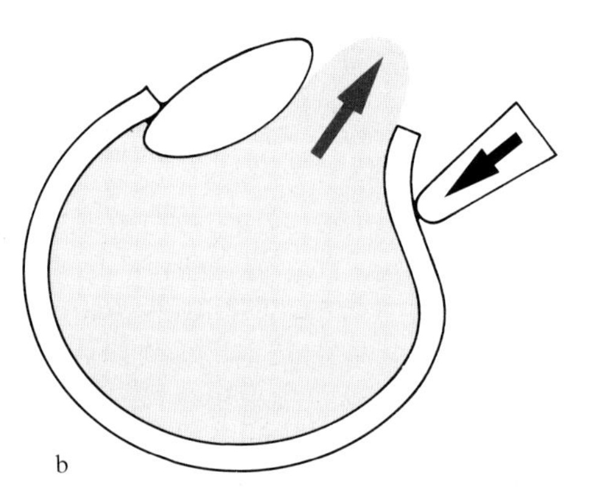

Fig. 306. **Pressure (expression) as a motor for lens delivery**

a The pressure is increased by deforming the vitreous chamber (this increase being independent of the site of the deformation, see Fig. 125). If the lowest resistance is in front of the lens, the lens is expressed.

b If the zone of least resistance lies elsewhere, extralenticular tissue will protrude when pressure is increased (e.g., vitreous prolapse due to inadequate tamponade)

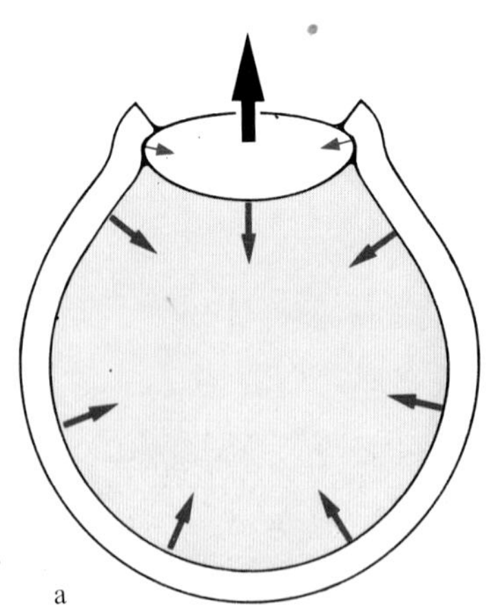

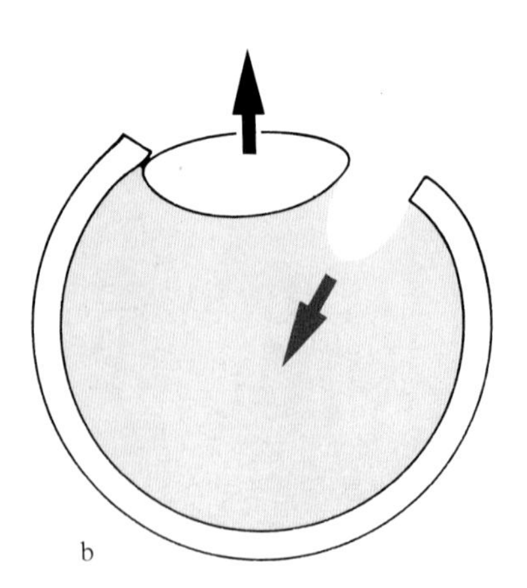

Fig. 307. **Traction (extraction) as a motor for lens delivery**

a Traction on the lens creates a vacuum in the pressure chamber which holds the lens back and hinders delivery.

b Gaps next to the lens allow pressure to equalize

of the diaphragm (tamponade). If control is imprecise, zones of low resistance may arise at undesired sites, and a pressure increase will cause extralenticular structures to prolapse while the lens itself remains stationary (Fig. 306b). In **extraction,** a *negative pressure* is created in the vitreous chamber by traction on the lens (Fig. 307). The lens is held back by this partial vacuum and can be delivered only if the pressure is equalized. This is done by creating pressure-equalizing "gaps" (e.g., basal iridectomy, localized rupture of zonule).[2]

Thus, **the control of resistances** has a diametrically-opposed purpose in each procedure. In *expression,* extralenticular gaps in the diaphragm are a source of complications, since pressure equalization is undesirable. It is the task of the surgeon to *tamponade* these gaps. In *extraction,* on the other hand, such gaps are essential for the maneuver to proceed smoothly. The surgeon must create these openings at the start of the extraction and *keep them clear* throughout the procedure.

The motor (pressure or traction) should be controlled so as to prevent the applied forces from being stored as potential energy, which may suddenly become kinetic in unforseen ways. In a properly controlled delivery, every application of force is followed by a corresponding movement of the lens. *Immobility of the lens* during pressure or traction is indicative of an obstruction which must be identified and eliminated.[3]

Locomotion alone, meaning simply the delivery of the lens through the pupillary and corneal opening, requires relatively little force. Most of the force applied is expended in freeing the lens from its zonular attachment.

[2] The negative pressure can also cause *pseudorigidity* of the iris by holding it so firmly against the lens that delivery is impossible. Unlike true iris rigidity, which is manifested even preoperatively by poor dilatation of the pupil, pseudorigidity is relieved at once when pressure is equalized.

[3] If the lens remains immobile during an *expression* despite increasing pressure, any further pressure increase will only heighten the risk of vitreous prolapse.

If the lens fails to move during an *extraction* despite traction on the lens, rupture of the capsule may result. The location of the obstruction is indicated by the direction of folds in the capsule ("arrows which point to the obstruction").

2.1 Zonulolysis

To limit the destruction of the diaphragm to the *zonule,* the applied forces are concentrated there while being distributed as broadly as possible over all the other parts of the diaphragm, especially the lens capsule.

The forces that must be applied locally can be reduced by preliminary **tensing of the zonule.** In *expression* this tension is created by the general stretching of the diaphragm. In *extraction* it results from the transmission of the traction on the lens capsule to the zonule. The more flaccid the lens capsule, the more traction is needed to make the zonule tense (Fig. 308). Because the capsule tends to become increasingly flaccid as zonule separation proceeds, the *amplitude* of the traction must be continuously increased during the course of the delivery (Fig. 308c).

The **local application of force** consists in engaging the fibers with an instrument (zonulotome)[4] and overstretching them either perpendicular or parallel to the vitreous surface (Fig. 309). Due to the deforming effects of perpendicular force vectors (see Fig. 129), a *perpendicular* thrust is made only to form the *initial gap* in the zonule,[5] but from then on the separation is continued entirely *parallel to the vitreous surface;* this allows large-amplitude movements without deforming the vitreous chamber.[6]

[4] A scleral indentation made with an expressor (Fig. 320b), an iris retractor (Fig. 321c) or a suitably-shaped special instrument can serve as a zonulotome.

[5] The instrument that makes the initial gap need not be inserted deeply, of course, for it must pass no farther than the posterior border of the zonule.

[6] The resulting gaps in the zonule act to equalize pressure and must be kept open or tamponaded, depending on whether this pressure equalization is desired or not (see Figs. 306b and 307b).

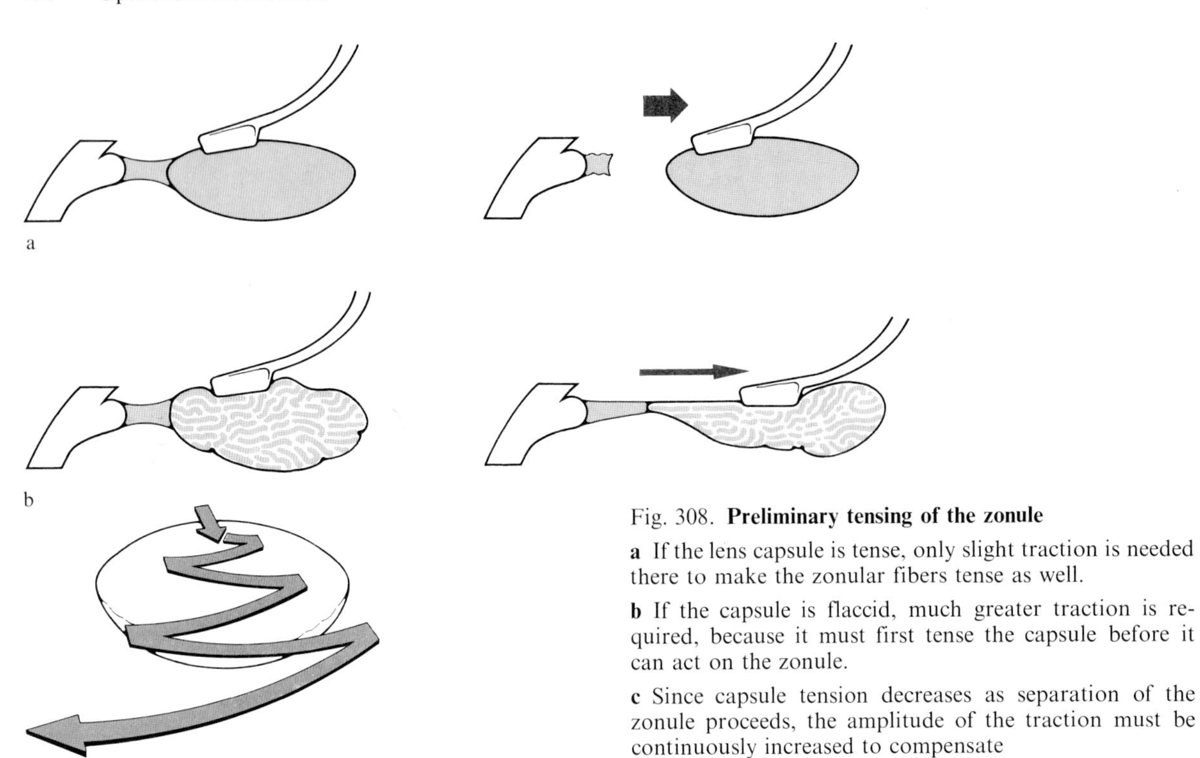

Fig. 308. **Preliminary tensing of the zonule**

a If the lens capsule is tense, only slight traction is needed there to make the zonular fibers tense as well.

b If the capsule is flaccid, much greater traction is required, because it must first tense the capsule before it can act on the zonule.

c Since capsule tension decreases as separation of the zonule proceeds, the amplitude of the traction must be continuously increased to compensate

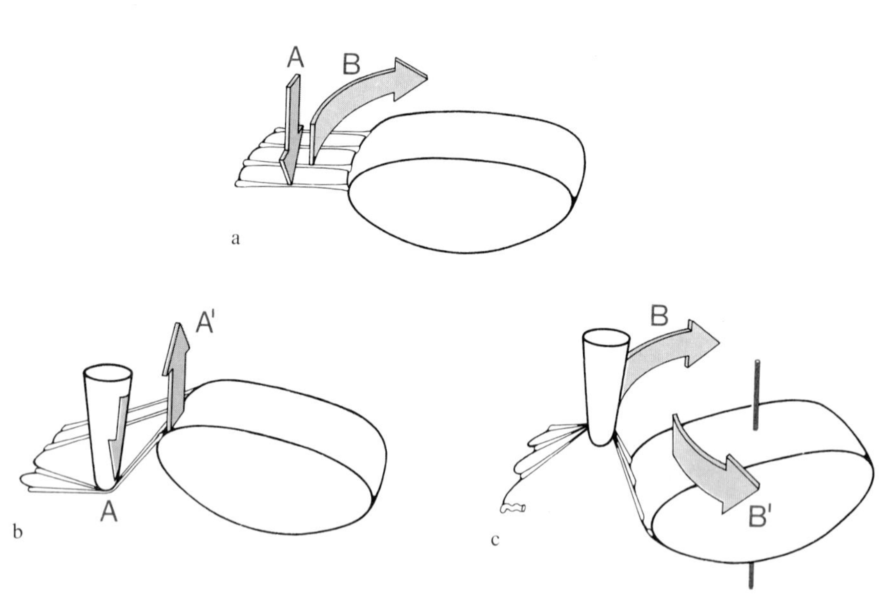

Fig. 309. **Mechanical separation of the zonule**

a Direction of fiber stretch: The fibers can be ruptured by overstretching them either perpendicular *(A)* or parallel *(B)* to the surface of the vitreous chamber.

b Perpendicular rupture is accomplished either by thrusting an instrument (zonulotome) into the zonule *(A)* or by lifting the lens *(A′)*.

c Parallel separation is accomplished either by passing a zonulotome along the border of the lens *(B)* or by rotating the lens about its sagittal axis *(B′)*.

Movements *A′* and *B′* stretch the entire zonule and are thus suitable for preliminary tensing.

Movements *A* and *B* create only a strictly localized tension

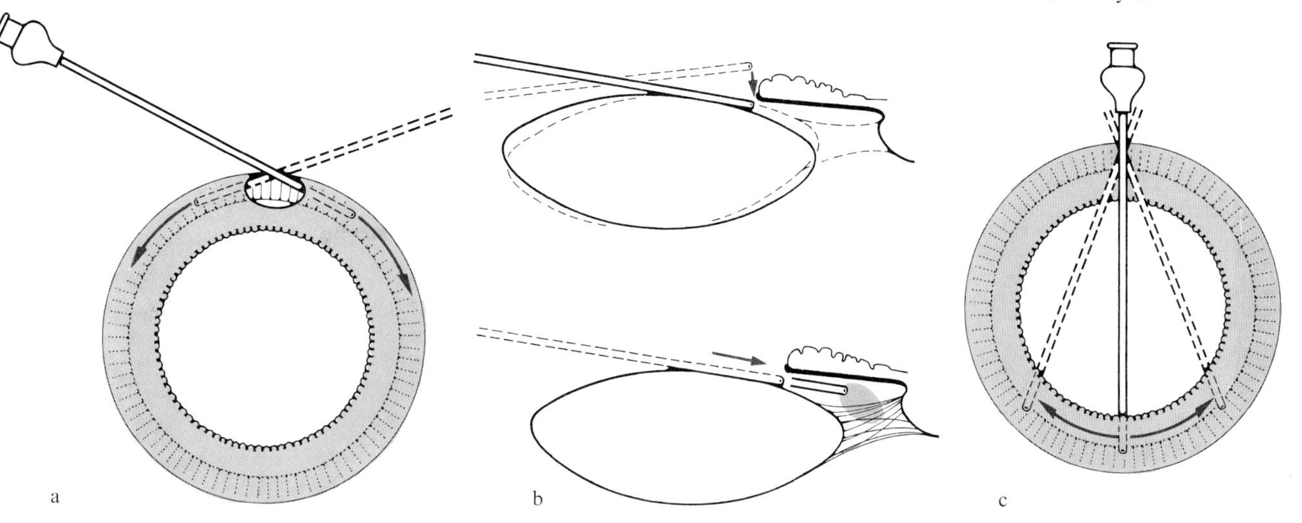

Fig. 310. **Application of zonulolytic enzyme**

a To apply the enzyme directly to the zonule, it is injected behind the iris. The upper circumference is accessible through a basal iridectomy.

b The lower circumference is reached by crossing the pupil. To avoid damaging the lens, the cannula is guided through the chamber without lens contact until the pupillary margin is reached. Only there is the cannula lowered and inserted beneath the iris. The end of the cannula now moves tangentially away from the anterior lens surface.

c The enzyme is distributed along the lower zonule by a pendular movement of the cannula

Chemical dissolution of the zonule with alpha-chymotrypsin [7] reduces the force needed during delivery to the small amount necessary for locomotion. However, a liquid enzyme is difficult to control both in terms of its desired action and side-effects.[8]

The enzyme dose can be reduced by combining chemical zonulolysis with mechanical zonulotomy. For example, alpha-chymotrypsin may be used only to produce the initial gap – the critical phase of the separation – while the remaining fibers are mechanically separated (parallel to vitreous surface).

The enzyme is applied as close as possible to the intended site of action (Fig. 310). On completion of zonulolysis (Fig. 311), residual enzyme and zonular debris are removed by irrigation of the anterior chamber. The lens is now *subluxated.*

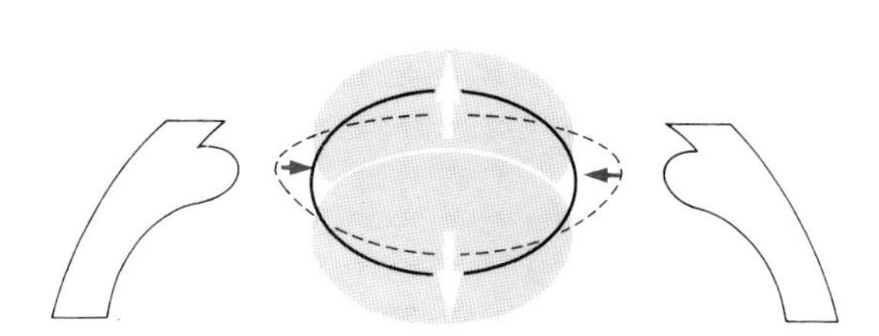

Fig. 311. **Signs of total zonulolysis.** Total zonulolysis is evidenced by the signs of absent lens suspension: The lens becomes more spherical *(red arrows)*; it moves somewhat outward if there is a slight overpressure in the vitreous, or sinks slightly inward from its own weight if the hyaloid membrane is relaxed *(white arrows)*

[7] Alpha-chymotrypsin is a proteolytic enzyme which dissolves the zonular fibers in concentrations of 1:5,000 to 1:10,000. In acts in 1–5 minutes at a temperature of 25–35° C, its time of action depending in part on whether the enzyme is cold or preheated when applied.

The enzyme is inactivated by acids and alkalis, serum and blood, DFP and chloramphenicol (can be used intraoperatively to inactivate the enzyme), detergents, disinfectants, alcohol (needles and cannulas must contain no residue from these substances and must be heat-sterilized), and temperatures above 40° C. The enzyme preparation can be sterilized only be filtration. No preservatives may be added. For this reason fresh solutions should always be used to lessen the danger of contamination.

[8] The major side-effect reported is a postoperative rise of intraocular tension. Also reported are damage to the cornea if the endothelium is injured, lesions of the hyaloid membrane, and retinal lesions if alpha-chymotrypsin enters the vitreous.

2.2 Locomotion

Displacements of the lens have effects on the vitreous chamber which must be taken into account when selecting the direction of motion. Motion vectors *perpendicular* to the vitreous chamber alter its volume and create a positive or negative pressure. On the other hand, motions about the *"vitreous center,"* the *center of curvature of the posterior lens surface* and the *sagittal lens axis* cause no volume changes (Fig. 312).

In **delivery by sliding** (Fig. 313), the pole of the lens nearest the opening (the superior pole) emerges from the chamber first. Additional zonular gaps besides the initial one are formed at other sites. This facilitates pressure equalization in *extraction,* but hinders tamponade in *expression* because a large area must be controlled.

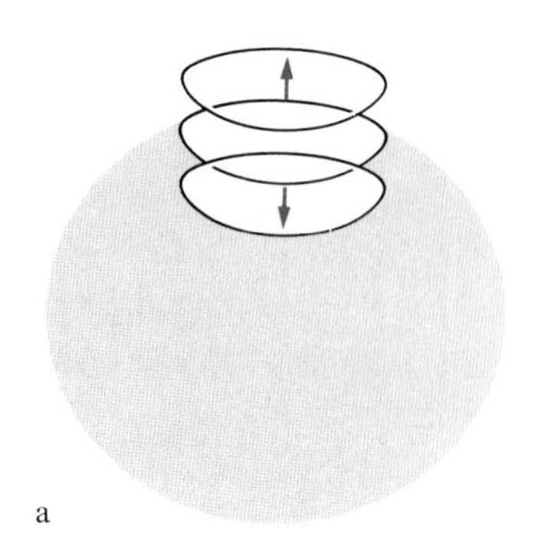

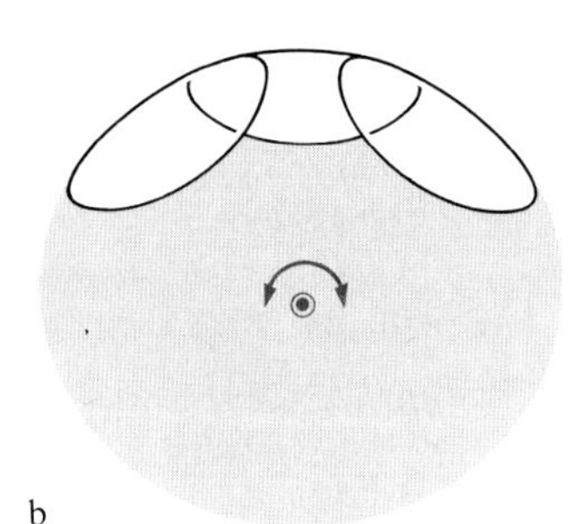

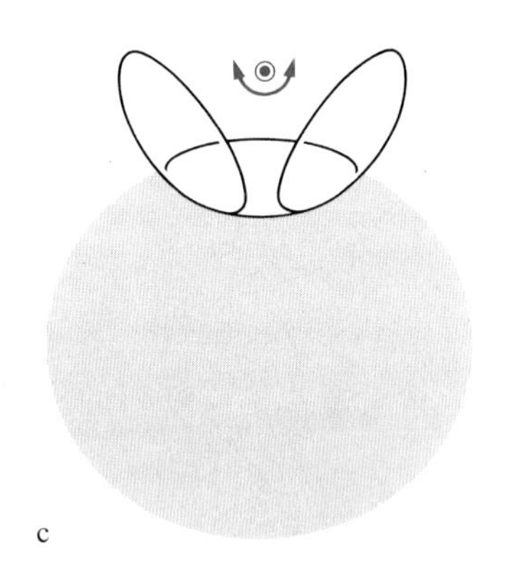

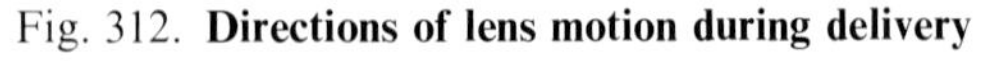

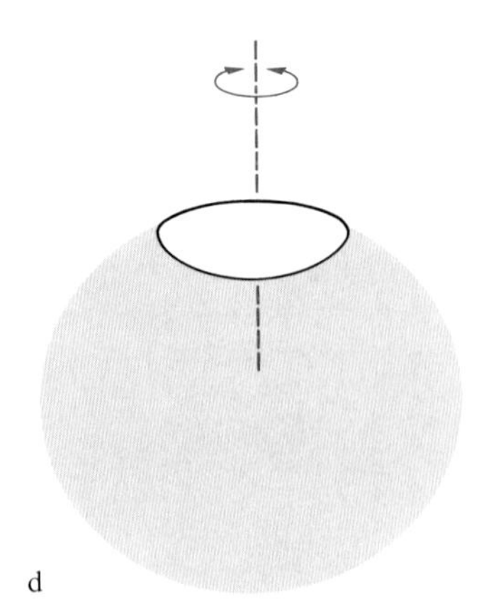

Fig. 312. **Directions of lens motion during delivery**

a Perpendicular (i.e., centrifugal and centripetal) vector components alter the volume of the vitreous body and thus create a positive or negative pressure.

b Movements along the vitreous surface cause shifts of vitreous substance but do not alter its volume.

c Movements about the center of curvature of the posterior lens surface alter neither the shape nor volume of the vitreous body.

d Rotational movements about the lens axis do not affect the shape or volume of the vitreous

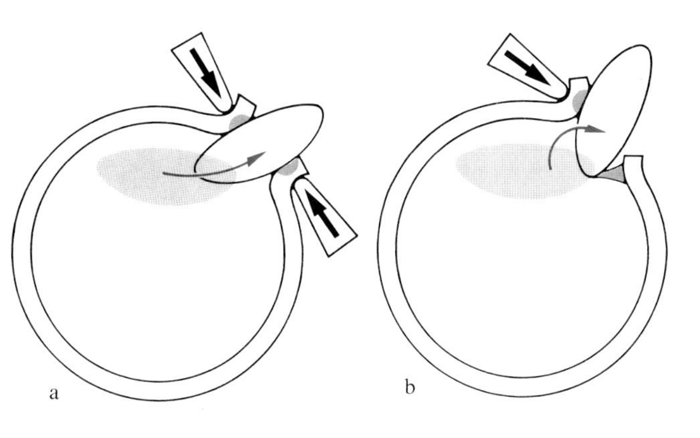

Fig. 313. **Lens orientation during delivery**

a Sliding: The superior pole of the lens passes first through the pupil and incision. Zonular gaps are present both on the side of the corneal opening and the opposite side. Therefore tamponade is difficult since it must involve both lips of the wound.

b Tumbling: The inferior pole of the lens emerges first. The initial gap is on the inferior side, and from this point separation of the zonule continues in the direction of the corneal opening. Tamponade is easier, since only one wound lip must be monitored

In **delivery by tumbling,** the opposite pole of the lens is first to emerge. Here only *one* gap is made in the zonule which can be tamponaded as soon as it forms. Various tumbling maneuvers are conceivable (Fig. 314). If the lens is rotated about its *superior* pole, the rotary movement contains a perpendicular component (Fig. 312a), and the lens presents its largest cross-section when passing through the pupil and incision. If the lens is tipped about an *intralenticular transverse axis,* some shifting of vitreous will occur. The more the lens deviates from a sphere, the greater the shift, and the greater the resistance to the rotary motion. If the lens is delivered by *reverse tumbling,*[9] the maneuver consists of two movements, neither of which significantly alters the vitreous volume; moreover, the lens can emerge in its smallest cross-section.

[9] The two separate movements about two different pivot points are comparable to the backing of an automobile.

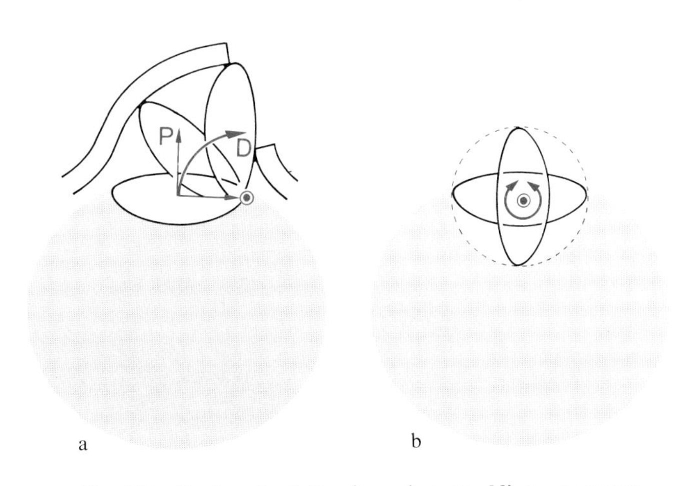

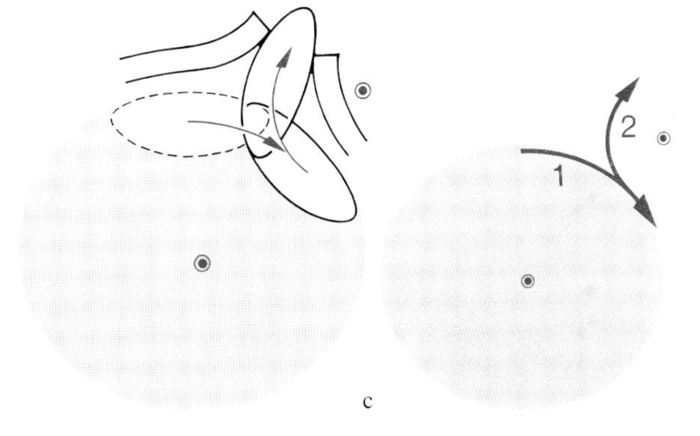

Fig. 314. **Center of rotation in various tumbling maneuvers**

a Tumbling the lens about an axis through its superior pole: The rotary movement *(D)* produces a vector component *(P)* perpendicular to the vitreous chamber. The lens presents its largest cross-section when traversing the pupillary and corneal openings.

b Rotation of the lens about its transverse axis. A spheroidal lens can be rotated in any direction, analogous to a spheroidal joint in a socket. The more the lens deviates from a sphere, however, the greater the shift of vitreous substance caused by its rotation.

c Reverse tumbling about extralenticular points. Tumbling in two phases: *1* Rotation of lens about the "center" of the vitreous body (analogous to Fig. 312b). *2* Rotation about the center of curvature of the posterior lens surface (analogous to Fig. 312c). The lens can be guided with its smallest cross-section through pupil and incision

2.3 Instruments for Lens Delivery

2.3.1 Expressors

The tension in the vitreous necessary for lens expression is created by an indentation formed in the wall of the eye with a blunt instrument *(expressor)* (Fig. 315). This may form a small indentation with relatively "sharp" properties or a broad bulge with tamponading properties, depending on the contact area.[10]

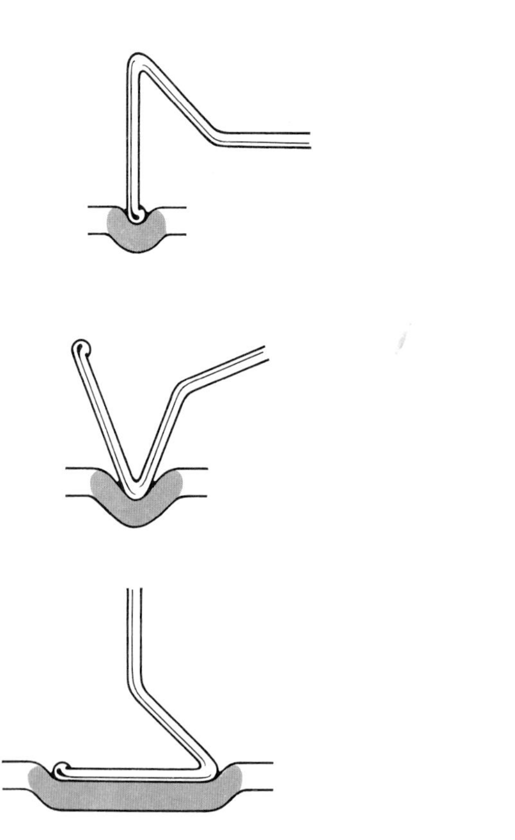

Fig. 315. **Expressors.** The scleral indentation *(pink)*, which actually is the "expressor," is always larger and blunter than the instrument which produces it. Many instruments offer the possibility of varying the area of contact and consequently the "sharpness" of the expressors (here: a squint hook)

2.3.2 Forceps for Grasping the Lens Capsule

Forceps grasp the lens by a *fold* made in the capsule (Fig. 316). To make this fold, the jaws of the forceps must be pressed so firmly against the capsule that the friction prevents slippage during closure of the blades. To prevent capsule lesions, the pressure of the jaws must be evenly distributed over the entire grasping surface.

2.3.3 Erysiphake

The erysiphake consists of a suction cup in which a *vacuum* is created which fixes the lens to the extraction instrument.

To spare the lens capsule, the cup is so constructed that the suction surface remains constant (Fig. 317). The anterior capsule partially prolapses into the cup, thereby making the entire capsule tense and, with it, the zonule.

Application of the instrument requires only minimal pressure, i.e., just enough so that the entire rim of the cup is in contact with the capsule.

2.3.4 Cryoextractors

Cryoextractors form an adhesion with the lens by means of an *ice ball* encompassing both the instrument and tissue. The fixation is optimal if the ice ball penetrates to the deeper part of the lens and thus does not tax the tensile strength of the capsule alone (Fig. 318b). Even if the capsule is damaged, complete extraction is possible if all edges of the lesion can be included in the ice mass (Fig. 318c).

The size and shape of the ice ball depend on the *shape* as well as *temperature* and *cold capacity* of the cryoextractor, and thus on instrument properties which are invariant in a given case. Its size also depends on the *thermal conductivity* of the various parts of the operative field, and thus on the fluid content in- and outside the lens.[11] Differences in thermal

[10] Formerly some surgeons even used their fingers as expressors, which allow fine control owing to the tactile sense.

[11] See Chapter I, 2.2.

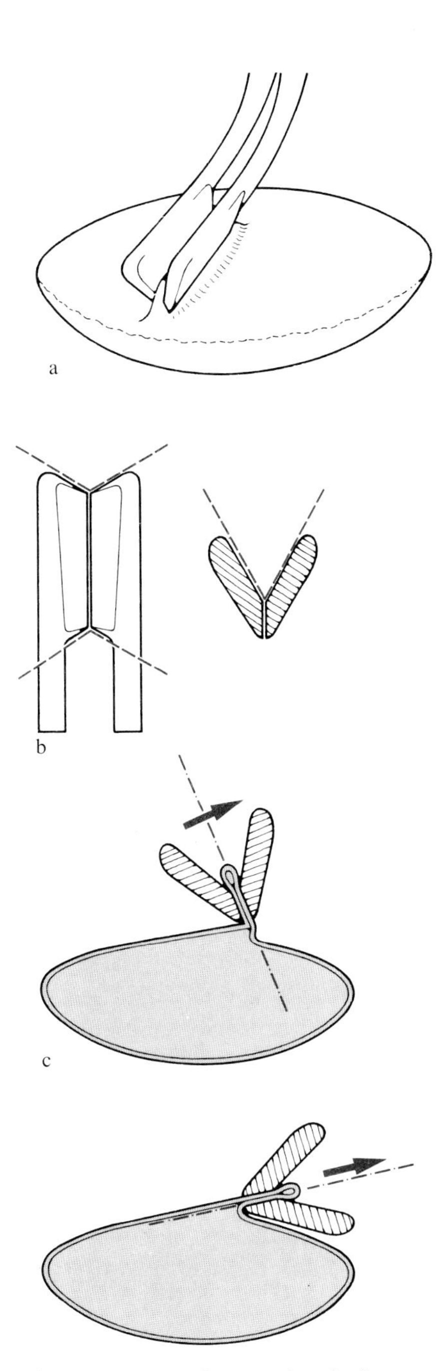

Fig. 316. **Forceps for grasping the lens capsule**

a The lens is grapsed by a fold in the capsule.

b Construction of jaws: To ensure a uniform pressure distribution over the entire grasping surface, the opposed surfaces must be flat and smooth, and their edges carefully rounded. When the blades are closed, the jaws must appose evenly for their full length (stabilization of grasping pressure, see Fig. 9). The jaws are designed to diverge where not in direct contact with the capsule in order to lessen the danger of including neighboring tissues in the grip (the iris, for example).

c Position of jaws during traction: If the fold is held in the direction of traction *(right)*, only the blunt grasping surfaces will act on the capsule, and not the edges. However, if the fold is perpendicular to the direction of traction *(left)*, one edge behaves as a sharp instrument, with possible lesion of the capsule

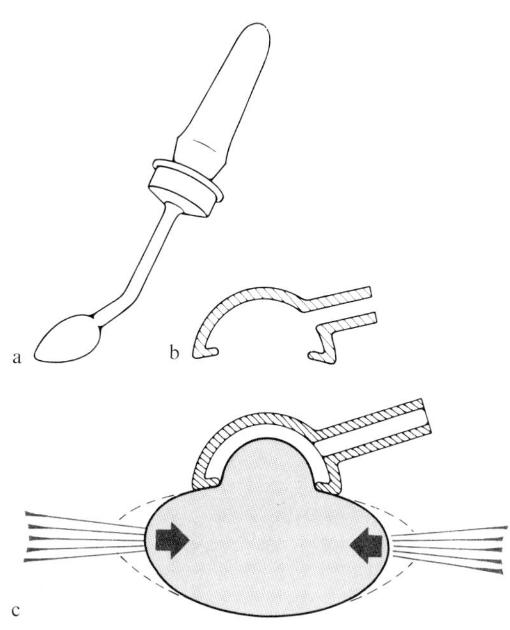

Fig. 317. **Erysiphake**

a Erysiphake with suction cup.

b Cross-section of suction cup. The rim is broad and shaped to conform to the lens surface so that it will not act as a cutting edge when suction is started; its edges are carefully rounded. The size of the cup is chosen so as to prevent contact of the lens capsule with the inside surface or vacuum tube (resulting in a reduction of suction surface).

c The suction leads to a general tensing of the zonular fibers

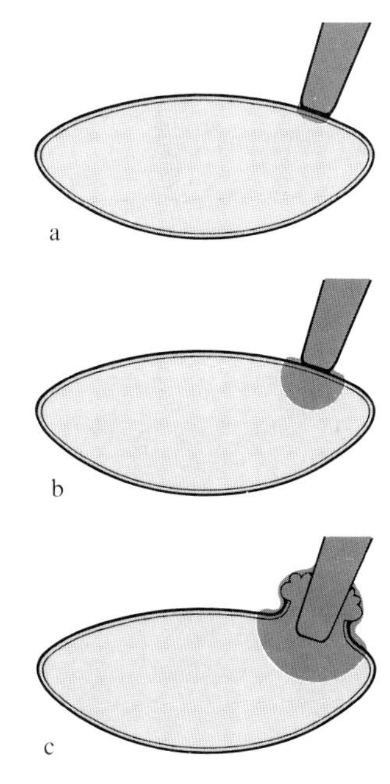

Fig. 318. **Cryoextractor**

a Superficial ice formation: includes only the capsule.

b Large ice ball: penetrates to the deeper part of the lens, encompasses the cortex and nucleus.

c Closure of a capsule lesion by a large ice ball

conductivity can even allow the freezing of a lens in a liquid film within the anterior chamber or in the fluid vitreous, since the ice ball forms more rapidly in a solid lens than in its liquid surroundings. On the other hand, if the lens contents are highly liquid (as in intumescent cataract), the ice ball forms only superficially in the dryer capsular tissue, and the cryoextractor only has grasping properties similar to a forceps (Fig. 318a).

2.3.5 Criteria for the Use of Extractors

The selection of an extraction instrument is based on such factors as its intrinsic volume, its contact area, and the lens deformation caused by the grasping mechanism (Table 3).

Table 3

	Forceps	Erysiphake	Cryo-extractor
Anterior chamber space required by instrument	small	very large	depends on quality of insulation (i.e. on danger of freezing of surrounding tissues)
Area of contact with lens	small	very large	depends on size of ice ball
Pressure on lens during grasping	high	low	very low
Deformation of lens during grasping	considerable	depends on extent of prolapse into suction cup	very slight

The **volume** of instrument that may be introduced into the anterior chamber depends upon the margin of deformation (depth of anterior chamber, vitreous pressure), for if the instrument is too bulky one has to press the lens inward, thereby *raising the pressure* in the vitreous chamber.

The **area of tissue contact** plays an important role with regard to the danger of *capsule rupture*. If the extractor behaves as a "sharp" instrument, it will tend to rupture the capsule rather than the zonule. The contact area further influences the *intrinsic mobility* of the lens. If the contact area is small ("point fixation"), the lens can adapt its position in response to all applied forces from the surgeon as well as from the zonule. If it is *large*, on the other hand, the surgeon's actions will have the predominant effect on the lens and are apt to be transmitted to surrounding structures.

The **pressure** which the instrument exerts on the lens during grasping also raises the vitreous pressure and must therefore be opposed by adequate resistance from the diaphragm. If the latter is damaged (e.g., subluxated lens), instruments with minimal grasping pressure must be used.

Deformation of the lens is possible only as long as the ratio of volume to surface area allows it. If the lens is practically spherical (as in intumescent cataract), any deformation leads to a generalized capsule tension which may proscribe the use of deforming instruments for grasping.[12]

2.4 The Phases of a Lens Delivery

Lens delivery is a continuous procedure in which various processes take place simultaneously and in succession. In broad terms, however, the delivery can be subdivided into four main phases according to the type of force applied:

1. *Application of the instruments*
2. *Formation of the initial gap in the zonule*
3. *Passage of the lens through the pupil and incision*
4. *Final phase.*

1. When the **instruments are applied,** the applied forces serve only to *engage the lens* with the delivery instrument. The amount of force applied thus depends on the type of instrument used (see Table 3).

[12] Forceps are then unable to produce a capsular fold (i.e., the lens can no longer be grasped) or will induce capsule rupture.

2. During **formation of the initial gap**, the applied forces serve to *initiate a rupture of the zonule*. Locomotion is employed only to the degree necessary to make the fibers tense. Since perpendicular forces are unavoidable in this phase (Fig. 309), great caution is warranted. If a zonulotome is thrust toward the vitreous to rupture the fibers, the pressure in the vitreous chamber will rise. On the other hand, if the lens is lifted and the zonule pulled past a stationary zonulotome, a negative pressure results which draws the hyaloid membrane back from the initial gap (Fig. 307b). The presence of a proper initial gap is essential for the next maneuver to proceed smoothly.

3. **Passage of the lens** through the pupil and incision represents the *main phase of the delivery*, for it is now that most locomotion occurs and most of the zonule is separated, and thus the *greatest force is applied*. It is important in this phase, therefore, that the relatively large forces be applied in safe directions, i.e., *parallel* to the vitreous face and not perpendicular. The nature of the force applied (pressure or traction) determines whether the developing zonular gaps must be tamponaded or left open.

4. The **final phase** begins as soon as the *largest lens cross-section* has traversed the corneal opening. At this point the lens will no longer sink back through the opening when the locomotive forces cease, and the delivery is practically complete. The forces can be reduced to the minimum required for separating the few remaining zonular fibers. This reduction of forces acting on the vitreous chamber is an important safety factor during the final phase, in which extensive zonular gaps are present.

2.5 Methods of Lens Delivery

We shall now discuss a few of the many delivery methods in context in order to show by *example* how the principles described can be combined.

2.5.1 Expression

In delivery by pure expression, as mentioned earlier, the vitreous chamber is deformed from the outside by expressors and the resulting pressure increase utilized to induce and control a prolapse (Fig. 319). The main problem is the danger of *undesired prolapses*.

The creation of the initial gap, which must be formed bluntly and thus with relatively large forces, is most successful if the lens is practically spherical. Such a lens can be rotated in any direction without altering the vitreous volume (see Fig. 314b), permitting extensive stretching of the zonule. A voluminous lens also leaves a large margin of deformation (Fig. 133c) after its removal, thereby reducing the risk of vitreous prolapse.[13]

An important advantage of pure expression technique is that *no instruments* need to be introduced into the anterior chamber. If this is the tactical goal, the risk of vitreous prolapse can be decreased by resorting to partial expression: The lens is expressed only until its superior pole appears in the wound. There the lens can be grasped with an extraction instrument[14] and finally delivered by a combined technique (expression and extraction).

2.5.2 Combined Extraction and Expression

If pressure as well as traction are employed during lens delivery, the most favorable "motor" can be selected in any given situation. *Traction* relieves stress on the vitreous body and is indicated if a *prolapse* threatens. *Pressure* relieves stress on the lens capsule and is employed if there is a danger of *capsule rupture*.[15] It is important to remember, however, that a rapid change in the type of force employed requires a correspondingly rapid ad-

[13] This suitability of spherical lenses for delivery by expression may explain why Smith's expression technique was so successful in India, but frequently failed elsewhere. The cataractous lenses of Indians are often large and spherical.

[14] If a cryoextractor is used to grasp the lens, care must be taken that the zonule is not frozen at its attachment.

[15] Impending capsule rupture is recognized by the formation of traction folds.

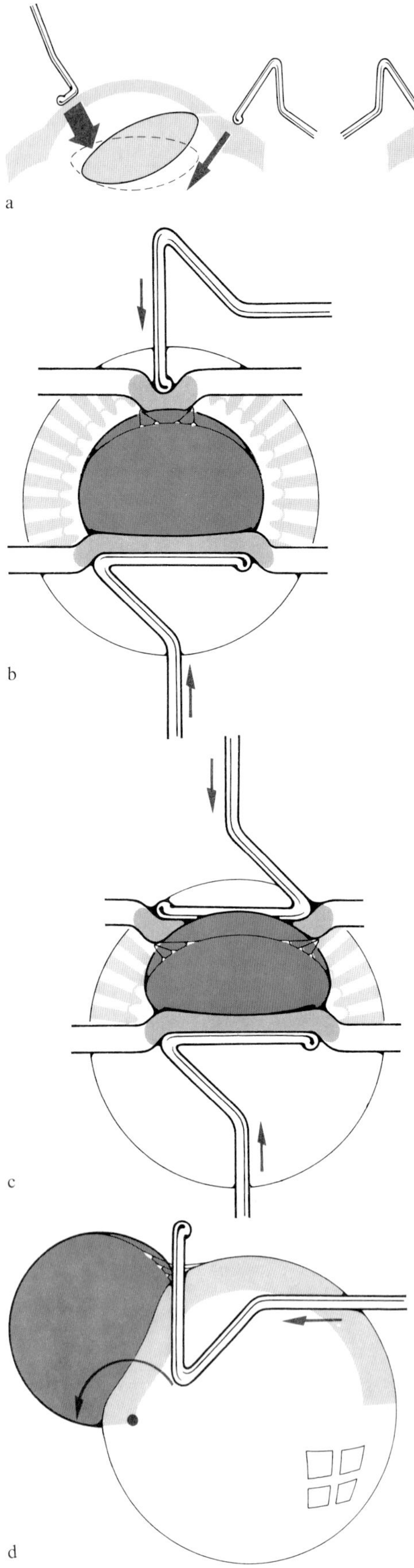

a

b

c

d

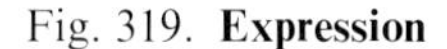

Fig. 319. **Expression**

a *Application of instruments* (*left:* sliding; *right:* tumbling). The position of the expressors determines which pole will be first to emerge: The expressor on the side of the leading pole is applied far enough from the lens border to permit its unrestrained movement (see Fig. 304). It acts as a zonulotome to make the initial gap and so is applied with its "sharpest" point. The opposite expressor is used to keep the lens from rising and is applied "bluntly" to avoid zonule rupture at that site.

b–c *Sliding*

b *Formation of initial gap.* The upper "sharp" expressor is pressed inward to rupture the zonule and simultaneously tamponade the resulting gap.

c *Passage of lens through pupil and incision.* Only when the leading pole is exposed (recognizable by its free edge), the pressure is increased to induce locomotion. Further separation of the zonule occurs as the lens slips past the upper expressor, which is now applied over a broader area to tamponade the expanding zonular gap.

d *Final phase.* All pressure on the vitreous is released as soon as the largest lens cross-section has passed through the corneal opening. The delivery is completed and the wound simultaneously closed by gentle stroking with the expressor. If the lens is wheeled out over the opposite wound edge, it will tamponade the corneal opening until the delivery is completed

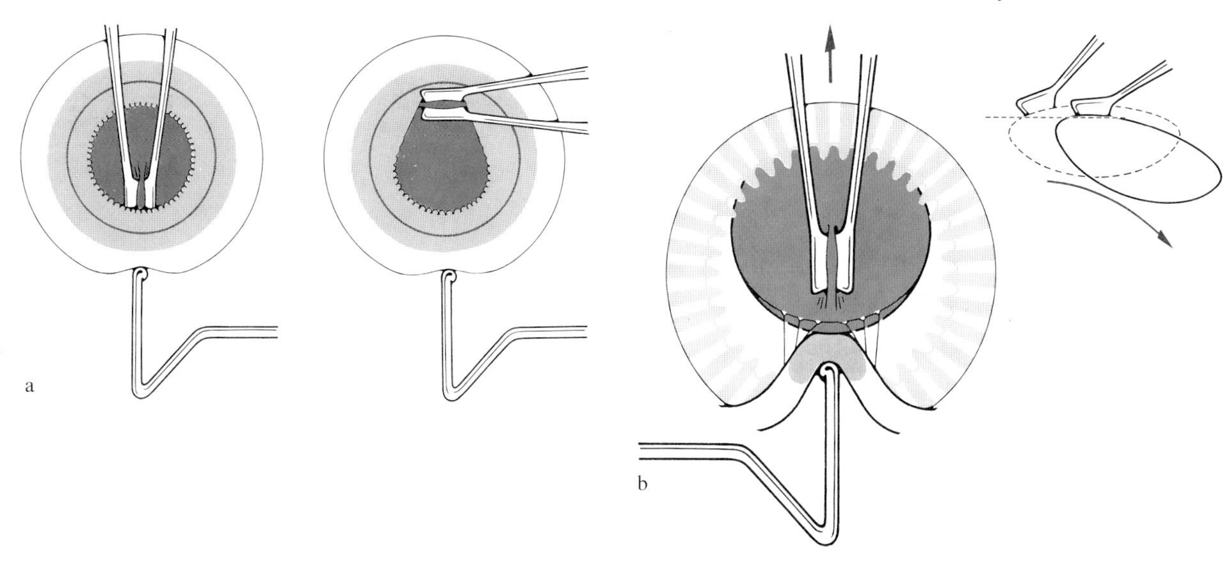

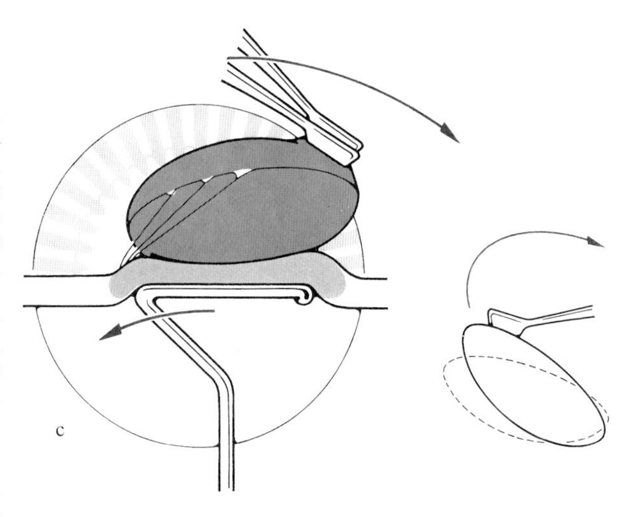

Fig. 320. **Combined expression and extraction (forceps)**

a *Application of instruments.* In delivery by *sliding (right)*, the forceps are applied transversely in the preequatorial zone (see Fig. 305), the iris being simultaneously pushed aside. In *tumbling (left)*, the forceps are passed closed beneath the iris to the preequatorial zone on the opposite side and then opened. The expressor is then used to raise the vitreous pressure until the lens is pressed against the forceps and a sufficient frictional resistance is created between the capsule and jaws. Then the forceps are closed. A grip on the capsule can be verified under difficult viewing conditions by the transmission of diaphragm tension to the forceps: The resistance to slight lateral movements of the forceps changes as the vitreous pressure is altered by the expressor.

b–c *Tumbling*

b *Formation of initial gap.* Traction on the forceps is straight toward the center of the pupil to make the zonule tense. If this traction is exactly *horizontal*, the first phase of the reversing maneuver has begun *(diagram at right)*. The expressor, applied as a zonulotome at its sharpest point, produces the initial gap and simultaneously tamponades it.

c *Passage of lens through pupil and incision.* The vitreous pressure is increased to initiate locomotion. The zonule is tensed by zig-zag movements (with gradually increasing amplitude, see Fig. 308c). Countermovements are made with the expressor to rupture the zonule (parallel to vitreous face, see Fig. 309c). Following separation of the zonule on the inferior circumference, the forceps are passed toward the corneal opening for the second phase of the reversing maneuver *(diagram at right)*. The expressor is applied with its broadest surface to tamponade the expanding zonule gap.

d *Final phase.* All pressure is released as soon as the largest lens cross-section has passed through the corneal opening. The lens is wheeled out over one edge of the wound. The wound is closed by tamponading with the expressor

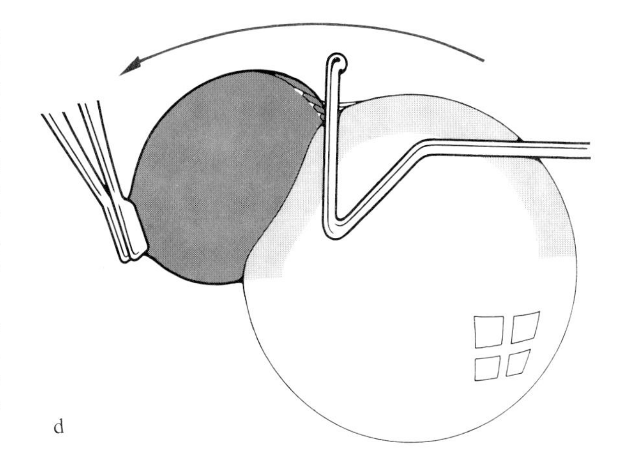

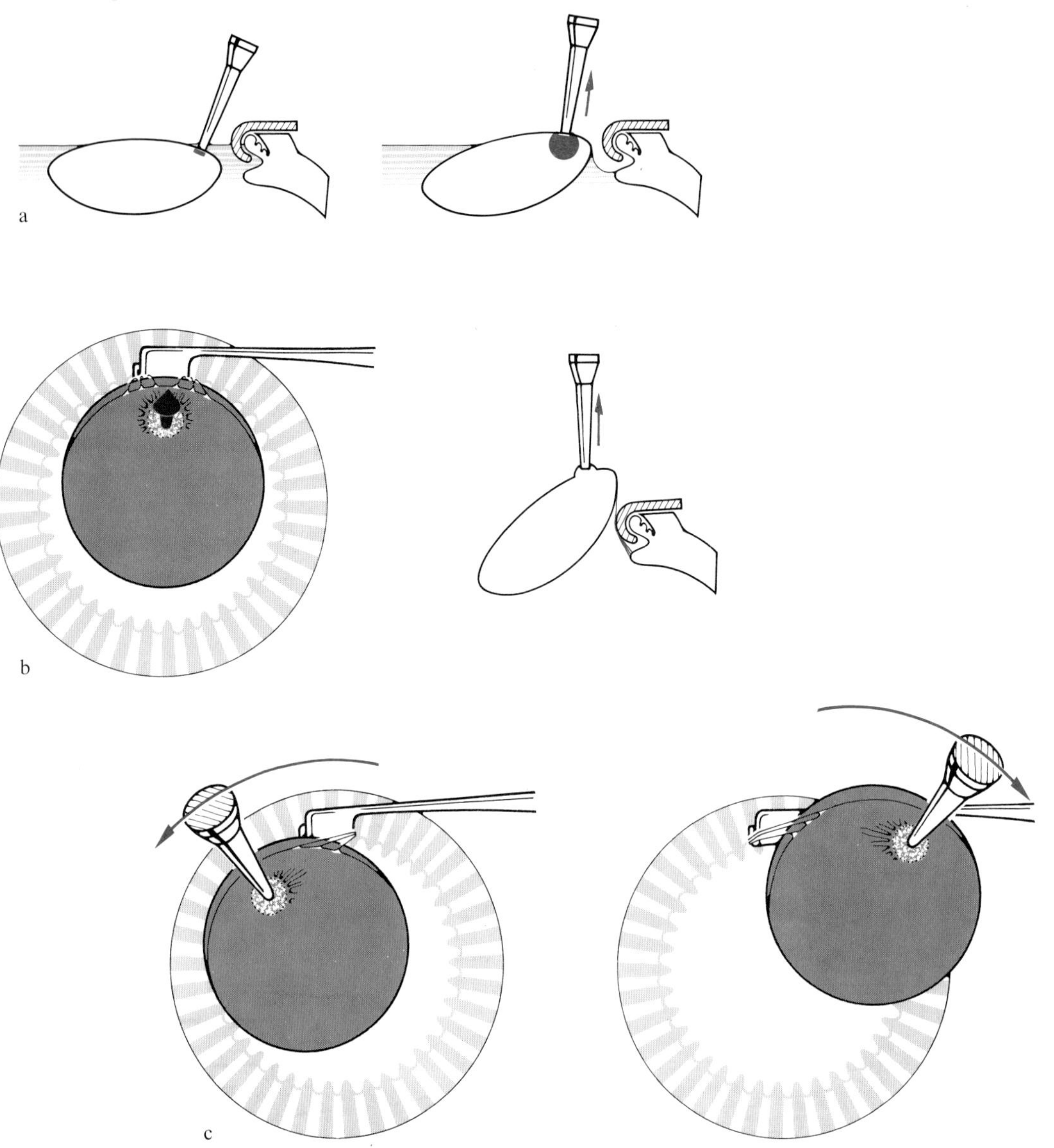

Fig. 321. **Extraction with cryoextractor**

a *Application of instruments.* The superior pole of the lens is exposed with an iris retractor. The cryoextractor is applied uncooled* *(left)*, is cooled, and the lens is immediately raised so as to remove the application site from the heat-conducting liquid layer *(right)*. The definitive ice ball is formed in the insulating air.

b *Formation of initial gap.* Upward traction brings the zonule in direct contact with the iris retractor, which acts as a "sharp zonulotome" to rupture the fibers.

c *Passage through pupil and cornea.* Traction is increased to initiate locomotion. At the same time, the rest of the zonule is separated by pulling the lens past the iris retractor in rotary motions (analogous to Fig. 309c).

d *Final phase.* The lens is wheeled out over one edge of the wound. Remaining zonular fibers are separated, and the wound is simultaneously closed with a blunt instrument (e.g., specially-shaped retractor handle)

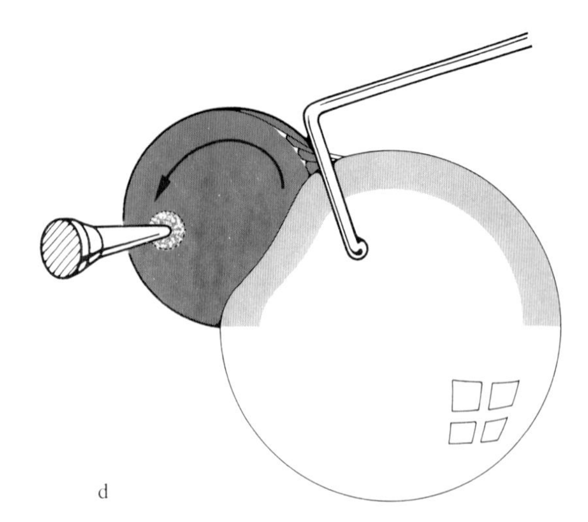

* See also Fig. 118

justment in the management of the resulting zonular gaps (see Figs. 306 and 307).

The accurate coordination of forces is aided if the lens can respond to them freely. This is facilitated by applying the grasping instruments in a *small area*, although this entails the risk of capsule rupture.

In delivery by *tumbling*, only a single zonule gap is created which is easily tamponaded; this facilitates expression. In delivery by *sliding*, on the other hand, several gaps are formed which are difficult to tamponade; this favors delivery primarily by traction.

Combined extraction and expression (Fig. 320) is in principle a controlled expression in which pressure serves as the principal motor while traction is used mainly for control.

2.5.3 Extraction

In delivery by pure extraction (Fig. 321), all applied forces are exerted on the lens capsule. The main problem in this technique, therefore, is to *relieve tension on the capsule* to prevent its rupture.

One means of accomplishing this is to use an extractor which is *applied over a large area* (possibly including the capsular contents) (see Table 3). Another means is to *reduce the force expended in zonule separation* (enzymatic zonulolysis, mechanical zonulotomy). If, despite such measures, signs of impending capsule rupture are observed (traction folds), the direction of traction is altered in an effort to relieve stress on the capsule by selective fiber tension (see also Fig. 339b).

The advantage of delivery by pure extraction is the absence of pressure on the vitreous chamber – a significant safeguard against the danger of undesired prolapse.

3 Extracapsular Cataract Extraction

Only the *contents of the capsular bag* are removed in extracapsular cataract extraction; the capsule itself remains a part of the diaphragm (Fig. 120b). In terms of operative technique, extracapsular extraction differs from intracapsular extraction mainly in that the part to be extracted is separated from the diaphragm in a separate step *(capsulotomy)* (Fig. 322) and not in combination with locomotion.

3.1 Capsulotomy

An *adequate anterior chamber depth* is essential for the use of sharp instruments. When **knives** are used (Fig. 323) which cut both the cornea and lens capsule, the chamber depth can be maintained by tamponading the opening with the shaft of the instrument itself. A *conical* shaft keeps the opening watertight only as long as the blade is advanced. A *cylindrical* shaft can seal the wound during withdrawal as well, provided its cross-section is equal to that of the blade (Fig. 323a). However, the shaft can effectively seal the wound only if the latter is not extended during *manipulations*. Thus, knives with two cutting edges are passed through the cornea precisely along their central axis (Fig. 324), while blades with only one cutting edge are directed along the blunt back of the knife (Fig. 325). During manipulations in the anterior chamber, moreover, care is taken that the center of rotation of blade movements lies at the entry puncture. If these conditions cannot be met, the anterior chamber must be maintained either by *irrigation systems* or by replacing the aqueous with viscous substances.

For *incision of the capsule*, the rules for the cutting of compliant, resilient tissue apply.

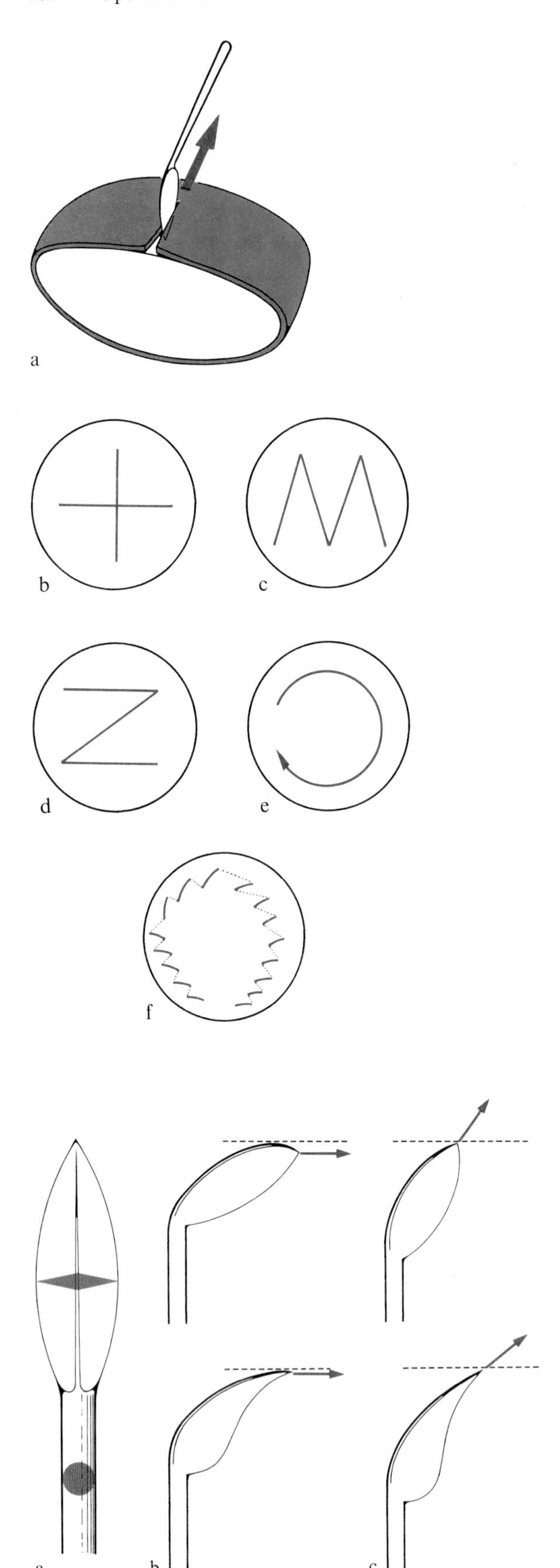

Fig. 322. **Opening the anterior lens capsule**

a Small knives produce a slit-shaped incision. Several incisions are required to open a surface. *Note:* To incise the capsule, a superficial cut is sufficient.

b–d Incisions for obtaining large surface openings by the retraction of flaps.

e Capsule opened by circular incision and removal of the excised piece.

f Excising a piece of the capsule in small steps ("can opener" technique)

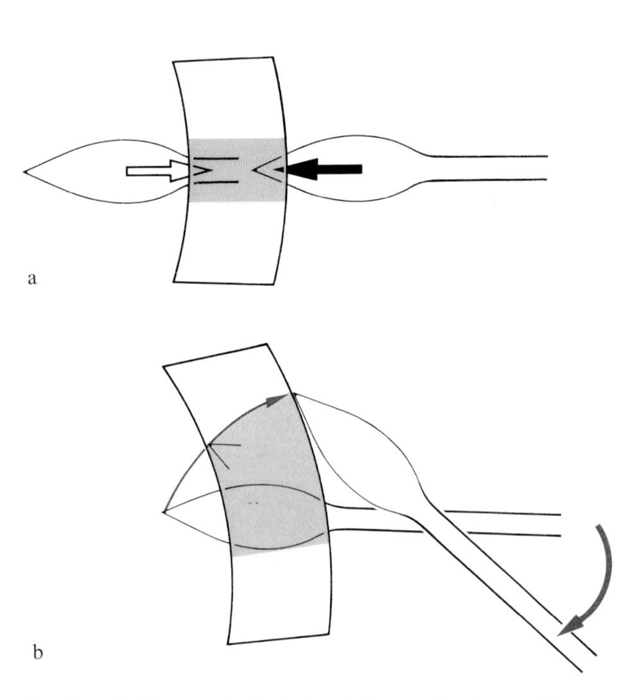

Fig. 324. **Guidance of discission knives with two cutting edges during keratotomy**

a The cross-section of the opening remains equal to that of the blade if the knife is guided precisely along its central axis through the tissue (forward and backward).

b Any slewing movement extends the corneal opening

Fig. 323. **Simple blades for opening the capsule**

a Discission knife with two cutting edges: The blade is an extremely narrow keratome and can cut both forward and laterally. It is "blunt" only during withdrawal. If the cross-sections of the blade and shaft are equal *(gray)*, the shaft can tamponade the corneal opening when moved forward or backward.

b, c Cutting blades with a blunt back. If no cutting parts are forward-directed *(left)*, the knives are blunt during forward and lateral movements and can be freely moved to and fro within the chamber; they are sharp only when moved backward. If the preferential path of the tip *(arrow)* is forward-directed *(right)*, the instruments are also sharp when advanced

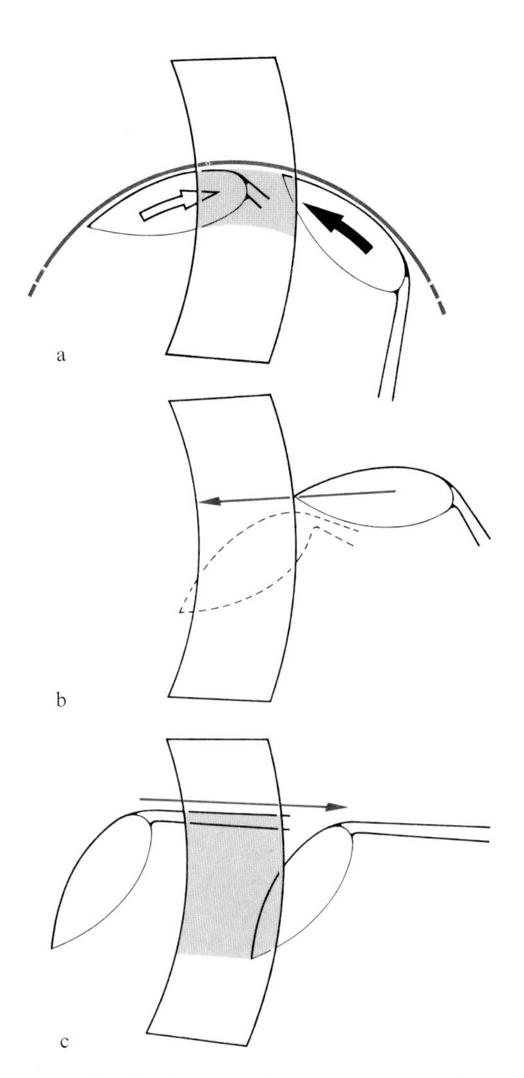

Fig. 325. **Guidance of discission knives with one cutting edge during keratotomy**

a The corneal opening is not extended if the blade is advanced and withdrawn along its blunt back. Note the oblique ("overcorrected") incidence angle during insertion.

b If the blade is advanced along its axis of symmetry (as in Fig. 324a), it is deflected along its back (see also Fig. 228). Any attempt to forcibly keep the blade on track will create a high resistance, and the blade will behave as a blunt instrument.

c If the blade is withdrawn in a straight path, the corneal opening is extended

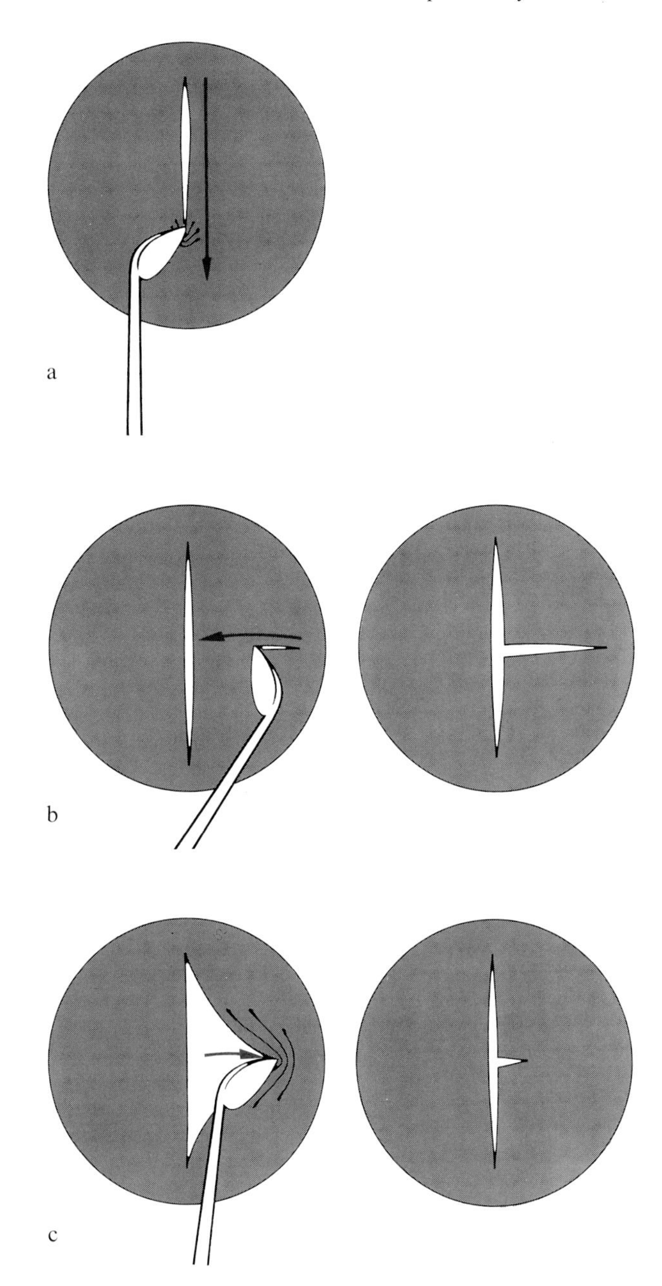

Fig. 326. **Shortening of capsular incision due to forward shifting tendency**

a The start of the incision is defined by the point of initial puncture. The end of the incision, however, cannot be predefined, since, the capsule shifts ahead of the cutting edge, and the resulting cut is shorter than the distance travelled by the blade.

b If the second incision is begun in the periphery and extended toward the first incision *(left)*, the length of the incision is determined by the point of insertion *(right)*.

c If the second incision is made from the original incision toward the periphery *(left)*, the capsule is already flaccid and will be displaced by the blade. The resulting incision is shorter than the amplitude of the guidance movement *(right)*

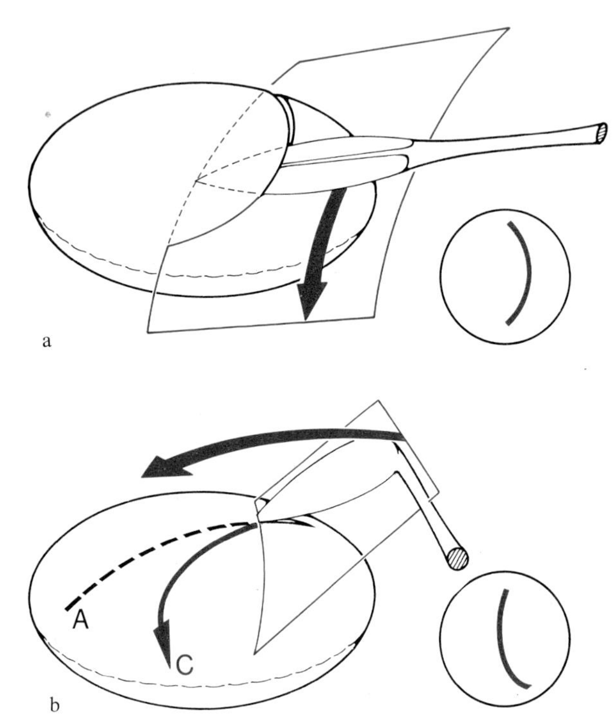

Fig. 327. **Deviation of incision during cutting by slewing movement**

a If the preferential path of the blade coincides with the guidance direction (slewing movement), the incision will be symmetric with respect to the slew axis.

b If the preferential path is at an angle to the guidance direction *(A)*, the incision will deviate *(C)* increasingly (in this example: toward the point of the corneal incision) (see also Fig. 37)

The shifting tendencies are most pronounced in soft cataracts, since the capsule tension decreases here as soon as it is incised. The shifting tendencies can be reduced to some extent through insufflation of air into the anterior chamber, thus exploiting the surface tension of the air bubble to stabilize the capsule. Nevertheless, the tissue will still tend to shift ahead of a blade (see Figs. 37, 39 and 40), making it difficult to produce carefully preplanned incisions, particularly since the possibilities for compensatory guidance movements are limited.

Forward shifting of the tissues shortens the length of the incision, particularly if capsule tension is low. Only the starting point of the incision can be accurately defined; its endpoint is indeterminate (Fig. 326). *Lateral shifting* becomes an important factor if the preferential path of the blade does not coincide with its guidance path, as during slewing movements of the blade (Fig. 327). Since lateral shifting is dependent on lateral resistance, it can be reduced by passing the blade *superficially* through the lens and utilizing it more or less as a "point" cutting edge.

Cystitomes (Fig. 328) are specifically designed to cut "at a point." They are blunt every-

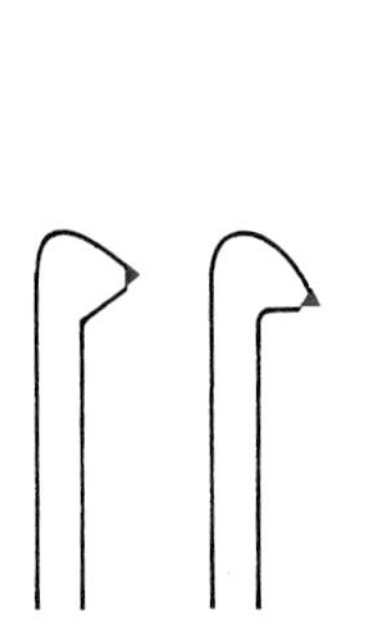

Fig. 328. **Cystitomes.** Cystitomes are blunt everywhere except at the tip and can therefore be used even in a shallow anterior chamber. *Left:* Cystitome which offers equal resistance in all directions. *Right:* Cystitome which is sharp mainly when pulled backward

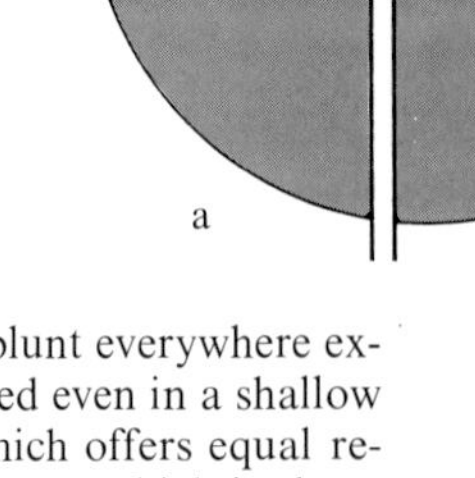

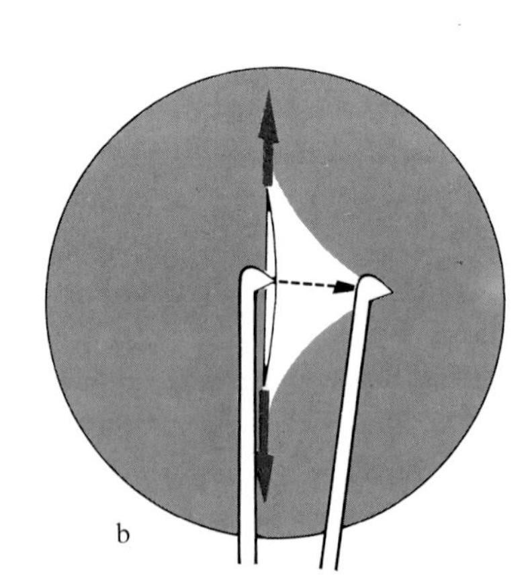

Fig. 329. **Tearing with cystitomes.** If a cystitome tears open the capsule instead of cutting it, the direction in which the tear propagates does not necessarily equal the guidance direction, but depends on local capsule tension.

a When the cystitome is pulled back from its entry puncture, the tear spreads at right angles to the guidance direction of the instrument.

b In the attempt to make a second, perpendicular incision from an initial one (analogous to Fig. 326c), it is merely the initial incision which is lengthened

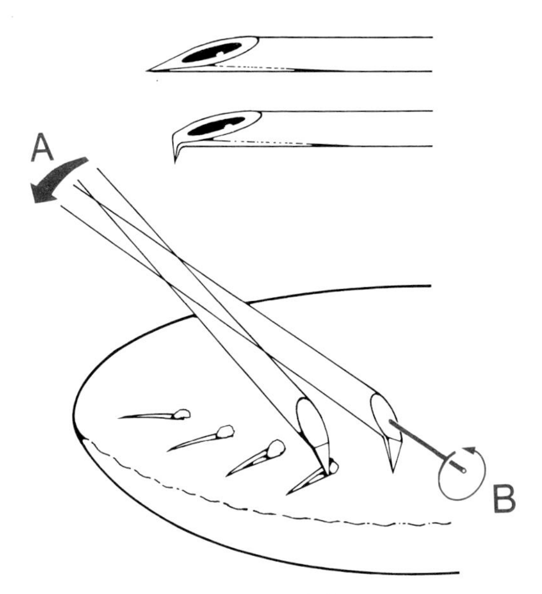

Fig. 330. **Small-step discission ("can opener" technique).** The effects of deviations of the cut (Figs. 326 and 327) can be minimized by tearing the capsule in repeated small steps. In this example a bent injection cannula is used *(above)*. The capsule is perforated by small incisions along the planned discission line. It is then ruptured similarly to a postage stamp.

Note: The working motion (incision) is a simple rotation about the axis of the cannula *(B)* and can be made independent of the guidance motion (moving the cannula to a new incision site *A*)

where except at their short cutting tip. Since they cannot themselves open the anterior chamber, a different instrument must be used for that purpose.[16]

When a sharp cystitome is used to incise the capsule, the shape of the incision will equal the guidance direction only if the instrument is guided superficially. Otherwise it will lose its sharpness at the capsule and tear rather than cut it.[17] The shape of the resulting tear then depends on the tissue resistance, and thus on capsule tension, and does not necessarily coincide with the guidance direction of the cystitome (Fig. 329).

Due to the tendency of the cut to deviate from the intended path, it is difficult to make accurate capsule incisions with knives (Fig. 327) or cystitomes (Fig. 329). However, since the amount of deviation depends on the distance travelled by the blade it is possible to approximate a preplanned shape by making the incision in several small steps ("*can-opener technique*," Fig. 330).

When **forceps** are used for the capsulotomy, the capsule is ruptured and a piece removed all in one step (Fig. 331). The *area of the extraction* is determined by the forceps blade spacing, which is in turn limited by the *width of the corneal opening*. To avoid lesions of other structures by the sharp teeth, the forceps is always closed when moved through the anterior chamber and is opened only when in contact with the capsule. After closure, the forceps is not withdrawn until the surgeon has made sure the piece of capsule is completely separated all around (danger of unintentional luxation of the lens).

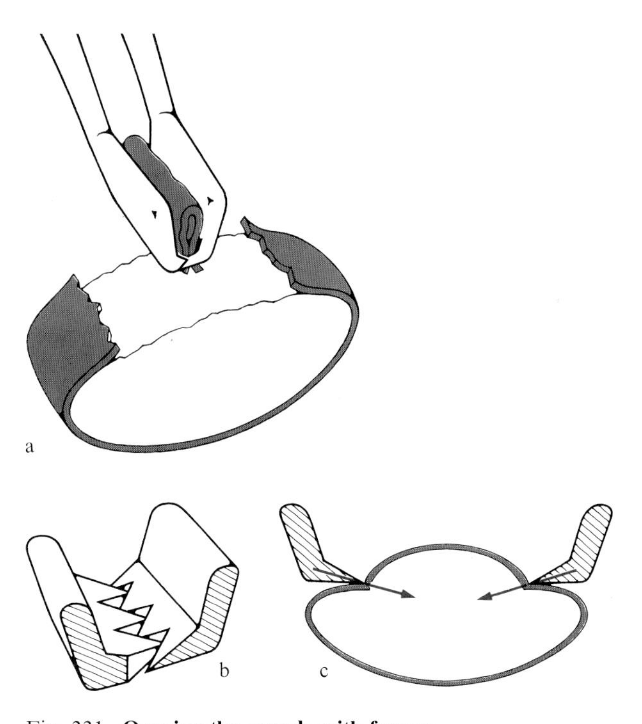

Fig. 331. **Opening the capsula with forceps**

a The forceps tears out the tissue included in its grip and removes it from the eye.

b When closed, the jaws are smooth externally and can be moved about safely within the anterior chamber.

c For grasping, the sharp teeth are pressed into the lens so that their preferential paths *(arrows)* are nearly perpendicular to the capsule surface

[16] This means that the anterior chamber may be flat when the cystitome is used. It is essential, therefore, that only the tip of the instrument (which is turned toward the lens capsule) is sharp; the rest must be blunt (tested by feel).

[17] If the cystitome is passed so deeply that it catches the nucleus, it will dislocate it.

3.2 Locomotion in Extracapsular Extraction

Only a small force is required for locomotion of the capsular contents because, unlike intracapsular extraction, no sectioning of the diaphragm is involved. On the other hand, control is difficult because the contents include irregularly-shaped particles which easily become lodged in surrounding structures (Fig. 332).

The most important *incarceration site* is the equatorial intercapsular sinus beneath the pupillary margin[18] (Fig. 333); particles can be removed from this space only if it is kept open.

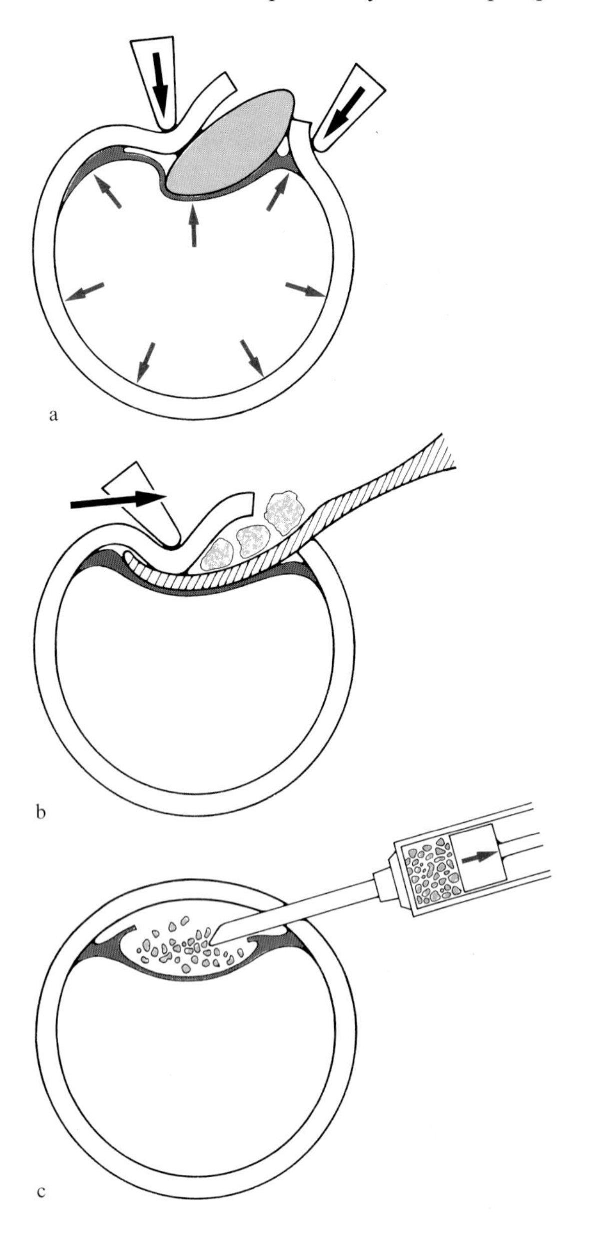

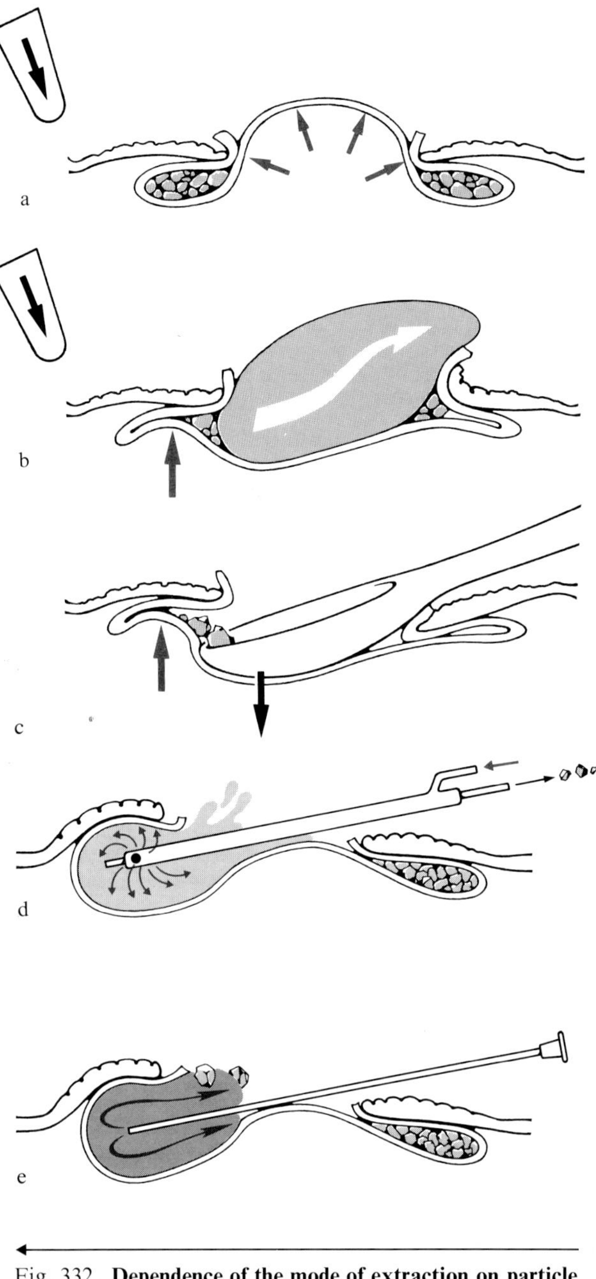

Fig. 332. **Dependence of the mode of extraction on particle size**

a A compact nucleus can be expressed with the aid of the protruding diaphragm. As in intracapsular expression, the expressors create the motor by raising the vitreous pressure.

b Small particles are pushed out of the eye over a smooth surface (a spoon, for example). This is not an expression maneuver. The spatula used to expel the lens material is not used as an expressor and is not pressed centripetally toward the spoon, but is directed horizontally *(arrow)*.

c If the particles are small enough to pass through the lumen of a cannula, they can be aspirated. The motor here is a vacuum

[18] Another incarceration site is the *basal iridectomy*, which for this reason is frequently made only upon completion of the delivery maneuver.

Fig. 333. **Incarceration of lens particles at the intercapsular sinus**

a In the attempt to remove small lens particles in an expression maneuver, i.e., by increasing the vitreous pressure, the diaphragm protrudes and traps lens material lying within the space between the peripheral anterior and posterior capsule at the pupillary margin.

b If a sufficiently large nucleus is present, it can prevent contact between the anterior and posterior capsule at the pupillary margin. Peripheral lens material can be massaged up against the nucleus and expressed along with it.

c Clearing the pupillary passage with a spoon. By depressing a spoon passed below the pupillary margin, the pressure on the vitreous chamber is increased, the posterior capsule is raised, and the material present there is pushed out onto the spoon.

d The opening of the equatorial intercapsular sinus with an irrigation-aspiration tip. The force for lifting the remnants of the anterior from the posterior capsule is produced by the stream of the injected liquid.

e Use of viscous material for opening the equatorial intercapsular sinus. The injected material keeps the space open through its ductility and brings the particles there afloat

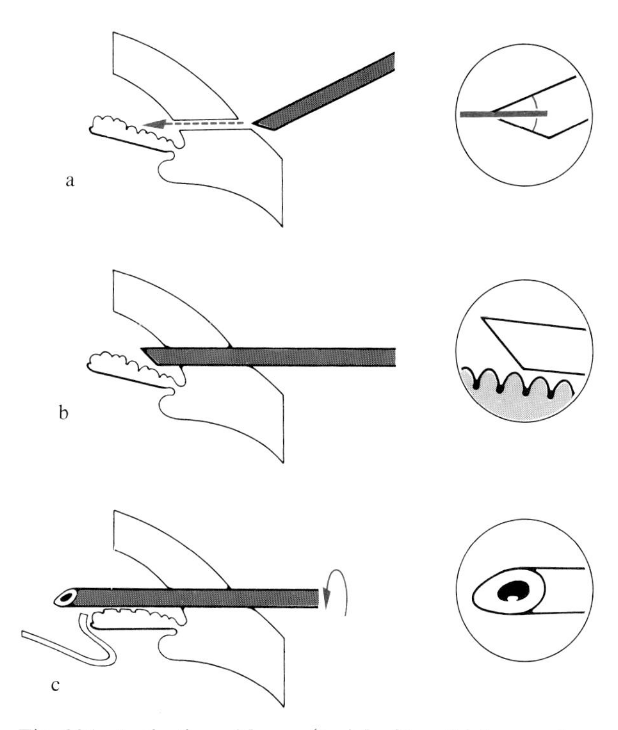

Fig. 334. **Aspiration of lens material with a thick cannula**

a The blunt cannula is inserted into the wound. The insertion direction with the least resistance is given by the bisector of the cannula tip (not by the direction of the cannula axis!).

b Guiding the cannula in the anterior chamber. The cannula glides smoothly over the iris surface if its blunt side is turned toward it (i.e., tip upward).

c During aspiration, the cannula tip is turned to the side to prevent injury to the inner corneal surface and posterior lens capsule. The opening faces slightly upward so that the aspiration process can be easily watched

If a **large nucleus** is present, it can be utilized to keep a passage clear for the smaller particles.

An artificial, rigid guide, such as a *spoon*, can also be used to prevent the incarceration of **small lens fragments** by the mobile diaphragm. In this technique the delivery is nearly independent of vitreous pressure. The pressure in the vitreous chamber is only raised in the initial phase to load the material into the spoon. Thereafter the applied forces serve merely to transport the lens particles over the spoon to the outside. If for this purpose a spatula is applied to the cornea, it is not moved concurrently with the spoon lest endothelial lesions result. *Liquids* can be injected

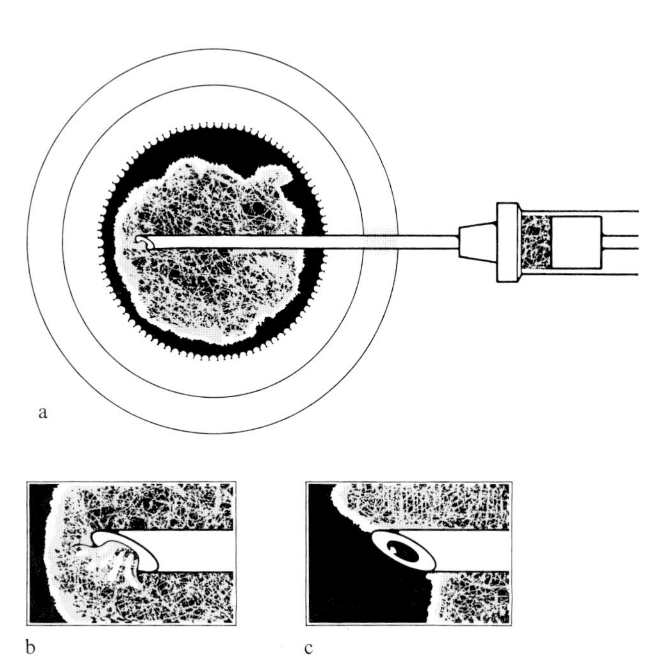

Fig. 335. **Control of the aspiration maneuver**

a The material lying directly before the cannular opening is aspirated, that with the lowest resistance being aspirated first.

b If only lens particles lie before the opening, only they are aspirated.

c Danger: If liquid material lies before the opening (aqueous fluid, vitreous fluid), this is aspirated first while the solid lens particles are left behind. As soon as the pupil appears black (or pure red in coaxial illumination) in front of the cannular opening the vitreous is threatened. The cannula must then be relocated to an area which still contains gray material (restoring the situation in **b**) to open the sinus while the particles are removed by flushing.

Cannulas are used to aspirate particles which are small enough to pass through the lumen (Figs. 332c, 334). Control of this maneuver aims to selectively aspirate the lens particles only and requires careful monitoring of the cannula opening (Fig. 335). The larger the *lumen*, the smaller the resistance to the lens particles, the lower the necessary aspiration pressure, and the simpler the control. With small cannula diameters, greater care must be taken due to the higher aspiration pressure and greater risk of inadvertant lesions.

Removal of particles by flush irrigation is described in Chap. VIII (Fig. 343).

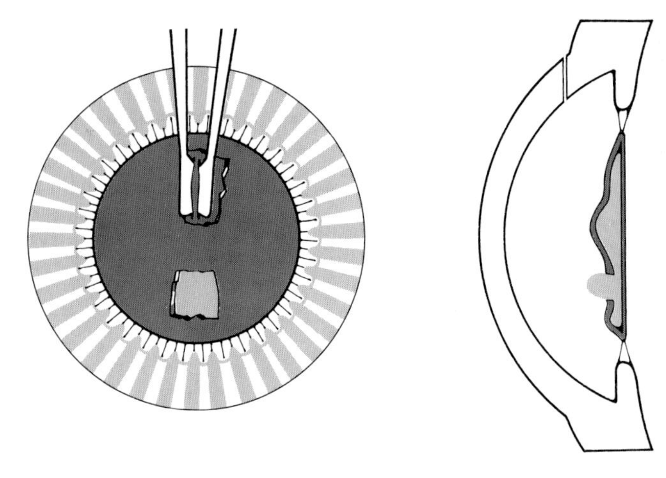

Fig. 337. **Rupture of the capsule on grasping.** The rupture lies at the site of extractor (here: forceps) application. The capsule is still made tense by the intact zonule

3.3 Extraction of the Capsule

If an extracapsular extraction is planned, the object of the operation is to leave the posterior capsule in the eye. However, if *rupture of the capsule* occurs during a planned intracapsular extraction – and one adheres to the original

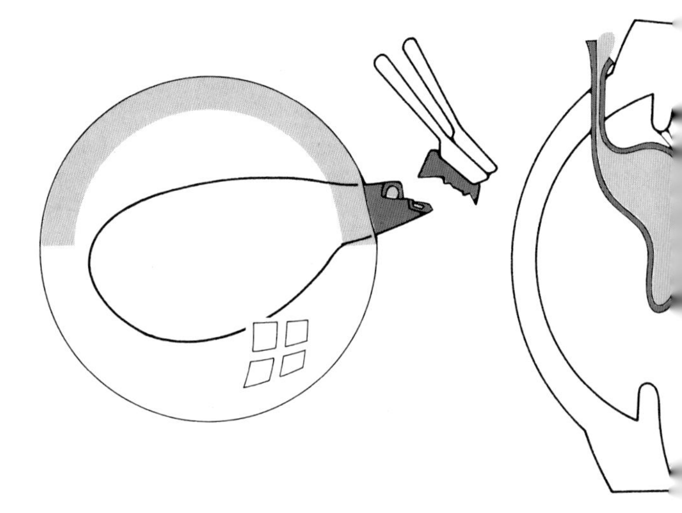

Fig. 338. **Rupture of the capsule on extraction.** If the capsule ruptures during the course of extraction, part of the capsule is already between the wound lips. The zonule is partially separated

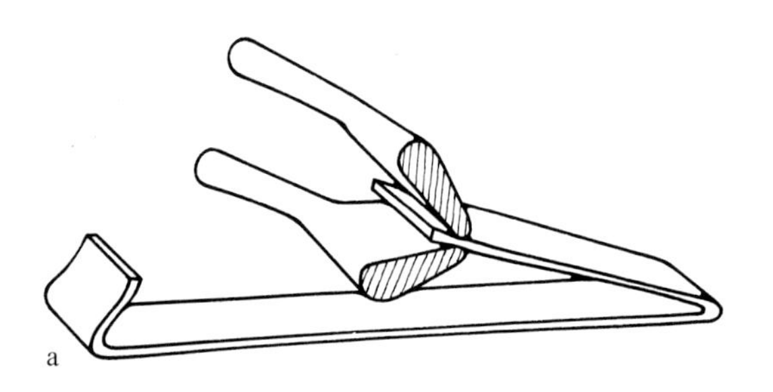

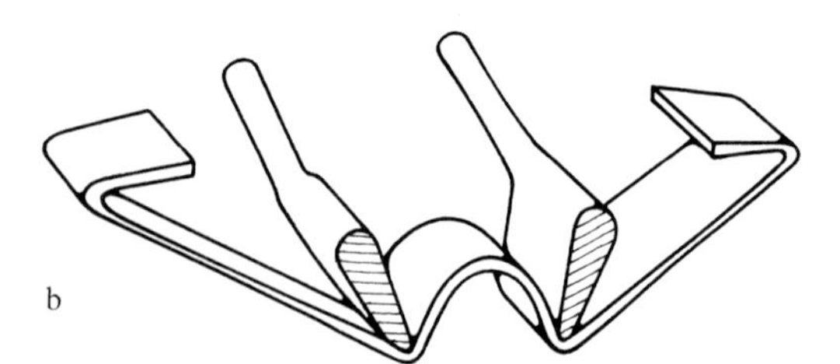

Fig. 336. **Grasping the capsule (here: with capsule forceps)**

a The edge of the capsule is grasped at the site of rupture. *Note:* The forceps is held at an angle.

b If the forceps were applied vertically, as is customary when grasping an intact lens (see Fig. 316a), it could grasp only by producing a fold. But this could result in rupture of the posterior capsule or incarceration of vitreous

operating plan – it becomes necessary to extract the capsule in a separate maneuver.

In *grasping the capsule*, first the *free capsule edges* are identified and then brought between the jaws of the forceps (Fig. 336). If the capsule is ruptured at the *start of the delivery* (Fig. 337), the lesion lies at the application site of the grasping instrument. Damaged capsule remnants can be recognized by their motion during irrigation of the anterior chamber. If the capsule ruptures in the *final phase* of the delivery (Fig. 338), capsule remnants are accessible at the lip of the wound. The zonule is partially separated by then and offers little resistance.

During **extraction of the capsule**, no generalized tension can be produced since the capsular bag is destroyed, and so forces are no longer transmitted to the entire zonule (see p. 153). Thus, the zonular fibers are tensed only if the forceps is applied *close to their insertion*. Since the distance between the forceps and remaining intact fibers increases as the extraction proceeds, the forceps must be continuously reapplied closer to the fibers to be separated *(taking alternate grips with two pairs of forceps)*. The applied forces are optimally utilized by employing selective fiber tension (Fig. 339).

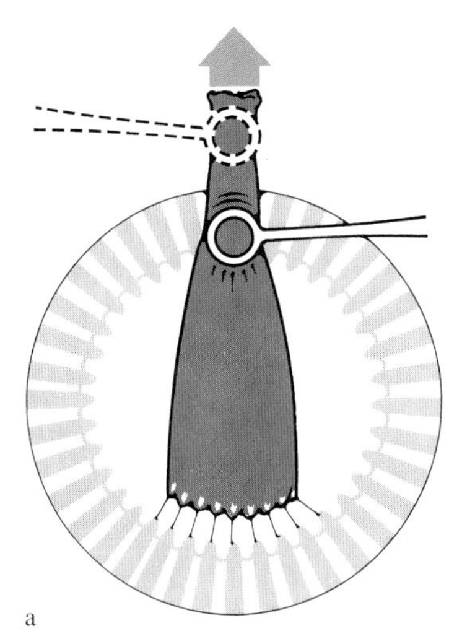

a

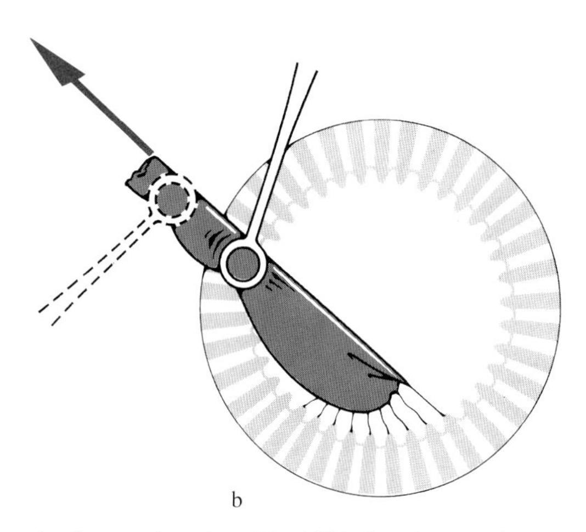

b

Fig. 339. **Extraction of the capsule (here: with ring forceps)**

a If the capsule is pulled in a direction parallel to the normal course of the zonular fibers, a diffuse tension is exerted. On each fiber it is relatively low compared with the force applied.

b By selective tension (see Fig. 32b), i.e., by traction at a large angle to the anatomic fiber direction, maximum tension is exerted on those fibers which are to be separated, while all other fibers are relaxed.

Note: The capsule is extracted by taking alternate grips with two pairs of forceps in a "hand-over-hand" manner

VIII Space-Tactical Procedures

1 General

Spatial strategy and tactics play an important role in eye surgery, since the globe mainly contains "empty" spaces which are filled with fluid and communicate which each other through circulatory orifices (Fig. 340).

Spatial **strategy** is aimed at final goals, is part of the general therapeutic plan and is taken into the account in the design of all surgical methods.[1] Spatial **tactics,** on the other hand, deal with intercurrent short-term goals related to a momentary situation during a surgical act. Tactical measures may be contrary to the strategic goal.[2] In such a case they must be discontinued at the end of surgery in order to restore all spaces and orifices in accordance with the strategic goal.

The principal tactical goal is the maintenance of spaces in spite of surgically produced openings. This requires that a **pressure** be created there which is higher than the pressure within adjoining structures. Thus, the pressure level which *must* be attained depends on the ambient counterpressure. The pressure which *can* be attained depends on the relation between the volume of inflow and the resistance to outflow.

The **outflow resistance** is determined by the geometry of the outflow opening (i.e. its length and cross-section) and by the viscosity (i.e. internal friction) of the fluid material.[3]

The *anterior chamber*, for example, is maintained or restored by producing an adequate counter-pressure to the vitreous pressure (see Fig. 124a). The *vitreous space* is maintained by a counterpressure to the elastic contractile forces of the adjoining tissues, to the pressure within the subchorioidal space,[4] or to the pressure of the orbita. The outflow resistance in both spaces is localized at the surgical wound. It can be increased by changing *geometric factors*, i.e. by selecting a suitable shape of the incision (see chapter V, 2.2), by the proper manipulation of injection cannulas (Fig. 341) and by partial or complete closure with sutures.

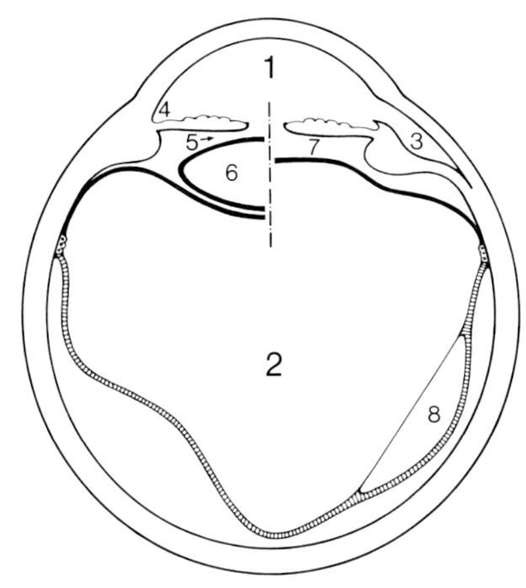

Fig. 340. Space-tactical goals in the intraocular chambers and their subcompartments

Space	Clinical indication for creation, maintenance or enlargement of the space
Whole chambers	
1. Anterior chamber	protection of deep portions during corneal incisions protection of corneal endothelium during complicated maneuvers at the iris-lens diaphragm
2. Vitreous chamber	smoothing of plicated retina
Subcompartements	
3. Subchoroidal space	maintaining patency of cyclodialytic opening
4. Chamber angle	separation or prevention of anterior synechiae
5. Iridocapsular space	protection of lens during suturing of iris
6. Intercapsular sinus	flushing of cortical masses; insertion of implants
7. Iridohyaloid space	insertion of implants; protection of anterior hyaloid during suturing of iris in aphakic eye
8. Retinovitreal interstices	facilitating vitrectomy of preretinal membranes by increasing distance from retina

[1] For example: Routine iridectomies in surgery of the anterior segment.

[2] For example: Blockade of circulatory openings to prevent the spread of fluid (blood, vitreous) during a surgical act will lead to glaucoma in the postoperative period if not removed at the end of surgery.

[3] Poiseuilles law.

[4] For example: Retrochorioidal hemorrhage ("expulsive" hemorrhage).

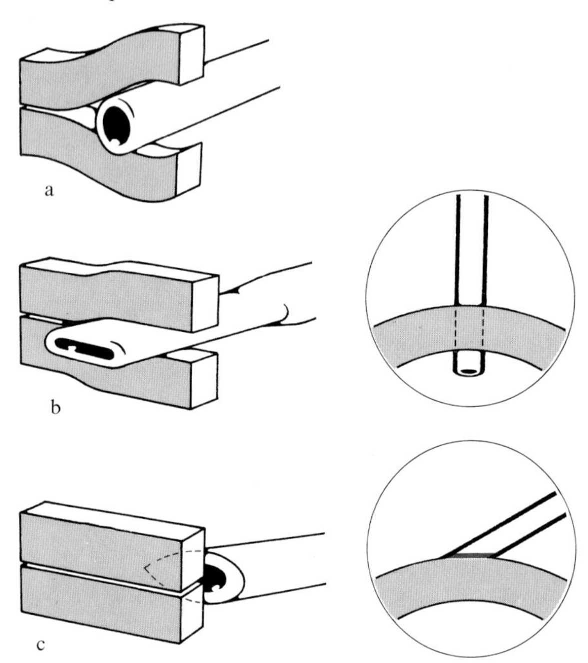

Fig. 341. **Cannulas for injecting liquid or gas into the anterior chamber**

a Open gaps are left next to cylindrical cannulas, allowing fluid to escape. Such cannulas can form a chamber only if a high injection pressure is used.

b A flattened cannula opens the wound little, and the greater drainage resistance requires a lower injection pressure.

c If a beveled ("sharp") cannula is applied to the wound such that its entire rim is pressed snugly against the tissue surface,* the fluid stream will open the wound without the necessity of inserting the cannula itself. The size of the resultant opening equals the diameter of the fluid stream.

Note: Whereas the cannulas in **a** and **b** can be introduced at any angle, only one angle is suitable in **c**, defined by the bevel angle of the cannula

* "The lips must meet as in a kiss" (Olivares)

If the outflow opening must be kept open for tactical reasons (e.g. for manipulations at open wounds) or cannot be closed at all (e.g. in intraocular subcompartments), the pressure is raised by varying *rheologic factors.* In this case the physical properties of the injected material play the main role. The surgeon decides which action must be exploited to achieve the tactical goal: The force of the injection stream (i.e., kinetic energy), the internal friction (i.e., ductile properties), or the surface tension (i.e., elastic properties).

Based on these criteria, the choice is made between 1) watery fluids, 2) viscous substances or 3) gas or oil.

2 Fluids with Low Viscosity ("Watery Liquids")

Watery liquids have the same physical properties as aqueous.[5] Owing to their low viscosity they will leak from any opening which is not watertight. Thus, when injected into open compartments, these fluids must be supplied in a continuous stream in order to maintain the space (i.e. pressure) necessary for operative manipulations. Control of this flow is no problem as long as the outflow opening and thus the outflow resistance remain constant.[6] If the opening, however, is deformed by the manifold intraocular manipulations and thus the outflow resistance is constantly changed, control of the flow will necessitate refined technology[7] or may be only partially effective.[8] This difficulty of control limits the applications of watery liquids.

One main indication of watery liquids is the use in situations where the kinetic energy necessary for building up the pressure is also exploited for additional tactical goals, i.e. for **flushing** (Fig. 343). For the removal of *fluid material* or liquid suspensions (blood), flushing signifies merely an exchange of volume. *Particles* still adherent to surrounding tissue, however, must first be mobilized by the direct application of forces. If flow resistance can be utilized, which is dependent on the cross-section of the particle, *low flow velocities* are sufficient.

At the surface of solids (i.e. at the surface of a firm tissue) the velocity of flow is always zero and particles remain fixed there. To mobilize them, force vectors must be produced

[5] Watery fluids for intraocular use should have a chemical composition as close to natural aqueous as possible (e.g. balanced salt solution).

[6] For example: Mechanically formed outflow channels in pars plana vitrectomy.

[7] For example: Phacoemulsification.

[8] For example: Maintaining sufficient chamber depth during intraocular implant insertion.

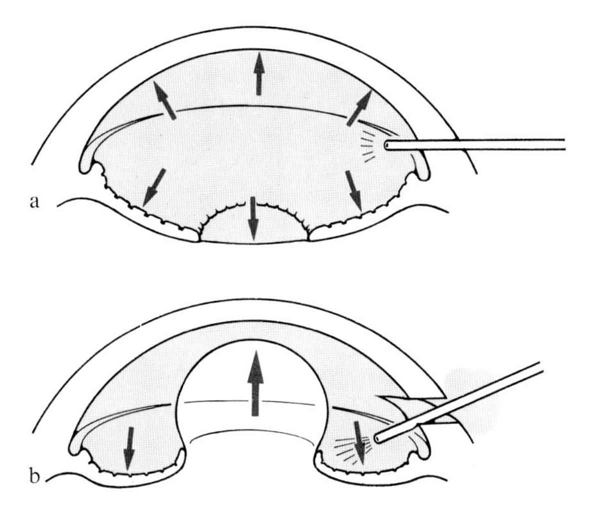

Fig. 342. **Injection of watery liquid into the anterior chamber**

a If the anterior chamber is a closed pressure chamber, its volume can be increased, and its pressure rises. The diaphragm moves as a whole, so that a recession of the iris also indicates recession of the anterior hyaloid membrane.

b If the chamber is open, the hydrostatic pressure cannot increase, and the total chamber volume remains unchanged. If the iris is pressed inward by hydrodynamic forces, a compensatory outward movement of the anterior hyaloid occurs (vitreous "mushroom")

which are perpendicular to the direction of flow. Such vector components are the result of dynamic lift[9] and require very *high flow velocities*.

The high flow energy which is necessary for mobilizing particles may cause *damage to vulnerable tissues*. Strict visual control of the stream action is mandatory, therefore. The efficiency of this control, however, is impaired by the transparency of the fluid (which in itself is invisible) and can only be judged by its effects on the tissue. If the tissue is transparent as well, inadvertant lesions may occur.[10] This applies especially to the highly vulnerable anterior hyaloid membrane (Fig. 342b), and special care is taken not to direct the liquid stream toward places where the membrane is exposed (pupil or iridectomy, Fig. 343).

Another important indication for the use of watery liquids is in situations where the difficulties of flow control no longer exist, i.e. in **restoring the fluid chambers** after wound closure (Fig. 342a). In case of high outflow resistance, watery liquids are ideal aqueous substituents since they have no side-effects and do not impair fluid circulation within the eye.

Visual control is not impaired by watery liquids as long as one observes through the optical surfaces of the globe. At the margins of open wounds, however, the surface becomes curved and distorts vision owing to prismatic effects.[11] This is not a major problem, since removing liquid with a sponge remedies such situations easily.

[9] Dynamic lift is the upward force which is produced by asymmetrical flow velocities on both sides of an object (e.g. an aircraft wing).

[10] Note that the usual method of deducing the position of the anterior hyaloid membrane from the iris position is unreliable under the action of a liquid stream. The anterior hyaloid (as part of the diaphragm) is on the iris plane only if the anterior chamber forms a pressure chamber, i.e., if the injected liquid cannot escape. If the anterior chamber is open, however, the hyaloid membrane surges forward while the iris is driven backward by the stream. This results in a "mushroom" of vitreous which may go unnoticed by the surgeon and may be damaged by a direct liquid stream (see also Fig. 301).

[11] For example: Optical distortion of the needle and the tissue edges by fluid in the wound interspace during suturing.

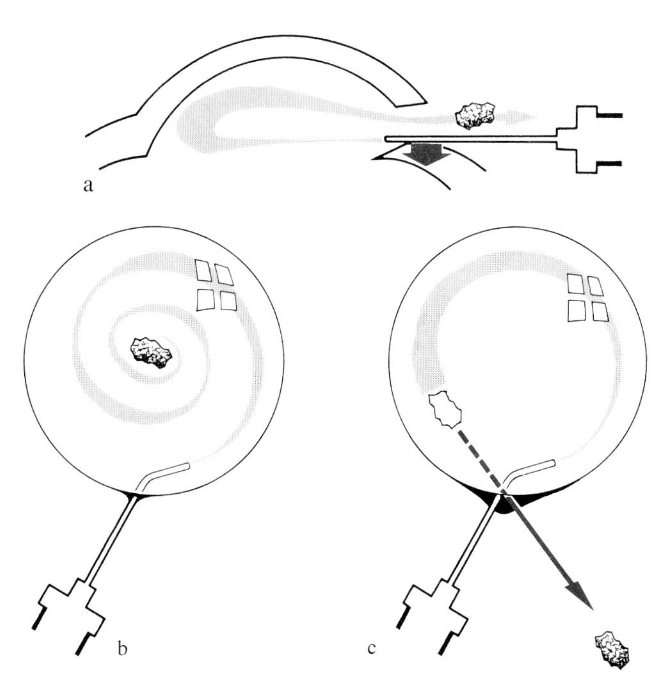

Fig. 343. **Irrigation of the anterior chamber**

a The cannula is lowered to open the wound and control the outflow of liquid.

b If outflow is insufficient, the injected liquid forms eddy currents in the chamber.

c When the wound is opened, the liquid flows out and carries loose material with it. The flow pressure required for this is lowest if the wound is opened not when the particle is directly before it, but somewhat sooner, i.e. when the particle enters a tangential path directed toward the opening

3 Fluids with High Viscosity ("Viscous Implants")

The viscosity, specific gravity and surface tension of fluids vary with the shape and concentration of their larger molecules.[12]

If the **specific gravity** of a viscous substance considerably exceeds that of the aqueous fluid, it may mobilize heavier particles which tend to sink in the aqueous. Whether this effect can be utilized tactically depends on the viscosity, which retards upward travel by the particles.

The **surface tension** of viscous substances in aqueous gives the implants elastic properties which can be utilized tactically for the *blockade* of orifices to prevent the passage of blood[13] or vitreous[14] (Fig. 345a and b). The pure surface effect lasts only for the moment of application, however, since the sharp boundary soon disintegrates due to dilution by the aqueous.

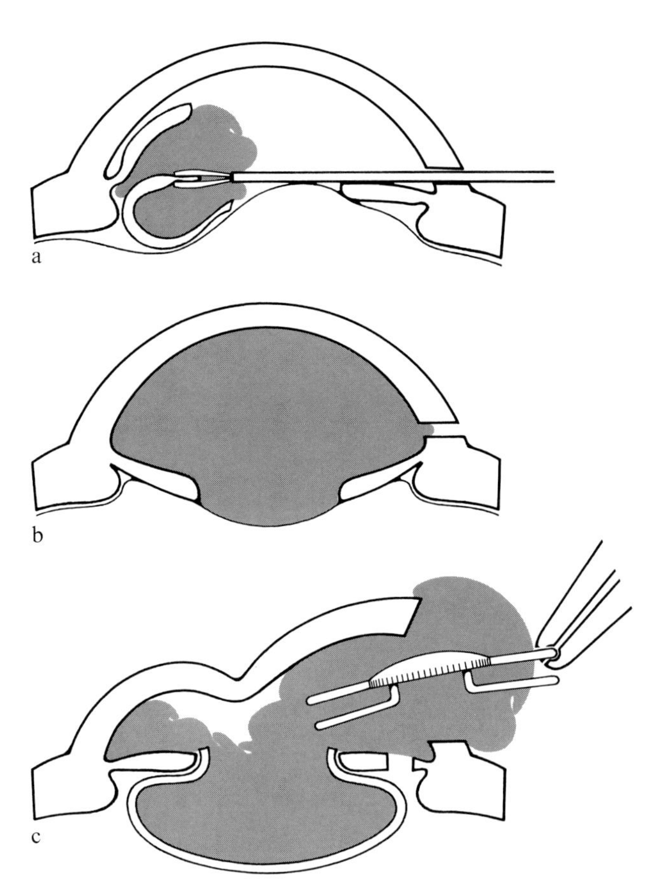

Fig. 344. **Use of viscous substances as space-tactical instruments**

a Use of viscous material to deepen subcompartments (here: for grasping capsule remnants with microforceps).

b Use of viscous material to deepen the entire anterior chamber. Despite the unsutured wound, a counterpressure to the vitreous can be produced, and the diaphragm displaced inward on account of the high resistance to outflow and to the formation of a hinge fold.

c Use of viscous material to raise the wound lip: The wound is kept open for insertion of an instrument or implant without touching the edges of the wound with forceps. Note: In contrast to **b** the chamber must not be filled to a degree that would hinder formation of the "hinge fold"

Consequently it is the **internal friction** which is the main advantage from the standpoint of spatial tactics. It provides the viscous implant with plastic properties and *decreases the velocity of all movements* – those of the substance's own molecules as well as of all material embedded within the viscous substance.[15]

[12] Viscous material for intraocular use must be atoxic, anallergic and absorbable without inflammatory reactions. The material must be transparent. Air bubbles trapped in viscous substances impair the visibility of the operative field. Since it is nearly impossible to remove these bubbles, viscous substances should be supplied by the manufacturer in ready-to-use syringes. The viscosity of material for multipurpose action should be high enough to maintain the shape of a viscous plug but should still permit the material to pass through an injection cannula of acceptable diameter (for example: Healon, Na-hyalonurate 1% with a viscosity of 340,000 centistokes as a thick jelly retains its shape in aqueous but can be injected through a 27 gauge cannula).

[13] The expansion of a hemorrhage can be prevented by filling the empty spaces around the source, so that bleeding is confined to the point of origin (e.g. to a lesion of the major circle of the iris or to a retinal vessel). Note: If much blood already has entered the anterior chamber, first the pupil is blocked with a viscous plug in order to prevent deeper spreading. Then the chamber is flushed with watery fluid and is completely filled with viscous material only after removal of the blood.

[14] To prevent vitreous prolapse in subluxation of the lens, the cannula is inserted from the opposite side in order to permit the safe evacuation of aqueous according to Fig. 347.

[15] Remember: Flow velocities are zero directly at the surface of solid tissue giving rise to a certain fixation effect there.

The plasticity, damping action and fixation effect of viscous materials provide spatial stability and precision in a type of surgery whose success depends on slight pressure changes in liquid-filled pressure chambers.

One of the consequences of high viscosity is **high outflow resistance.** If there is virtually no outflow, pressure can be produced without a continuous inflow. Thus, even in spaces with unsealed openings, i.e. in a chamber with an open wound or in subcompartments, all tactical goals of Fig. 340 can be achieved without the devices necessary for the control of watery liquids.

For example, by filling the anterior chamber with viscous substances, the corneal tissue can be shielded during manipulations in the deeper parts and vice versa (Fig. 344). The corneal endothelium is thus protected during *operations on the iris and the lens*[16] even when instruments without infusion systems are used. This allows smaller instrument diameters, which provides a significant safety factor during long and complicated manipulations.

Moreover, when the chamber is filled with viscous substances prior to *sectioning of the cornea*[17] it is possible to obtain conditions of high "sharpness" while avoiding the dangers inherent in incising a hard eye. As mentioned earlier, the sectility of tissue is increased by raising the intraocular pressure (see Fig. 33b) and the precision of the cut is improved. If this pressure is raised by replacing aqueous with viscous material, the chamber will not drain suddenly when opened and the iris and lens will not surge forward to meet the cutting edge and thus are protected from inadvertant damage.

The **damping action** of viscous substances is utilized tactically to stabilize mobile structures. This provides an additional means for maintaining the anterior chamber, because the viscous material resists the formation of the hinge fold essential for the opening of a wound by rotating a flap (Fig. 344, see also Figs. 202, 205). Moreover, viscous substances can be used widely for stabilizing displaceable

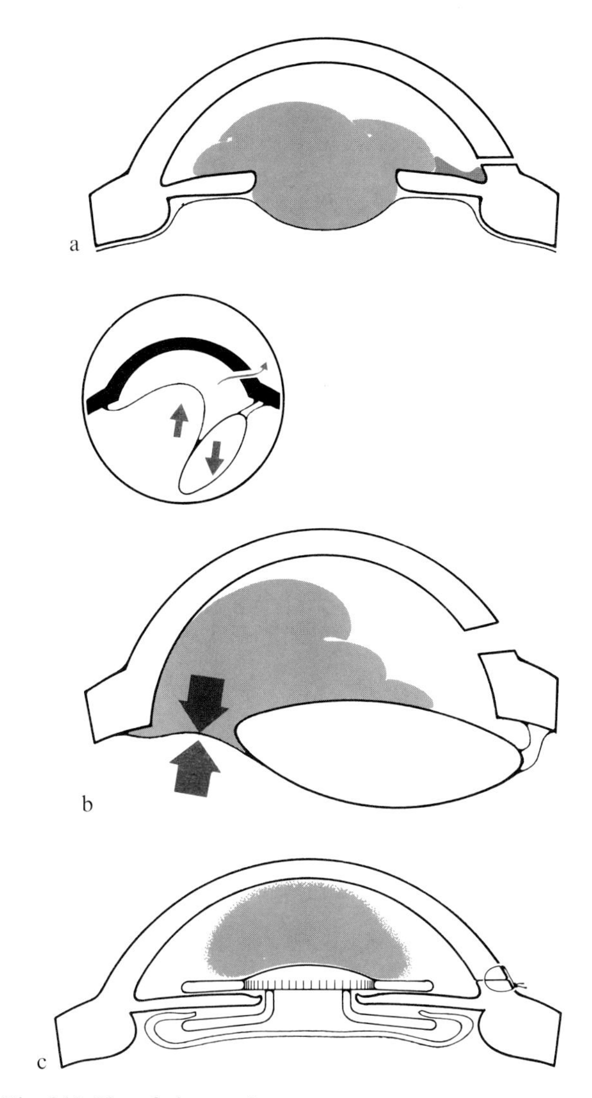

Fig. 345. **Use of viscous plugs**

a Viscous plug used to block a hemorrhage at its source. Spreading of the hemorrhage within the chamber or to deeper levels is prevented.

b Viscous plug used to obstruct an opening in the zonule. A subluxated lens tends to sink into the vitreous with an accompanying upward shift of vitreous substance as soon as the anterior chamber is opened and the counterpressure there removed (inset). A viscous plug can compensate for the lost aqueous counterpressure and stabilize the vitreous, thereby preventing the lens from sinking.

c Viscous plug for fixation of an implant. A viscous depot is left in front of the artificial lens to prevent its dislocation. This allows early dilatation of the pupil in case of extracapsular lens extraction.
Note: The chamber angle area is flushed clean before the surgery is completed.

---

[16] For example : Circumcision and removal of the anterior lens capsule; grasping of foreign bodies; insertion of intraocular implants; suturing of the iris.
[17] For example: Trephination (see page 122).

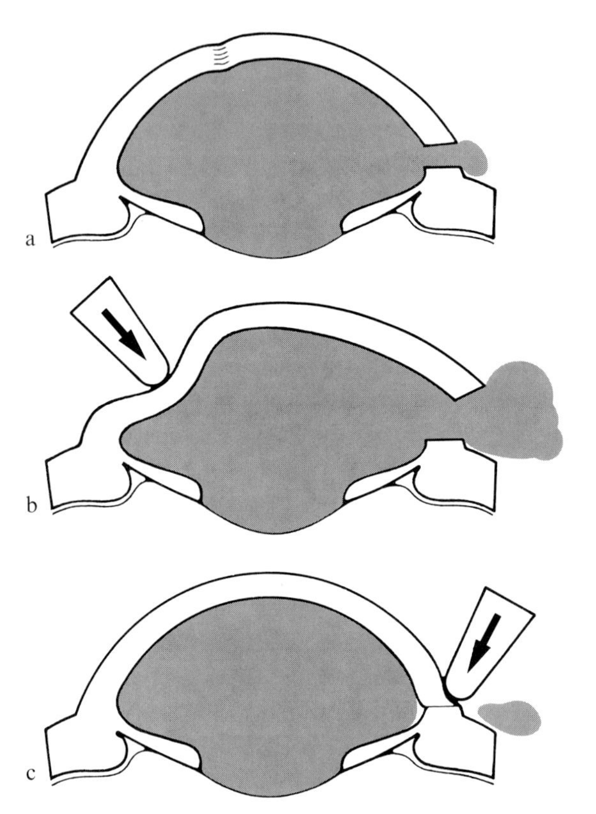

Fig. 346. **Impairment of valvular function by viscous substances**

a Viscous material between the wound edges interferes with valvular closure. The wound gapes; yet it will not open by rotating a flap on account of the resistance to the formation of a hinge fold.

b A pressure increase which normally would close the valve (see page 100) causes it to open. The partial evacuation of viscous material now permits the formation of a hinge fold.

c Valvular function can be restored by removing the viscous material from the wound area (e.g., by compression)

tissues,[18] the motion of instruments[19] or foreign bodies.[20] This action is effective not only during surgery but in the early postoperative period as well (Fig. 345c).

The slowness of the stream provides little kinetic energy for **irrigation.** Particles are mobilized more effectively by utilizing the plastic properties of viscous material as a means of rupturing tissue connections by the distension of tissue interstices and compartments. For removal, particles are pushed outward by the surface of the viscous plug. If during this maneuver particles are brought into contact with adjacent tissue surfaces, they will become affixed there due to zero flow velocity at such locations. To prevent this, all adjoining surfaces are coated with viscous material before the "viscous irrigation" is started. Since slow motions are easy to control, viscous material is suitable for moving particles for short distances, i.e. for displacements within the eye.[21]

When using viscous substances, one must bear in mind that the physical properties differing from aqueous which are useful tools for achieving specific *tactical* goals, may be contrary to *other* goals. In other words: the desired tactical effects are linked with **side-effects.**

The properties which are utilized to maintain the patency of spaces and orifices will *prevent the function of valves* and hinder wound closure. Therefore, viscous material must be carefully removed from wound edges (Fig. 346), unless the strategic goal is to keep then open.[22]

The damping action of viscous substances *decreases the mobility of the iris.* Reposition of the pupil by elastic or muscular forces is impeded. On the other hand, sectility is increased and the iris becomes more prone to inadvertant lesions.[23]

The ability of viscous substances to obstruct orifices may cause a *rise in intraocular pressure.* Since the viscous material is gradually diluted, blockade of the pupil is not a major

[18] For example: Stabilizing the iris to facilitate suturing of a rupture or dialysis; stabilizing the iris position in the early postoperative period to avoid the formation or recurrence of anterior synechiae.

[19] For example: Damping inadvertant movements of an implant; damping the transmission of vibrating instrument motion to surrounding tissues.

[20] For example: Stabilizing a foreign body for grasping with forceps. Stabilizing the position of an implant in the early postoperative period.

[21] For example: Transport of particles situated behind the iris into the anterior chamber to be grasped there under visual control (see Fig. 333c).

[22] Example: Glaucoma operations.

[23] Care must be taken when enlarging a corneal section with scissors in an anterior chamber which has been filled perviously with a viscous substance. The iris cannot yield if trapped by the inserted blade, and may be torn or cut.

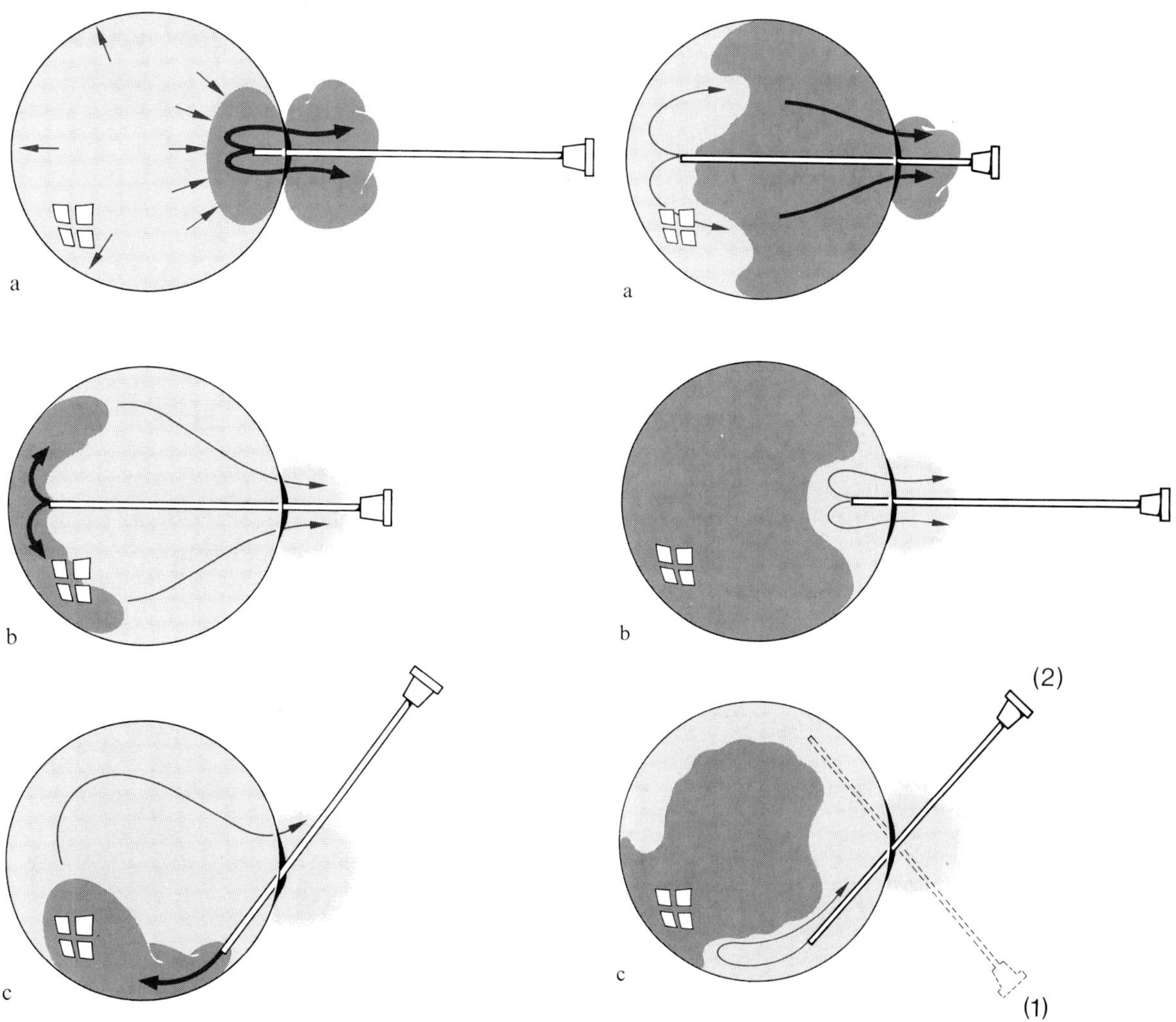

Fig. 347. **Injection of viscous material into a chamber filled with watery fluid**

a The injection of viscous material directly at the entry site produces a viscous plug which prevents aqueous drainage. But without this compensatory drainage, the intraocular pressure rises during the injection and prevents the entry of further viscous material.
b Injection opposite the entry wound permits compensatory aqueous escape.

c Injection in lateral direction. The cannula enters the chamber at an oblique angle, thereby keeping the wound open and facilitating aqueous escape

Fig. 348. **Injection of watery fluids into a chamber filled with viscous material**

a Evacuation of the whole viscous plug from the chamber: If the watery fluid is injected opposite the entry wound, the viscous plug obstructs the outflow and is ejected with minimum rinsing.

b and **c** Evacuation of viscous material from the chamber angle while retaining a central plug (see Fig. 345c): The task now is to prevent the obstruction of the outflow opening by rinsing first the adjoining portion (**b**) and then enlarging the drainage tunnel to both sides (**c**). The rinsing action of the watery fluid is dilution of the viscous material rather than expulsion

problem; but the outflow through the fine trabecular meshwork is impaired even at low viscosity, and the danger of increased intraocular tension persists until the material is completely reabsorbed. The obstructive tendency requires proper procedures to avoid or exploit *blockade of the entrance opening* when injecting (Fig. 347) or evacuating (Fig. 348) viscous material.

The decrease of fluid motion also *decreases thermal convection.* As a result, over-effects can occur if thermal energy is applied according to the same rules followed for aqueous. Cryodes produce larger ice balls in viscous material than in watery liquids, and the danger of inadvertant freezing increases. Heat generated by instruments activated by high frequency vibration is poorly dissipated, the temperature rises, and adjoining tissues may be coagulated.

Optical effects of viscous substances depend on the index of refraction, which may be higher than aqueous. Transparent tissues with the same index of refraction will become completely invisible.[24] Other optical effects are caused by the deformation of free surfaces when viscous material interfaces with air in an open wound. The surfaces becomes convex, and the visual control of topographic relations is impaired.[25] This surface can again be flattened by rinsing with watery liquids (i.e. through dilution of the superficial layers and consequent decrease of surface tension).

When using viscous substances one has to bear in mind that owing to their strong effects and side-effects they are not were substituents of aqueous meant to remain within a chamber once introduced there. Rather they are to be treated as mechanical instruments which are applied precisely at specific sites, removed and reapplied according to momentary needs.

4 Substances with a High Surface Tension ("Membranous Implants")

Surface tension plays a role wherever two immiscible fluids are separated by a sharp boundary. This occurs between fluid and gas media or between water-soluble and fat-soluble liquids.

As a result, gas and oil behave as *impenetrable foreign bodies* when immersed in aqueous fluid ("membranous implants"). The viscoplastic properties in the interior of such implants are of little practical importance.[26] The tactical value of the implants depends, rather, on their interaction with the surrounding fluid, i.e. on their *surface tension* (responsible for elastic properties) and *specific gravity* (responsible for direction of motion under the influence of gravity).

A single bubble tends to assume the shape of a sphere and owing to its elastic properties imposes this shape upon its surroundings. A *single large bubble* can therefore be used to force a collapsed ocular space back into a spheroid shape.[27]

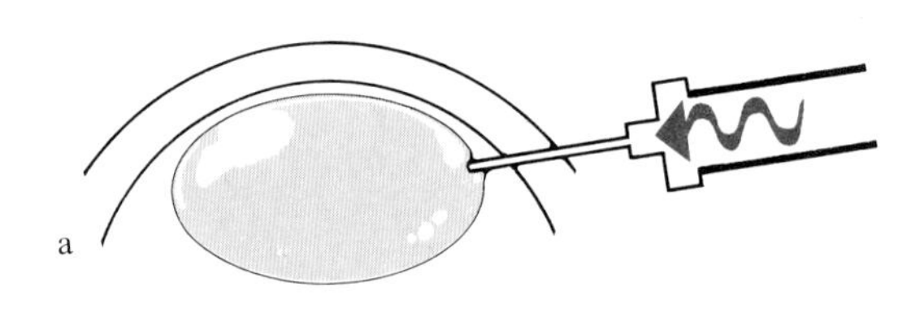

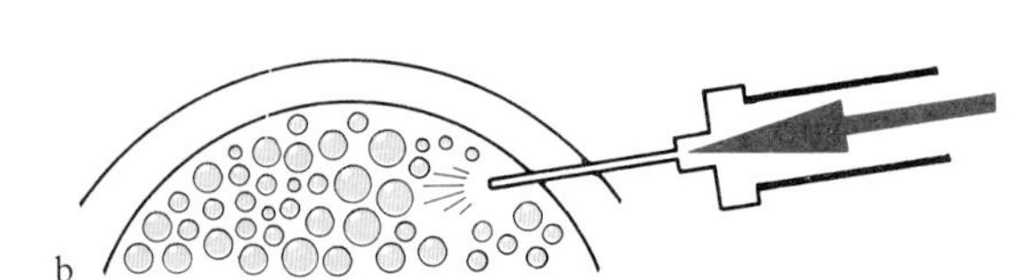

Fig. 349. **Gas injection to maintain the anterior chamber**

a Large bubbles are formed by slow injection.

b Many small bubbles have a larger total surface area, a higher surface tension, and must be formed by a correspondingly greater force: rapid, forceful injection

[24] For example: The lens capsule and anterior hyaloid are indiscernible if observed in 1% hyaluronic acid.

[25] The optical distortions can cause errors when grasping or suturing the iris or an implant in an "open sky" technique.

[26] The chemical composition of the implants is important to the extent that it determines the absorption time. Gas (e.g. air, SF_6) is reabsorbed relatively quickly and is therefore more of a tactical instrument. Silicone oil, on the other hand, is non-absorbable and is therefore a strategic tool.

Multiple small bubbles have a larger total surface area and thus a higher surface tension than a single large bubble (Fig. 349). A greater force is needed to produce them; but they can also withstand a higher counterpressure and are therefore used to maintain irregularly shaped spaces under such conditions.

The boundary surface acts as **a membrane** which can effectively seal small openings.[28] The membrane, however, is unstable when it comes in contact with another surface of the same medium. Small bubbles with a high surface tension will then coalesce with larger bubbles. Thus, gas bubbles are particularly unstable when exposed to the outside air in an open wound. They are easily broken when manipulations take place at wound edges and are unsuitable as tactical tools in such circumstances.[29]

The difference in **specific gravity** can be utilized tactically to move bubbles to the desired site and to exert pressure on surrounding structures. The *chemical nature* of the enclosed material determines the absorption time and thus the duration of this pressure. The difference in the *specific gravity* of the bubbles and surrounding fluid determines whether the bubbles will exert *upward*[30] or *downward*[31] pressure.

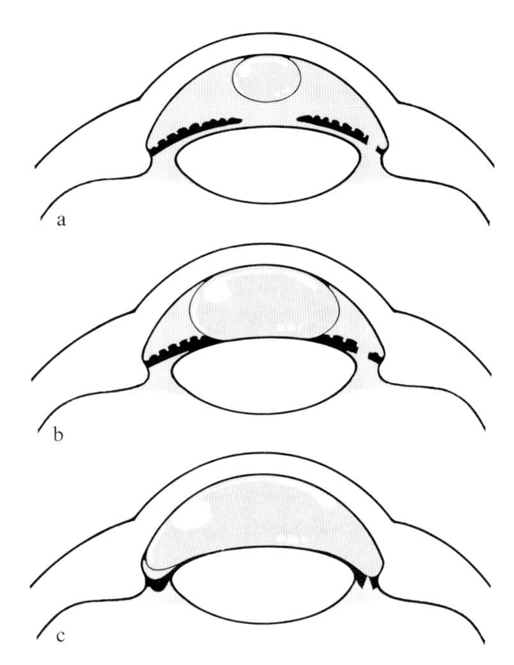

Fig. 350. **Obstruction of aqueous circulation by gas bubbles**

a Small bubble does not impair aqueous circulation.

b Pupillary block. The basal iridectomy is still clear. Holding the head erect would block the basal iridectomy while freeing the pupil.

c Total gas block: pupil, iridectomy and trabeculae are blocked by the gas bubble. The block cannot be relieved by repositioning the patient

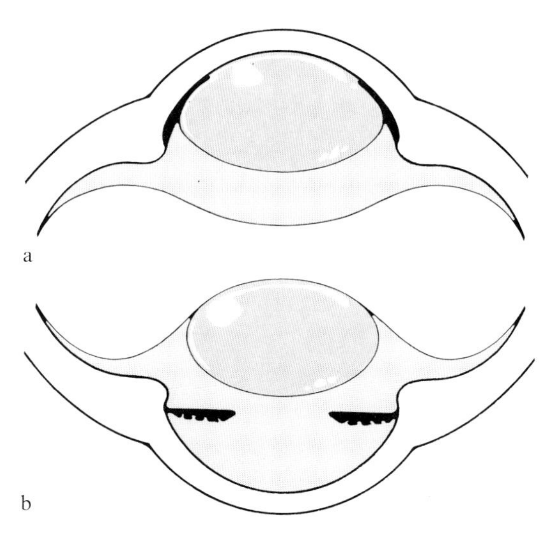

Fig. 351. **Gas block in the aphakic eye**

a In aphakia, gas can enter the space behind the iris. The pupil is blocked, the iris is pressed against the posterior corneal surface, and the iridectomy opening and chamber angle are obstructed.

b Treatment by repositioning the patient: In the prone position, the gas bubble rises and frees the openings for aqueous circulation

[27] For example: Filling the *anterior chamber* with gas restores the corneal curvature and facilitates precise apposition during suturing. Filling the *vitreous space* after vitrectomy with gas (for tactical purposes) or silicone oil (for strategic purpose) pushes a detached and plicated retina back against the spherical eye wall.

[28] Examples: Sealing of small wound dehiscences in traumatology until closure by biological processes takes place; sealing of retinal tears.

[29] The collapse of bubbles at an open wound is of no consequence *when the counterpressure is low*, since then the bubble has no tactical function. Note: The *spontaneous invasion* of air on opening of the anterior chamber in case of low vitreous pressure is not related to problems of surface tension but is merely the result of a communication with the outside air. The absence of chamber drainage in such a case is a sign that vitreous pressure does not exceed atmospheric and is to be distinguished from the tactical use of gas bubbles as a tool to create counterpressure.

[30] Examples of material lighter than aqueous are gas (air, SF_6) or light-weight silicone oil.

[31] Example of a material heavier than aqueous is heavy silicone oil.

Even after wound closure, therefore surgical actions can be performed. To apply the bubble to the desired site, it is necessary to place the patient in a precisely defined position. Any deviation from this position will displace the bubble, thus losing the desired effect and possibly creating adverse effects: blockade of the pupil (Fig. 350) or shifting of mobile tissue into undesired positions.[32] Such situations can be remedied by repositioning the patient, of course (Fig. 351). But do draw the maximum benefit from membranous implants, the patient should maintain the necessary position as long as the bubbles remain within the eye.[33]

The requirement of absolute immobility can be relaxed somewhat if the bubbles are placed into *viscous substances*, as these will have the effect of slowing the rate of bubble motion. Thus, by the proper choice of the surrounding substance, it is possible to produce absorbable **intraocular balloons** which are easy to control (Fig. 352).

Optically, membranous implants have marked effects owing to their well defined surface. Gas bubbles act as strong negative lenses and impair vision of the eye interior. Nonabsorbable material (e.g. silicon oil) should have the same index of refraction as aqueous, because it is nearly impossible to produce bubbles with ideal optical properties.[34]

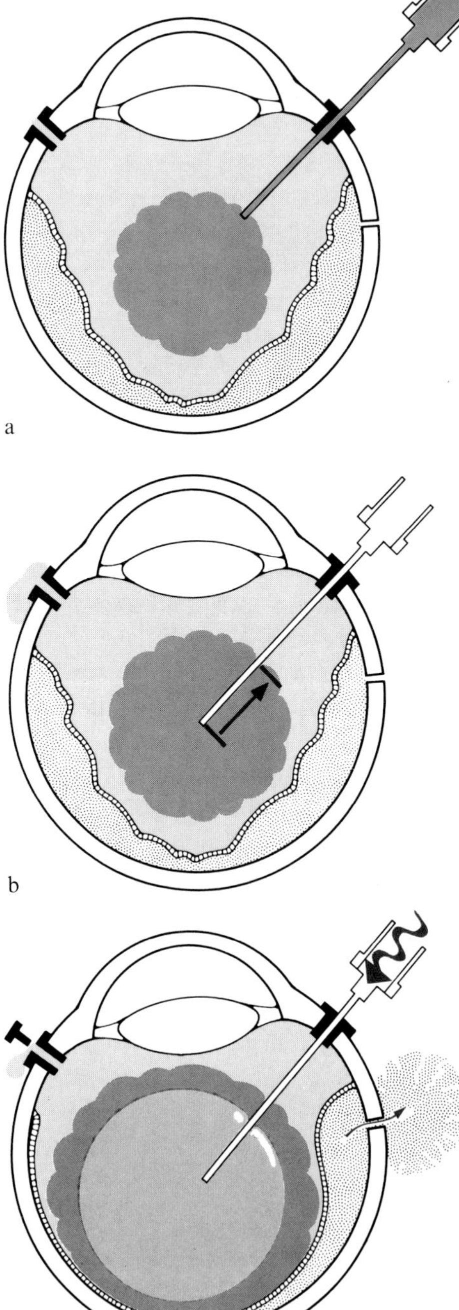

Fig. 352. **Combining viscous substance with gas ("intraocular reabsorbable balloon")**

a A viscous plug is placed into the vitreous cavity (after vitrectomy). If then gas is injected at once, it will most likely escape into the watery portion within the cavity where the resistance is lower.

b To avoid this, the cannula is advanced deeply into the viscous plug prior to the injection of gas.

c The vitreous plug is inflated by gas.

Note: Compensatory drainage of intraocular fluid may involve the intravitreal, retroretinal or retrochorioidal space depending on the tactical goal

[32] For example: Gas bubbles displaced behind the iris will push the latter against the inner corneal wound edge and cause anterior synechiae.

[33] This requirement limits the use of materials with a very long absorption time. Unabsorbable materials can be used only if their specific gravity is equal that of the aqueous and thus no shifting occurs, or if the shifting does not interfere with strategic goals (e.g. use of silicone bubbles trapped in vitreous framework).

[34] Severe optical distortions occur if optically active implants do not have regular spherical surfaces and are not precisely centered about the optical axis.

5 Control of Space-Tactical Measures

At the end of the surgery all space-tactical measures must be checked with regard to their impact on the strategic goal, which is to restore the shape of the intraocular spaces and to remove obstacles to fluid circulation. Substances with properties different from aqueous are withdrawn or at least reduced in size so as not to obstruct circulation openings. All spaces involved in fluid circulation should contain only watery aqueous substituents.

Before the intraocular pressure chambers can be restored by filling with watery liquid, a watertight wound closure must be achieved. The quality of wound closure is tested by the attainable intraocular tension.[35] When wound closure is checked by the injection of watery fluid, it must be remembered that complete watertightness allows the intraocular pressure to rise to the point where the retinal blood flow is severely impaired.

One of the principal means of verifying that the space-strategic goals have been achieved is by **checking the intraocular pressure** at the end of surgery as well as during the postoperative period.

---

[35] Only watery fluids provide a reliable means of verifying closure. Viscous substances or gas may simulate watertightness even in presence of leaks. These may become apparent once the aqueous substituents have been absorbed (unless sealed in the mean time by biologic response).

IX Combining Space-Tactical and Tissue-Tactical Procedures with Miniaturized Instruments

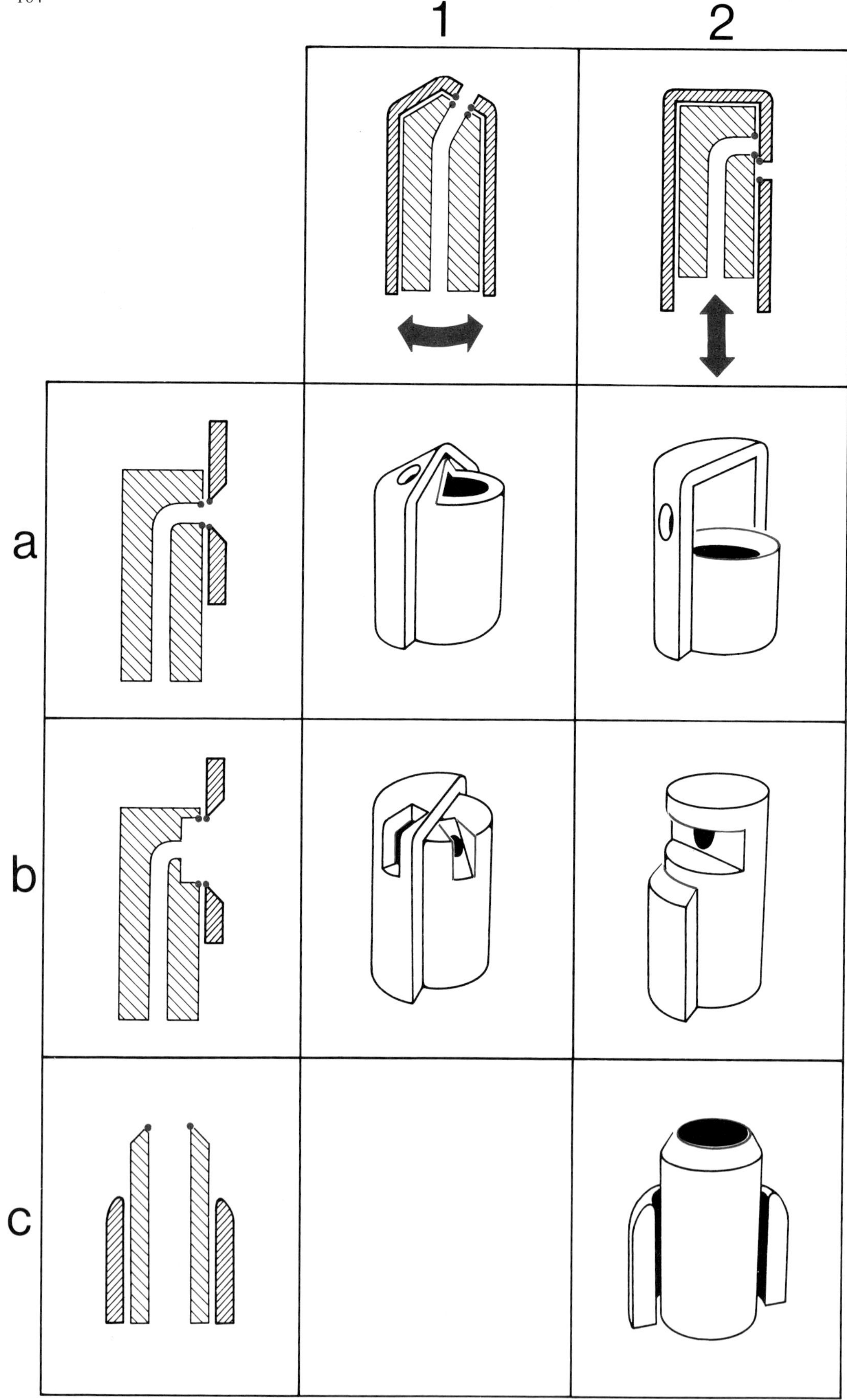

1
2
a
b
c

The grasping and cutting of tissue as well as the injection and removal of fluid can be executed all in one cycle with special miniaturised instruments called fragmentation cannulas. These instruments are characterized by a small diameter, short travel and long aspiration path – properties which permit a variety of manipulations in the eye through very small access openings.[4] The short travel of the working motions during both grasping and cutting allow the targeted structures to be approached in situ, a particularly great advantage in operations on deep-lying structures which are dangerous to bring out of the eye due to concomitant movements of adjacent tissues.[5]

The **head of the cannula** (Fig. 353) contains an aspiration port, a resection port (and possibly an infusion port). The *aspiration port* is that part of the suction system which is completely sealed by the material to be aspirated. The *resection port* is the opening over which the cutting edge moves. The two ports may be identical, if the resection port has the same cross-section as the aspiration tube (Fig. 353a). But they may also be separated by an antechamber so that the resection port can be made larger than the aspiration port (Fig. 353b).[6]

The selection of the type of cannula head is determined by the consistency of the material to be resected.

Grasping: *Pliable material* can be grasped by suction alone (Fig. 355). Small suction ports are best for this "sipping" action, for they can be completely sealed by the material with little difficulty. *Rigid material* (Fig. 356) that cannot be "sipped" into the aspiration port requires a large, curved ("embracing") resection port. If a rigid particle is too bulky, its inertia can be exploited for grasping by employing an ultrahigh-speed cutting motion (high-frequency vibrators, Fig. 357).

Division: Tissues are divided by the passage of the cutting edge close past the opposing edge of the resection port.

The *motion of the cutting edge* may be either about the cannula axis (rotary) or along its axis (reciprocating) (Fig. 354). Rotary cannulas have an infinetely long "travel" and can attain extremely high speeds.[7] Oscillating cannulas have short travels; for technical rea-

Fig. 353. **Fragmentation cannulas**

Column 1: Cannulas with a rotary cutting motion (continuous or oscillating).
Column 2: Cannulas with a reciprocating (axial) cutting motion.
Row a: Cannulas in which the resection port and aspiration port are identical ("sipping" cannulas).
Row b: Cannulas in which the resection port is separated from the aspiration port by an antechamber ("nibbling" cannulas).
Row c: High-frequency vibrators (emulsifiers).
red: cutting edges

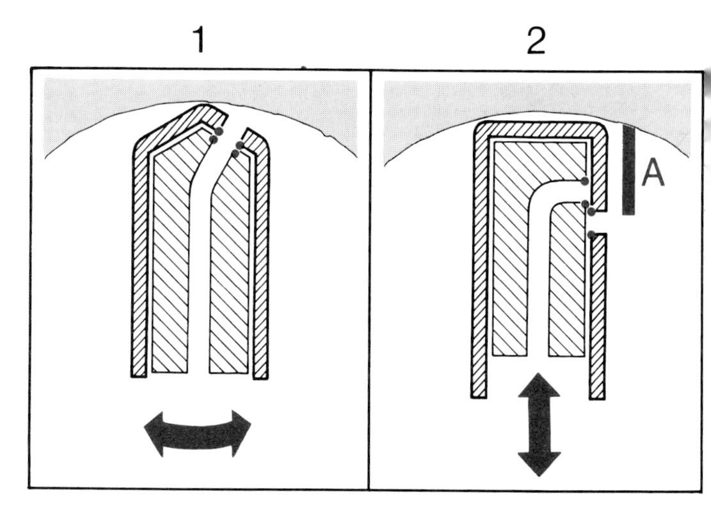

Fig. 354. **Position of cannula opening**

Left: In cannulas with a rotating cutter, the opening can be located near the cannula tip. This makes it possible to cut close to tissue surfaces lying *ahead of* the tip.
Right: In cannulas with a reciprocating cutter, the opening is located on the side and at some distance from the tip. The minimum distance A depends on the amplitude of the cutting motion

[1] Indications: Operations in which immediate, secure wound closure is desired, as in phacoemulsification.
[2] Indications: Operations on the vitreous (vitrectomies) in which traction entails the risk of retinal lesions.
[3] A discrepancy between the aspiration and resection port is present in "nibbling" cannulas with a built-in infusion channel. In order to keep the total cross-section small enough, the aspiration channel must be made thinner than the relatively large resection port.
[4] The maximum attainable speed is limited by inertial effects involved in stopping a moving object and reversing its direction. The associated technical problems can be easily solved only for axial reciprocating (forward-and-backward) motion.

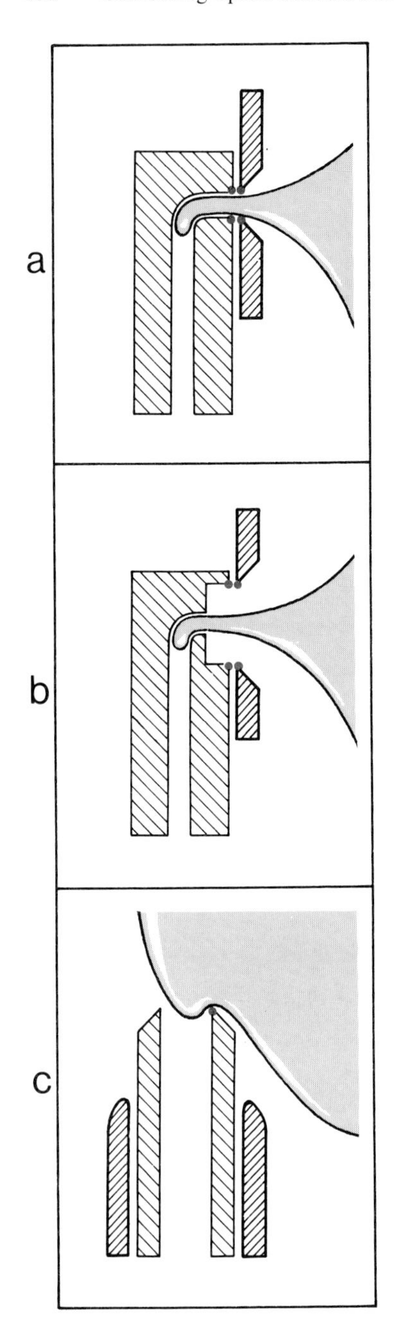

Fig. 355. **The grasping of pliable material**

a In "sipping" cannulas the material is grasped by suction. Sharpness can be improved by increasing the tension of the tissue at the resection port, i.e. by increasing the suction.

b In "nibbling" cannulas, pliable material is also held in place by suction. However, the material remains flaccid at the resection port and cannot be made tense even by increasing the suction. The "sharpness" of the instrument can be improved only by increasing the speed of the cutting motion.

c High-frequency vibrators are ineffective on pliable material unless it can be affixed to the edge by its own inertia (e.g. pulsatile aspiration [7])

sons, high speeds can be achieved relatively easily in reciprocating cannulas, but are quite difficult to achieve with rotary oscillating cannulas. [8]

The tissue is sectioned by the *punch principle*. A good cutting action based on this principle is obtained only if the cutting edges come into contact with equal pressure for their full length – a condition which calls for extreme precision in the manufacture of fragmentation cannulas. If its sharpness is inadequate, the instrument exerts only traction on the partially-divided tissue, whether by suction or the movement of the cutting edge. Instead of cutting the tissue (sharp dissection), the cannula merely tears it (blunt dissection). The process can no longer be controlled, and the section proceeds in the direction of least tissue resistance. [9]

This danger can never be fully avoided, because "sharpness" is largely a function of tissue sectility. Since this can seldom be judged in advance, it should be assumed from the start that the sectility is poor, and corresponding technical precautions should be taken. Generally, instruments with a short cutting stroke are safer to use than continuously rotating ones. In addition, one can try to *improve the sharpness* by increasing the sectility of the tissue or the cutting ability of the instrument.

Sectility is especially poor in pliable tissues. It can be improved by increasing the suction to make the tissue more tense. This effect is present only at the aspiration port, however. If this port is separated from the resection port by an antechamber, this mechanism is useless for improving sectility. Then the only recourse is to improve cutting ability by increasing the speed at which the cutting edge is moved past the port. Note: The decisive factor here is the speed of each stroke, which is not necessarily associated with an increase in frequency.

---

[5] Example: Rupture of the retina in vitreous surgery, avulsion of the iris at the base in iris resection.

[6] Inertial effects are helpful for maintaining regular motion.

[7] Note: Efficient only if the aspiration port can be sealed completely by the material to be sectioned.

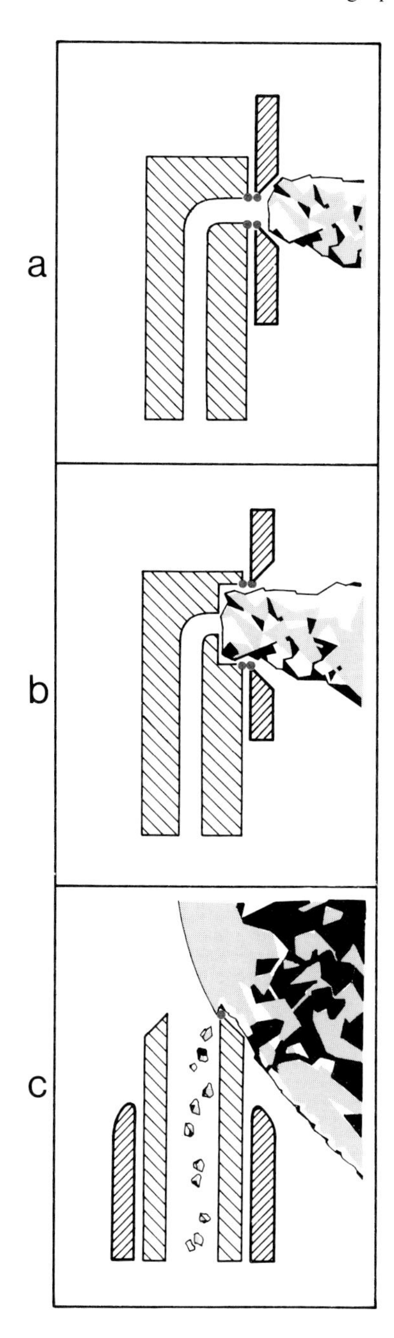

Fig. 356. **The grasping of rigid material**

a "Sipping" cannulas cannot cut rigid particles with a diameter greater than that of the aspiration port.

b "Nibbling" cannulas can grasp material which fits into the resection port. Increasing the suction does not raise the tension of the tissue. Sharpness is improved only by increasing the speed of the cutting motion.

c High-frequency vibrators can seize material whose inertia keeps it from shifting away from the cutting edge

Changes in frequency always require a corresponding adjustment of the suction. If suction is excessive, too much tissue is drawn into the cannula, and the danger of tearing is increased. If the suction is too low in relation to the frequency of the cutting motion, there is insufficient time for enough tissue to be drawn into the port, and no cutting action is obtained.

Cutting edges which oscillate at extremely high frequencies (**ultrasonic vibrators**) represent a special case. Here, the speed of the cutting motion is so high that it is the sole criterion for the cutting action; the shape of the cutting edge is of little importance. The "grasping" action derives from the inertia of the tissue itself. Thus, no suction is required to hold it in place, and the aspiration port does not need to be completely sealed. Accordingly, the control of amplitude and frequency is geared toward the mass whose inertia must prevent the vibration from being transmitted through the rigid material to its surroundings and inflicting damage there. Ultrasonic vibrators require a special *working technique* to ensure that the cannula tip will not become lodged in unyielding tissue. The instrument must be guided in such a way that the cooling fluid has free access to the operative site, and sufficient space is created for thicker parts that follow (Figs. 357 and 358).

It is important that the aspirated material be replaced by an equal volume of fluid, which is introduced either through the fragmentation cannula itself or by a separate **infusion**. Constancy of volume not only guarantees constant positional relations of the internal structures; it is especially important for maintaining the shape of the optical surfaces through which the interior of the eye is viewed.

Visual monitoring is essential for the successful use of fragmentation cannulas. Due to the short travel of the cutting edge, the surgeon receives no tactile feedback on tissue resistance. Moreover, the action of the cutting edge is far too fast to be directly followed with the eye. The cutting process can be judged only by watching its effect on the tissue. If the tissue contains transparent parts, these must be visualized by suitable illumination.

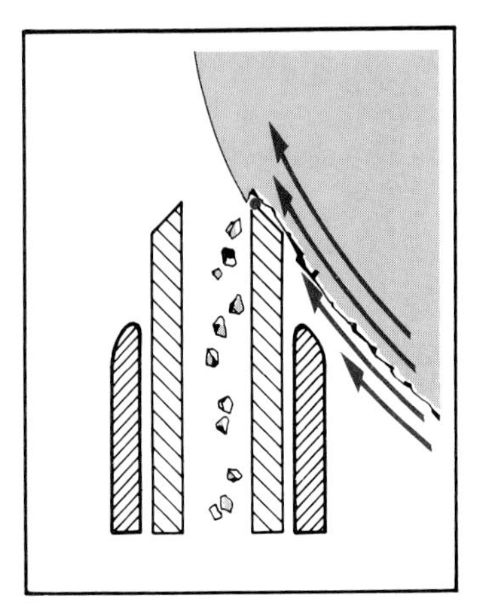

Fig. 357. **Working technique with high-frequency vibrators**

Chipping off rigid material parallel to the surface: The shape of the "cutting" edge is unimportant. The opening need not be sealed by the material to be aspirated. Access of cooling fluid to the operative site is ensured.

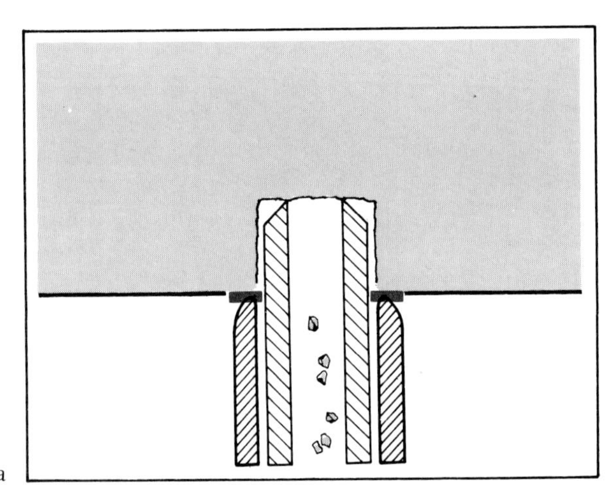

a

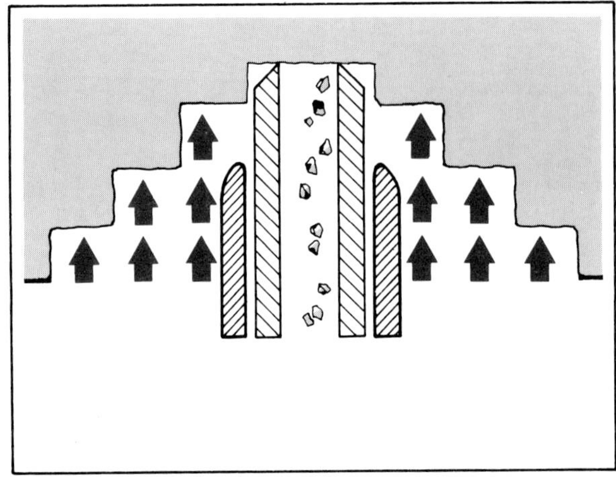

c

b

Fig. 358. **Working technique with high-frequency vibrators**

Perpendicular boring:

a If the instrument is advanced along a straight line, there is a danger that trailing parts with a larger diameter will be unable to fit through the narrow borehole, and further movement of the cannula will dislocate the particle as a whole. The supply of cooling fluid to the cannula tip would also be blocked.

b Splittable tissue (e.g. lens) will split if the displacement in front of the advancing edge is impeded by a resistance on the opposite side (danger of lesions there through the transmission of vibration!).

c To avoid these complications, the diameter of the tunnel is continously enlarged by repeated application in a lateral direction

High-quality optical aids are mandatory during surgery, therefore. The observation system must include means for adequate magnification. Supplementary optics (e.g., contact glasses) are necessary for deeper viewing. The illumination is either coupled to the observation system (coaxial or slit lamp) or provided by a separate instrument introduced into the eye (fiber optics). Which system is preferred depends on whether the surgeon simply wishes to illuminate opaque structures or must make transparent structures visible, and whether spatial orientation by the observation system (stereoscopy) is adequate or must be created by the illumination (slit lamp).

The control of the entire technical arsenal, the cutting motion, the aspiration pressure, the infusion of fluid, the observation system (focussing and change of magnification), the illumination system (incidence angle, size of light spot, etc.) as well as other auxiliary devices presents the surgeon with entirely new problems, for his hands are already busy controlling the position of the eye and the surgical instruments. Which functions should be controlled by foot switches, which by verbal communication with assistants and which by the automation of certain functions is a question of technical resources, and this is a field of rapid, intensive development.

Recent trends point to increasing reliance on instrumentation, with fewer alternative techniques available in case of instrument failure. The responsibility for controlling the course of the operation is thus shifting more and more from the surgeon to the technicians, who not only design and construct the apparatus but must also guarantee its reliable operation.

In ophthalmic surgery as in other fields, the transition from craftsmanship to automation has begun.

A. H. Chignell

Retinal Detachment Surgery

1980. 50 figures. X, 166 pages
ISBN 3-540-09475-X

Contents:

This book describes a practical and sequential approach to the management of patients with rhegmatogenous retinal detachment. It fills the gap between simpler accounts of retinal detachment found in larger ophthalmology textbooks and more specialized journal articles while avoiding the repetition that often occurs in books with multiple authorship. Chapters deal with the examination and assessment of patients, descriptions of the various types of detachment, operating planning and operative techniques – with emphasis on the simplest, safest and most effective techniques – prophylactic treatment and postoperative management and complications. The book is intended primarily for training ophthalmologists, and will serve as a useful guide for experienced professionals as well.

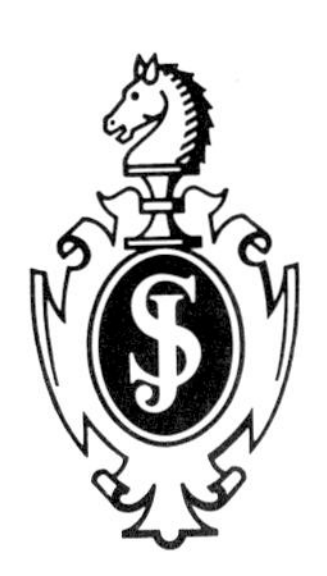

Springer-Verlag
Berlin
Heidelberg
New York

B. Barsewich

Perinatal Retinal Haemorrhages

Morphology, Aetiology and Significance
Foreword by O.-E. Lund
1979. 64 figures, 13 plates, 29 tables.
XII, 184 pages
ISBN 3-540-09167-X

Current Research in Ophthalmic Electron Microscopy 2

Editor: M. Spitznas
1978. 175 figures, 14 tables. IV, 216 pages
ISBN 3-540-09160-2

Current Research in Ophthalmic Electron Microscopy 3

Editor: W. R. Lee
1980. 109 figures, 3 tables. VI, 160 pages
ISBN 3-540-09953-0

G. Eisner

Biomicroscopy of the Peripheral Fundus

An Atlas and Textbook
Foreword by H. Goldmann
Drawings by W. Hess
1973. 121 partly colored figures.
XI, 191 pages
ISBN 3-540-06374-9
Distribution rights for Japan:
Maruzen Co. Ltd., Tokyo

Glaucoma Update

International Glaucoma Symposium,
Nara, Japan. May 7–11, 1978
Editors: G. K. Krieglstein, W. Leydhecker
1979. 48 figures, 27 tables. XII, 224 pages
ISBN 3-540-09350-8

S. N. Hassani

Real Time Ophthalmic Ultrasonography

In collaboration with R. L. Bard
1978. 423 figures. XXI, 214 pages
ISBN 3-540-90318-6

S. S. Hayreh

Anterior Ischemic Optic Neuropathy

1975. 139 figures, 16 stereoscopic illustrations. VIII, 145 pages
ISBN 3-540-06916-X

Recent Advances in Glaucoma

International Glaucoma Symposium,
Prague 1976
Editors: S. Řehák, M. M. Krasnov,
G. D. Paterson
1977. 77 figures, 46 tables. XIII, 295 pages
ISBN 3-540-07944-0
Distribution rights for the socialist
countries: Avicenum, Verlag für Medizin,
Prague

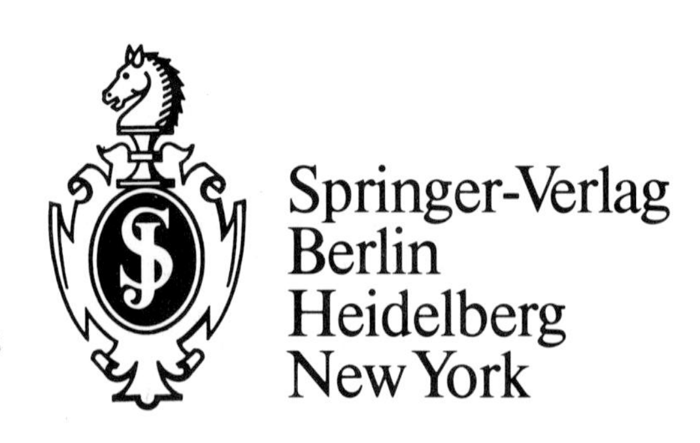